D1057994

CONSERVING HUMAN LIFE

PART I
THE MORAL LAW IN REGARD TO THE ORDINARY
AND EXTRAORDINARY MEANS OF CONSERVING LIFE
by
Daniel A. Cronin, S.T.D.

PART II
FEEDING THE HOPELESS
AND THE HELPLESS
An Application Of the Principles
by
Orville N. Griese, S.T.D., J.C.D.,
Former Director of Research, Pope John Center

PART III
THE MORAL OPTION NOT TO CONSERVE LIFE
UNDER CERTAIN CONDITIONS
An Application of the Principles
by
Albert S. Moraczewski, O.P., Ph.D.
Director, Regional Office of Pope John Center, Houston

Russell E. Smith, S.T.D.
Director of Education, Pope John Center
Editor

Pope John XXIII Medical-Moral
Research and Educational Center

Nihil Obstat: Rev. James J. O'Donohoe, J.C.D.
            Censor Deputatus
Imprimatur: Bernard Cardinal Law
            Archdiocese of Boston
    The Nihil Obstat and Imprimatur are a declaration that a book or pamphlet is considered to be free from doctrinal or moral error. It is not implied that those who have granted the Nihil Obstat and Imprimatur agree with the contents, opinions, or statements expressed.

Copyright 1989
by
The Pope John XXIII Medical-Moral
Research and Educational Center
Braintree, Massachusetts 02184

Library of Congress Cataloging-in-Publication Data

Conserving human life / Russell E. Smith, editor.
    p. 329   cm. xxiv
    Bibliography: p. 320
    Includes index.
    Contents: pt. I. Moral law in regard to the ordinary and extraordinary means of conserving life / by Daniel A. Cronin—pt. II. Feeding the hopeless and the helpless / by Orville N. Griese—pt. III. Moral option not to conserve life under certain conditions / by Albert S. Moraczewski.
    ISBN 0-935372-26-1
    1. Terminal care—Moral and ethical aspects. 2. Terminal care—Religious aspects—Catholic Church. 3. Life and death. Power over—Moral and ethical aspects. 4. Life and death, Power over—Religious aspects—Catholic Church. I. Smith, Russell E. (Russell Edward) II. Cronin, Daniel Anthony, 1927-   Moral law in regard to the ordinary and extraordinary means of conserving life. III. Griese, Orville N. Feeding the hopeless and the helpless. IV. Moraczewski, Albert S., 1920-   Moral option not to conserve life under certain conditions.
    [DNLM: 1. Catholicism. 2. Enteral Feedings. 3. Ethics, Medical. 4. Euthanasia. 5. Life Support Care   W 50 C755]
    R726.C67 1989
    174'.24—dc20
    DNLM/DLC
    for Library of Congress   89-16155
                                                          CIP

TABLE OF CONTENTS

+ + + + + + + + + + +

PART TWO—An application of the basic concepts of
Conserving Human Life to

FEEDING THE HOPELESS AND THE HELPLESS
By Rev. Msgr. Orville N. Griese, STD, JCD

PART THREE—THE MORAL OPTION NOT TO
CONSERVE LIFE UNDER CERTAIN
CONDITIONS

By Rev. Albert Moraczewski, O.P., Ph. D.

CONCLUSION, 274

DEDICATION

"Hail, Holy Queen!"
The Authors of This Publication
Join the Pope John XXIII Center
In Dedicating This Theological
Defense of Conserving Human Life
To The
BLESSED VIRGIN MARY
"The Perfect Example
Of . . . Spiritual and
Apostolic Life . . . ,
Queen Of Apostles."

Cf. Vatican II
Laity, n. 4

Preface to *Conserving Human Life*

In May, 1956, Father Daniel A. Cronin, a priest of the Archdiocese of Boston, defended his doctoral dissertation. It was published in 1958. The thesis topic was the history of the theological distinction between extraordinary and ordinary means of conserving life. This issue is as current now as it was in the mid-fifties. Since Father Cronin defended his dissertation in 1956, much has changed. "Father" Daniel Cronin was consecrated a bishop on September 12, 1968. And he is now the Bishop of Fall River, Massachusetts.

Medical science has undergone incredible progress as well. The development of medical knowledge on the one hand, and technological capability on the other have together produced a harvest of diagnostic, curative, preventative and resuscitative possibility that staggers even the most jaded observers of world events.

Because of the manifold changes in medical capability and hardware, one thing remains unchanged: the necessity of ethical reflection. Indeed, this necessity is all the more urgent today. Integral to the advancement of humanity and the progress of civilization, there is a thought process at work beyond the mere accumulation of knowledge. Within the sphere of human activity—religious or otherwise—there has been an attempt to examine and understand the meaning of human activity. In every age there has been a basic need to put "the music with the words" of life, to use Mark Twain's phrase. There has been an attempt to ascertain a quality beyond effectiveness and skill. This has been the pursuit of moral standards, a reflection upon our activity to determine the qualities we call "right" and "wrong." People take up ethical reflection to make sure that their lives meet the test of reasonableness. This kind of reflection has been undertaken in every age and in every culture. In the face of any practice or development in the sphere of human action, the question of morality, "Is it reasonable?" has always been found to be appropriate.

The Shape of this Presentation

Conserving Human Life was originally intended to be only a publication of Bishop Cronin's doctoral dissertation. But, in light of the advances in medicine since 1956 and the resulting moral controversies, two other monographs are included as well; one by the former Director of Research, the late Monsignor Orville Griese, and the other by the Director of the Pope John Center in Houston, Father Albert Moraczewski, O.P.

The Cronin Dissertation

Bishop Cronin's dissertation is a study of the extraordinary/ordinary means distinction in Catholic theology. This entails an historical and substantive examination of the distinction, from its grounding in the precept to conserve one's life, the explicit articulation of the distinction in the sixteenth century and its application from that point in the realm of pastoral medicine. Cronin demonstrates a clear development of this theological distinction in light of the pivotal developments taking place in medicine, e.g., the introduction of anesthesia and antiseptic procedure, and the resultant survivability of drastic medical intervention.

Cronin's doctoral studies predate the famous address of Pope Pius XII to the International Congress of Anesthesiologists of November 24, 1957. It was this address that articulated the ordinary/extraordinary means distinction at the level of papal teaching for the first time. Cronin presents a theological distinction applicable to a number of different types of illnesses: terminal illness, chronic illness and illnesses that are life threatening if left untreated but which perhaps require a certain therapeutic heroism. Pope Pius XII applied the richness of this theological tradition to the specific questions of resuscitation.

Since the Holy Father's address, the question of the ordinary or extraordinary nature of particular medical practices has been raised in innumerable contemporary cases. The Karen Quinlan case ended our technological honeymoon with the realization even at the popular level that the "technological imperative" ("If we *can* do it, we should") can and should be questioned. And so, for example, the difficult question of how aggressively to treat the

PVS (persistent vegetative state) patient is one contemporary forum in which we now hope to apply the distinction between ordinary and extraordinary (morally obligatory and morally optional) means. Starkly put, when is enough enough?

Because of the perennial recurrence of this question, the two additional monographs are added to the original Cronin work. Each picks up where Cronin left off. Monsignor Griese and Father Moraczewski approach the contemporary application from different perspectives and in different ways.

The Griese Monograph

Griese focuses attention on the issue of the artificial provision of nutrition and hydration [AN/H]. The crux of his argument can be stated as follows: There is a distinction between the *prolongation* of life (which is not morally imperative in all situations) and the *conservation* or sustaining of life (which is always morally obligatory.) This distinction, says Griese, echoes that made by the members of the Pontifical Academy of the Sciences which stated that medical *treatment* is not always morally obligatory, but ordinary *care* is always obligatory and may never be interrupted.

Griese then proceeds to say that the artificial provision of nutrition and hydration (e.g., by NG or gastrostomy tube) are morally obligatory forms of ordinary care (not medical treatment.) These means are obligatory in all circumstances except in cases in which the patient is physically unable to absorb the nourishment being directly placed in the alimentary canal, the imminence of death or the greater actual suffering induced by the feeding procedures themselves.

The reason for the obligatory nature of this artificial provision of nutrition and hydration rests on the further distinction between *supplementing* and *substituting* a vital function. When technically possible, the former is morally obligatory, the latter is not in all cases. Therefore, for Griese, the IV is always ordinary means (page 162) and "total parenteral nutrition [TPN] provided by the subclavian entry for a patient with a totally non-functional alimentary system would make it an extraordinary or disproportionate means of providing sustenance." (page 123.)

The moral methodology Griese employs is an explicitly "theocentric" methodology which may be described as deriving from a formulation of "dominion" and "stewardship" as moral coordinates. God has full dominion ("rulership") over what He has created. Humanity is given stewardship of creation. The theme of "conservation" is therefore quite resonant with this perspective. God is the ultimate explicit focus of ethical reflection in Griese's theological method. This too, derives from the traditional understanding of the definition of moral theology: "the scientific exposition of human conduct so far as it is directed by reason and faith to the attainment of our supernatural final end." (Jone/Adelman, I.1.)

In addition to the substantively moral evaluation of AN/H, Griese states that the courts equate artificially provided nutrition and hydration with a medical treatment which one can legitimately forego. Griese counters that AN/H is not therapeutic, that is, it cures no disease; therefore, it is not a medical treatment, but part of normal care. Further, the court's assumption that AN/H is optional medical treatment dovetails with a larger euthanasia strategy. Reassessment of this legal/medical trajectory is crucial, he says. The issue of AN/H is not a weighing of burdens and benefits. "The prime and formal focus is not on *burden as burden,* but on factors (costs, difficulties, etc.) which combine to constitute a virtual impossibility." (page 203).

Griese's section closes with four appendices: The Declaration on Euthanasia of 1980, a report from the Pontifical Council on Health Affairs [Cor Unum], a report of the Pontifical Academy of the Sciences and the allocution of Pope Pius XII to the International Congress of Anesthesiologists.

The Moraczewski Monograph

Part Three of *Conserving Human Life* is a contribution of Dominican Father Albert Moraczewski, director of the Pope John Center in Houston, and editor of *Ethics & Medics.* Moraczewski and Griese both focus attention squarely on the issue of nutrition and hydration, but each does so from a different perspective and with different conclusions. If one may describe Griese's examination of the material as "incisive," because of it primarily concentrates on the actual provision of nutrition and hydration as a process, Moraczewski's treatment of the same data may be described as "expansive," inasmuch as he concentrates primarily on the sweep of theological tradition as the horizon in which AN/H appears as one object of evaluation among many others.

Moraczewski's thesis can be summarized as follows: the Catholic theological tradition has consistently resisted any rigid identification of the terms "extraordinary" and "ordinary"—precisely as *moral* terms—with any given form of life-sustaining intervention. Therefore, it would be theologically improper to say, for example, that this or that life-conserving intervention is *always* ordinary means. Traditionally as well, food was considered to be a means to conserve life which in certain circumstances would be considered as morally optional. In other words, the distinction between ethically ordinary and extraordinary means articulates a "relative norm" which at times applies even to food and drink.

The duty to conserve life, then, is a positive precept of the natural law. Positive precepts oblige *"semper sed non pro semper."* That is, they do not bind in the presence of a proportionately grave difficulty. Negative precepts of the natural moral law such as "Thou shalt not kill" oblige *"semper et pro semper"*— always and in all circumstances.

The pivotal moral question becomes: "Is it of benefit to maintain a person indefinitely in a profound and permanent comatose condition? Would not the removal of food and hydration from this individual constitute direct killing?" Moraczewski parts company with Griese at this point. Moraczewski says "no." For purposes of *moral* evaluation, Moraczewski maintains that the physical and basic cause of death for this patient is the "concurrent pathology" of a severely damaged brain. It is this underlying irremediable pathology which prohibits the patient from being able to chew and swallow properly.

In the presence of irreversible and profound coma or in the PVS, Moraczewski maintains that there is no moral difference between providing the nutrition of calories by AN/H, and providing the nutrition of oxygen by artificial respiration. Moralists generally agree that there are situations in which the respirator can be considered extraordinary means of prolonging life. The same principles of such evaluation apply to AN/H as well. Throughout this consideration, the presence of PVS or profound and permanent coma is not a negligible factor in moral discernment about treatment and care. One cannot act as though this condition is not present.

Like Griese, Moraczewski is also sensitive to the moral climate being addressed by this "conversation" among Catholic theologians. Nevertheless, his premise can be summarized in the traditional maxim: *abusus non tollit usum*, the possibility of abuse cannot abolish the legitimate use of the subtle principles discussed in scholarly exchange. Despite real concerns about political manipulation by pro-euthanasia strategies, the theological dialogue must continue until the Holy See makes a definitive declaration on the matter of the artificial provision of nutrition and hydration.

* * * * *

The Pope John Center hopes to make its contribution to the ongoing discussion of these issues. In this volume the reader will find a comprehensive summary of the tradition until 1956 in Part I, the dissertation of Daniel Cronin. In Parts II and III, one will find two aspects of theological reflection on the development of the teaching on extraordinary and ordinary means vis-a-vis the tremendous progress in medical science and technological capability. Relevant documents are reprinted as appendices to Part II.

The present volume is intended to help clarify the issues and the vocabulary of some contemporary issues which medicine and moral theology discuss together. The precise "shape" the ordinary/extraordinary means distinction takes today can be stated this way: Can the artificial provision of nutrition and hydration be considered a morally optional involvement in the overall care of one who is not imminently dying but is unreachable and irretrievable because of the persistent vegetative state or profound and permanent coma? This book is intended for a variety of reading audiences, professionals, students and anyone interested in the vital issues of contemporary health care.

Anyone who studies this topic and reflects on the multifaceted issues involved and the complexity of contemporary health care potential and dilemmas is not engaged in a merely philosophical exercise. Rather, one is engaged in extended reflection about issues that confront real human beings, patients and those who care for and love them. One is, in this way, involved in the very *care* of the sick themselves, and in keeping company with those who have suffered great tragedy. And so, even in this academic forum, one is actively engaged in the mission of the Church and in the mystery of Christ.

In his Apostolic Letter on the *Christian Meaning of Human Suffering* (*Salvifici doloris*), the Holy Father, Pope John Paul II, offers these thoughts which may help the reader working through the text which follows:

"The parable of the Good Samaritan belongs to the Gospel of suffering. For it indicates what the relationship of each of us must be towards our suffering neighbor. We are not allowed to 'pass by on the other side' indifferently; we must 'stop' beside him. The name 'Good Samaritan' fits every individual who is sensitive to the sufferings of others, who 'is moved' by the misfortune of another . . .

"[T]he Good Samaritan of Christ's parable does not stop at sympathy and compassion alone. They become for him an incentive to actions aimed at bringing help to the injured man. In a word, then, a Good Samaritan is one who brings help in suffering, whatever its nature may be." [#28]

Father Russell E. Smith, S.T.D.
Director of Education
Feast of the Annunciation, 1989
Boston

Conserving Human Life
Part I

by
DANIEL A. CRONIN

A Doctrinal Dissertation
Orginally Published Under the Title of
THE MORAL LAW IN REGARD TO THE ORDINARY
AND EXTRAORDINARY MEANS OF CONSERVING LIFE

Dissertation Approved By
The Faculty Of the
Pontifical Gregorian University,
Rome, Italy
On May 30, 1956

Approved For Publication,
January 25, 1958

Foreword

At the request of the Pope John XXIII Center, I have made my dissertation, "The Moral Law In Regard to the Ordinary and Extraordinary Means
of Conserving Life," available for publication under its auspices. As a young
priest of the Archdiocese of Boston, I was privileged to be assigned for graduate studies in Moral Theology at the Gregorian University in Rome where I
had already obtained in 1953 the degree of Licentiate in Sacred Theology.
The research for my dissertation was begun in the Fall of 1954. It was defended in May 1956 as part of the requirements for the Doctorate in Sacred
Theology and was later published in 1958.

Frankly, I just worked seriously at what I had been assigned to do by the
Archbishop of Boston, the then Most Reverend Richard J. Cushing. It has
since emerged as a surprise to me that my dissertation contains research of
very important significance to those engaged presently in the ethical implications of certain medical and surgical procedures.

Though the insistence of staff members at the Pope John Center, I became convinced that what I had researched and deliberated upon concerning
the centuries old teaching of Catholic theologians could be of immense value
to modern day theologians and ethicists. Little did I realize that what I wrote
over thirty years ago as a young student, could be helpful today.

I would ask all who read this work to understand that it is presented as it
was put forward in 1956 with only minor annotations. It has not been rewrit-
ten. The reason for this is that I have been assured that the important contribution of the dissertation is the research and the resulting information which I
presented in the one work. I am happy to make this available to those who
will attempt to apply the age-old and consistent teaching of moral theologians
to the many, and at times intricate, practical cases occasioned by modern
medicine. It must be remembered, however, that apart from the teachings
over the centuries of the cited moral theologians, the views expressed by me
were those of a young student writing a doctoral dissertation, even though the
same work is hereby republished some thirty years later.

In reiterating my thanks to those mentioned in the original publication of my dissertation, I now add my expression of gratitude to all at the Pope John XXIII Center. In particular, I thank Monsignor Orville Griese whose insistent encouragement is the main reason for my agreement to the republication of "The Moral Law in Regard to the Ordinary and Extraordinary Means of Conserving Life" under its new title, "Conserving Human Life."

Monsignor Griese has written an insightful study about the means of conserving life, entitled "Feeding the Hopeless and the Helpless." This work, which is entirely his own, is printed as Part II of the Pope John XXIII publication: "Conserving Human Life."

Most Reverend Daniel A. Cronin, STD
Bishop of the Diocese of Fall River, Massachusetts

May 1988

1958—ORIGINAL INTRODUCTION—1958

This dissertation is a study of the moral law in regard to the ordinary and extraordinary means of conserving life. The moral principles of the natural law which govern the actions of men are immutable. However, as years pass, the conditions of human life change and present new circumstances in which these moral principles must be applied. But before these principles can be applied to the new conditions, it is very often necessary to investigate the meaning and implications of the principles. When the principles themselves are thus understood, an application of them to practical cases in new circumstances is not only easier, but also more exact.

This is particularly true in regard to the moral teaching on the ordinary and extraordinary means of conserving life. The advance of medical science presents in these days moral problems never before envisioned. Yet, these modern problems can be solved with the correct application of basic and changeless moral principles, if these principles are well understood. Very often medico-moral problems concern the licitness of a particular method of medical procedure. The moral solution in these cases concerns an action which may or may not be posited. However, the moral law in regard to the ordinary and extraordinary means of conserving life centers about a positive obligation. It concerns the definite duty incumbent on all men to care for their lives and health.

Modern medical science has advanced greatly. Today, it provides many artificial methods of preservation and prolongation of life. Very often, these methods are successful; often they are accompanied by serious danger and risk; often they are unsuccessful. Hence, an obvious question arises in regard to the moral obligation of using these means of conserving life. This moral question is especially pertinent when medical science is unable to cure a particular disease, but is able to postpone the death caused by the disease.

The textbooks and manuals of Moral Theology distinguish the ordinary means of conserving life from the extraordinary means of conserving life. The ordinary means are morally obligatory means, and the extraordinary means are usually not morally obligatory. The discussions on this question found in the manuals of Moral Theology, however, are quite brief. In general, they merely summarize the teaching found in the writings of the moralists of the sixteenth and seventeenth centuries, and very few authors have made any attempt to study this problem in the light of modern medical progress.

Before any licit application of the teachings of the moralists in this matter can be made to present day problems, one must clearly understand what the moralists meant by the terms, «ordinary means of conserving life» and «extraordinary means of conserving life». The early moralists did not define these terms, and they rarely, if ever, explained them. Frequently, however, they gave elements which constituted for them ordinary means and extraordinary means. Frequently too, they gave examples of ordinary and extraordinary means.

In the first chapter of this dissertation, the reader will find a study of the basic duty that binds all men to conserve their lives. This study is a necessary prerequisite to any discussion of the ordinary and extraordinary means of conserving life.

The second chapter contains an historical report of the opinion of the most noteworthy moral theologians in regard to the ordinary and extraordinary means of conserving life. Since many of these treatments cannot be found in the modern manuals of Moral Theology, they are given in Chapter Two as a basis for the discussion of these opinions, which follows in Chapter Three.

The first part of Chapter Three contains an analysis of the opinions of the moralists in regard to the ordinary and extraordinary means of conserving life. With the aid of this analysis, an attempt is then made to determine the nature of the ordinary and extraordinary means of conserving life. In the second part of the third chapter, a discussion of the moral obligation of using the ordinary and extraordinary means of conserving life is found.

The fourth chapter contains practical considerations in regard to the teaching on the ordinary and extraordinary means of conserving life, particularly with reference to modern medical and surgical procedures, and the obligation of the doctor in regard to supplying the ordinary and extraordinary means when he is treating a patient.

This dissertation is not a medical study of the ordinary and extraordinary means of conserving life. Rather, it is a study of the moral law in regard to these means. Hence, this dissertation contains discussions on the history of the moral teaching in this matter, the nature of ordinary and extraordinary means, and the moral obligation of using these means. Since the manuals of Moral Theology present only a very limited treatment of this problem, and since the concept of the nature of the ordinary and extraordinary means of conserving life is not always clear, and finally, since the determination of the moral obligation of using these means can sometimes be involved, it is hoped that this dissertation will present some clarification in regard to this very interesting and timely moral problem. In this way, it is also hoped that the theological investigation of the moral teaching on the ordinary and extraordinary means of conserving life will have been furthered and any future applications to practical cases, occasioned by medical progress, will thus be facilitated.

The author wishes to express his sincere gratitude to His Excellency, the Most Reverend Richard J. Cushing, D.D., Archbishop of Boston, for the opportunity of undertaking graduate studies in Sacred Theology. Thanks are also due to Thomas P. Linehan, Jr., M.D. of London, England, whose advice and suggestions have been of great assistance. The author is particularly indebted to the late Reverend Edwin F. Healy, S.J., Professor of Moral Theology for many years at the Pontifical Gregorian University in Rome, for his generous and expert guidance in directing the writing of this dissertation.**

Daniel A. Cronin
1958

**The author holds in prayerful remembrance his mother and father to whom the original dissertation was dedicated.

Conserving Human Life
Part I

by
DANIEL A. CRONIN

A Doctrinal Dissertation
Originally Published Under the Title of
THE MORAL LAW IN REGARD TO THE ORDINARY
AND EXTRAORDINARY MEANS OF CONSERVING LIFE

Dissertation Approved By
The Faculty Of the
Pontifical Gregorian University,
Rome, Italy
On May 30, 1956

Approved For Publication,
January 25, 1958

CHAPTER I

The Duty To Conserve One's Life

Human life is at once a gift and a responsibility—a gift, because man could never create himself; a responsibility because man must use this gift properly. God, Life itself, is the source of all other life and to Him alone, therefore, belongs every power over it. Christians have ever appreciated this truth and none perhaps better than the Apostle, Paul: "None of us lives as his own master and none of us dies as his own master. While we live we are responsible to the Lord, and when we die we die as his servants. both in life and in death we are the Lord's."[1]

Among the natural gifts with which the Most High God has favored man, there is none so excellent as that of life, because it is life that is the basis for all that man has or can hope to attain.

The human person exists as a composite: the immortal soul by which he is endowed with an intellect and free will, (this makes him similar to God Himself); the body through which his soul acts to satisfy man's natural needs and to acquire merit in the supernatural order.

Human life then is a gift, the fuller meaning of which becomes more evident elsewhere in Catholic theology. For the moral theologian, however, the aspect of main concern is life as a responsibility. This dissertation will

---

[1]Romans: 14, 7-8. The translation was taken from *The New American Bible* (Nashville—New York, Thomas Nelson, Publishers, 1971).

treat of one point under that aspect; namely, the extent to which man has the duty of conserving his corporeal life here in this world. In other words, pre-supposing the fact that on earth the body is a necessity in order that «the man» can act, this investigation will continue on then to determine just what responsibility man has to conserve his bodily life and health prior to that final hour which God alone knows and He alone will divulge.

1.1   THE MALICE OF SUICIDE

Interestingly enough, the reasons traditionally assigned to prove the duty of self-conservation are the very same ones by which the theologians have consistently exposed the basic malice of suicide. To explain, therefore, that suicide is evil is by that very fact a virtual demonstration of an equally true proposition: self-conservation is a duty.

It is quite apparent that there exists deeply embedded in the human fiber a strong drive which urges man on to self-conservation. Gradually, it also becomes clear that there is coupled together with this human urge a very definite duty to conserve one's life. Nonetheless, however forceful the natural drive may be, or however clear the duty of self-conservation may become, one seeks an explanation of the underlying reasons and this can be involved.

Quite often it happens that before any process of reasoning takes place, one recognizes the truth of the conclusion. It is only when the intellect brings forth the arguments that the difficulty begins. This detail did not escape the eminent Cardinal De Lugo;[2] it is precisely in his discussion of suicide that he mentions it. For de Lugo, the intrinsic wickedness of suicide is immediately apparent; the basis of this truth, however, is not quite so obvious.

A—The teaching in Sacred Scripture, the Fathers
and Church Documents

Properly speaking, suicide, as understood here, is the direct killing of a man, perpetrated by the man himself and on his own authority.[3] Suicide, thus understood, is always gravely illicit.

---

[2]«Tota difficultas consistit in assignanda ratione huius veritatis: nam licet turpitudo haec statim appareat, non tamen facile est eius fundamentum invenire: unde, quod in aliis multis quaestionibus contingit, magis certa est conclusio, quam rationes, quae variae a diversis afferuntur ad eius probationem».—J. de Lugo, *Disputationes Scholasticae et Morales* (ed. nova; Parisiis, Vivès, 1868-1869), VI, *De Iustitia et Iure,* Disp. X, Sec. I, n. 2.

[3]Later in this discussion, the broader definition, as given in E. F. Regatillo et M. Zalba,

That God alone has the power of life and death, the Book of Deuteronomy clearly states—«Learn then that I, I alone, am God, and there is no god besides me. It is I who bring both death and life,»[4] and again in Wisdom: «For you have dominion over life and death; you lead down to the gates of the nether world, and lead back.»[5]

To God then, belongs the power of life, and man must never fancy that he may determine the hour of death—Thou shalt not kill.[6] By this fifth injunction of the Decalogue, God forbids not only homicide but also suicide. How cleverly St. Augustine caught the full import of the fifth commandment:

It is not without significance, that in no passage of the holy canonical books can there be found either divine precept or permission to take away our own life whether for the sake of entering on the enjoyment of immortality or of shunning or ridding ourselves of anything whatever. Nay, the law, rightly interpreted even prohibits suicide where it says, Thou shalt not kill. This is proved specially by the omission of the words, «thy neighbor», which are inserted when false witness is forbidden . . . how much greater reason have we to understand that a man may not kill himself, since in the commandment, «Thou shalt not kill», there is no limitation added nor any exception made in favour of anyone, at least of all in favour of him on whom the command is laid . . . The commandment is «Thou shalt not kill man»—therefore neither another nor yourself, for he who kills himself still kills nothing else than man.[7]

Theologiae Moralis Summa (Matriti, Biblioteca de Autores Cristianos, 1953), II, p. 257, will prove more accurate. Zalba, the author of this second volume defines suicide as: «actio vel omissio quae ad mortem propriam causandam natura sua ordinatur ».

[4]Deuteronomy: 32, 39. This translation, and all translations of the Holy Scriptures cited herein, are taken from The New American Bible (cf. note 1).

[5]Wisdom: 16, 13.

[6]Exodus: 20, 13.

[7]S. Augustinus, *De Civitate Dei*, Liber I, Cap.20 (Migne, *Patrologiae Cursus Completus*, Series Latina [Parisiis, 1844-1864], XLI, col. 34-35). Henceforth, this series will be referred to as MPL. The translation from St. Augustine is taken from the *City of God*, Modern Library Edition (New York, Random House Inc., 1950).

Such has been the tradition among ecclesiastical writers down through the ages, as these excerpts testify:

Lactantius:

For if the one guilty of homicide is wicked because he destroys a man, the same crime is to be leveled on him who kills himself because he also kills a man. Indeed, we must consider this crime greater, the revenge for which lies with God alone. For, just as we did not come into this life of our own free-will, so also we must leave this domicile of the body, which was given to us to watch over, by the command of the same person who placed us in this body to inhabit it until such time as He orders us to depart from it . . . [8]

St. Jerome:

It is not up to us to seize death but to accept it willingly when inflicted by others.[9]

Rabanus Maurus, the Abbot of Fulda:

Excepting those whom either a generally just law or the very source of justice, God, in a special way commands to be killed, anyone who would kill another man or himself is guilty of the crime of homicide.[10]

Peter Abelard also discusses the problem of suicide, giving many famous examples from ancient times in chapter 155 of his *Theologica et Philosophica*.[11]

---

[8]« Nam si homicida nefarius est, quia hominis exstinctor est, eidem sceleri obstrictus est, qui se necat, quia hominem necat. Imo vero maius esse id facinus existimandum est, cuius ultio Deo soli subiacet. Nam sicut in hanc vitam non nostra sponte venimus, ita rursus ex hoc domicilio corporis, quod tuendum nobis assignatum est, eiusdem iussu recedendum est, qui nos in hoc corpus induxit, tamdiu habituros, donec iubeat emitti . . .»—Lactantius, *Divinarum Institutionum*, Lib. III, Cap. 18 (MPL. VI, col. 407).

[9]« Non est nostrum, mortem arripere, sed illatam ab aliis libenter excipere».—S. Hieronymus, *Commentaria in Jonam*, Cap. 1, ver. 12 (MPL. XXV, col. 1129).

[10]« His ergo exceptis quos vel lex generaliter iusta vel ipse fons iustitiae Deus specialiter occidi iubet, quisquis hominem vel seipsum vel quemlibet occiderit, homicidii crimine innecitur . . .»—Rabanus Maurus, *Commentaria in libros Machabaeorum*, (MPL. CIX, col. 1255).

[11]Petrus Abelardus, *Theologica et Philosophica*, (MPL. CLXXVIII, col. 1603-1606). The reader can confer also MPL., Index de suicidio, CCXX, col. 858-861, for a concise list of other references to the crime of suicide in the writings of the ecclesiastical authors.

6

The teaching of the Church has been no less constant. Even in the sixth century, the Church legislated against suicide in the Council of Orleans.[12] It was decided at that time not to accept the offerings of a man who died by his own hand. In the Catechism of the Council of Trent, one reads: « No man possesses such power over his life as to be at liberty to put himself to death. Hence we find that the Commandment does not say: Thou shalt not kill another, but simply Thou shalt not kill».[13] More recently, Pope Leo XIII reiterated the Church's doctrine when writing to the Bishops of Germany and Austria in regard to duelling.[14] Add to this also, the sanctions placed on the one who has attempted suicide ("sibi vitam adimere tentaverit") by the laws of the Church in the present Codex Iuris Canonici[15] and it then becomes quite clear that the teaching of the Church holds suicide to be a grave sin.

B—The teaching of St. Thomas and subsequent theologians

Catholic theologians have ever been mindful of the problem of suicide and in their writings have constantly censured it as base and despicable, always and everywhere to be condemned. The arguments employed by the theologians have their foundation in Sacred Scripture, the writings of the Fathers and Doctors of the Church, the practice of the Church, and also in reason itself.

St. Thomas had an extraordinary understanding of metaphysics and thus produced an equally extraordinary treatment of ethics.[16] Hence, his tract on suicide in question 64, article 5 of the Secunda Secundae of his *Summa Theologica* has been the basis for the subsequent theological discussions on the subject down through the years.

After introducing the article, as is his wont, with five arguments in favor of the opposite opinion, St. Thomas proceeds then to demonstrate by a three-fold argument the malice of suicide. First of all, suicide is against the natural

---

[12]J. Mansi, *Sacrorum Conciliorum Nova et Amplissima Collectio*, vols. 1–31, (ed. novissima, Phil. Labbeus-Cossaritius-Coleti; Florentiae-Venetiis, 1759–1798), VIII, 837.

[13]« Neque vero seipsum interficere cuipiam fas est; cum vitae suae nemo ita potestatem habeat, ut suo arbitratu mortem sibi consciscere liceat, ideoque huius Legis verbis non ita praescriptum est, Ne alium occidas, sed simpliciter, Ne occidas».—*Catechismus ex Decreto SS. Concilii Tridentini* (Patavii, 1758), Pars Tertia, Cap. VI, de Quinto Praecepto, N. 10.

[14]Leo XIII, *Pastoralis officii*, epistola ad episcopos Germ. et Austr., 12.Sept. 1891. Cf. H. Denzinger, *Enchiridion Symbolarum*, ed. J. Umberg (Friburgi, Herder & Co., 1942), n. 1939. Hereafter this work will be referred to by the letter D.

[15]*Code of Canon Law*, Latin-English Edition (Washington, D.C.: Canon Law Society of America, 1983), Canons 1041.5 and 1044.3.

[16]Cf. G. Gustafson, *The Theory of Natural Appentency in the Philosophy of St. Thomas* (Washington, Catholic University Press, 1944), p. 99.

inclination and charity with which everyone should love himself. In the second place, since every man is a part of the community and in that sense belongs to the community, he does an injury to the community when he destroys himself. Lastly, since God alone, according to Scripture, causes a man to live, and He alone should decide the hour of death, the one who deprives himself of life by suicide is actually usurping the judgment of a matter over which God actually never gave him jurisdiction.[17] St. Thomas, replying to the first objection, adds that suicide has a double aspect: in relation to the man himself, the guilty party has sinned against charity; in relation to God and the community, he has sinned against justice.[18]

Is man the master of himself? If so, it would seem that he might choose to live or die. Hence, any attempt on his part to appoint the hour of death would not only be licit, but sometimes, might even be laudable; e.g., he could select the time when his soul would be best prepared to meet God and thus insure his salvation. At least, one must admit that by suicide, if it were licit, it would be possible to avoid further sin.

Contained in the above reasoning is a fallacy which the Angelic Doctor exposes in his reply to the third objection:

We must say that man is constituted master of himself by his free will. Of his own free will, therefore, man is allowed to dispose of things of his life. But the passage from this life to a happier life, does not lie within the power of man's free will but, rather, within the power of Almighty God.[19]

Theologians subsequent to St. Thomas were heavily influenced by his argumentation. Some, in fact, were content with either a direct quoting of his words or a mere rephrasing.[20] Others, however, began to consider the full import of the reasoning, and thus, have left in their works a heritage of further thought on the subject. For example, the notion of justice existing between God and man was the point that Molina found troublesome. For him, our relationship with God is not one of justice; at least it does not fulfill

---

[17]S. Thomae Aquinatis, *Summa Theologica* (Taurini, Marietti, 1950), Pars II: II, q. 64, art. 5. For a very good commentary on this article, confer *Somme Theologique—Saint Thomas D'Aquin* (Editions de la Reveu des Jeunes, Paris, Desclée, 1934), II, La Justice, pp. 146 ss.

[18]St. Thomas, op. cit., II:II, q. 64, art. 5, ad 1.

[19]« Ad tertium dicendum quod homo constituitur dominus sui ipsius per liberum arbitrium. Et ideo licite potest homo de seipso disponere quantum ad ea quae pertinent ad hanc vitam, quae hominis libero arbitrio regitur. Sed transitus de hac vita ad aliam feliciorem non subiacet libero arbitrio hominis, sed potestati divinae»—Ibid., ad 3.

[20]Cf. D. Soto, *De Iustitia et Iure* (Lugduni, 1582), Lib. V. Quaes. I. Art. V.

8

the complete notion of justice because we are never in the position of being able to render to God the equivalent of what He gives us. However, Molina feels that even though there is something of higher value than justice which binds us to God, nevertheless, we can speak of justice in the less strict sense,[21] and thus condemns suicide as a sin against justice with respect to God.[22] This is true because man does not possess dominion over his own life; the Author of nature has reserved this dominion to Himself.[23]

When one is said to have dominion over anything, the implication is that he has supreme authority over it.[24] Hence, when theologians repeat again and again that the dominion over life belongs to God, they mean that He alone has the supreme and ultimate power over it.[25]

On this notion of dominion, theologians have built their argument from reason. Cardinal de Lugo develops it nicely. The Cardinal cites the statement of St. Thomas in the *Summa Theologica,* 2:2, q. 64, art. 5, that man is not the master of his life. Then, de Lugo proceeds to praise Molina for a very fine exposition of the consequence of this statement. Since man is not the master of his life, he can not dispose of it at will; much less can he destroy it, because to destroy something implies an act which is proper only to the one having supreme mastery over it. This is all well and good, but for de Lugo, the problem is not explaining the consequence, but rather, proving the fact that man is not master of his own life. Very cleverly, de Lugo goes to the heart of the argumentation. For him, therefore, once it is proved that man does not possess supreme authority over his life, then everything else fits into place— but first, prove the point.

Now we prove that man is not the master of his life this way: although man can receive dominion over things which are extrinsic to himself or which are distinct from him, he cannot, however, receive dominion over himself, because from the very concept and definition, it is clear that a master is something relative, for example, a father or a teacher; and just as no one can be father or teacher of himself, so neither can he be master of himself, for to be master always denotes superiority with regard to the one over whom he is the master. Hence, God Himself cannot be master of Himself, even though He possesses Himself most perfectly. There-

---

[21]Cf. St. Thomas, op. cit., II;II, 1. 58, art. 2.
[22]Cf. L. Molina, *De Iustitia et Iure* (Coloniae Agrippinae, 1614), IV, Tract. 3, Disp. 1, n. 1.
[23]Ibid., Disp. 9, n. 2; also St. Thomas, op. cit., II:II. 1. 59, art. 3, ad 2.
[24]Cf. word «dominion», *Webster's Collegiate Dictionary* (Springfield, Merriam Co., 1942), p. 299.
[25]Cf. Deuteronomy: 32, 39.

fore man cannot be master of himself, however, he can be master of his operations, and therefore, he can sell himself and thus, improperly speaking, we might say he gives mastery of himself to another but, he really does not give over mastery of himself basically or radically, but only mastery over certain of his operations, . . . therefore a man can dispose only of his own operations of which he is the master, not of himself, (or to say the same thing) not of his own life over which he is not master, nor can he be.[26]

A study of these words of de Lugo revels that fundamentally, he bases his reasoning on the notion of relativity contained in the concept of dominion, and ultimately on the relation which man, the creature, has to God, his Creator. For de Lugo, to have dominion necessarily implies something extrinsic to the one having dominion. Over and above that, dominion implies superiority, so that not even God has dominion over Himself, properly speaking. Since it is obvious that no man can be extrinsic or superior to himself, it follows that neither can he be basically master or lord of himself in regard to his life.

While it is true that man possesses a mastery over the actions of his life, which after all proceed from his own free will, he does not possess any like mastery over his life radically. Therefore, lacking the mastery, he must not act the part of a master and perform an act proper to the master alone—destruction. Hence, because of the lack of dominion in the strict sense, direct suicide is gravely illicit.[27]

Who, then, has the supreme dominion? The implication is rather simple for de Lugo. God is the only one who is both extrinsic and superior to man—it is from God that man came—and therefore, He alone has supreme dominion. This becomes clear from de Lugo's reply to the first objection where he reasons that it would be licit for a man to kill himself in virtue of a precept or

---

[26]«Porro hominem non esse dominum suae vitae, probari potest, quia licet homo potuerit accipere dominium aliarum rerum, quae sunt extra ipsum, vel quae ab ipso distinguuntur; non tamen potuit accipere dolminium sui ipsius, quia ut ex ipso conceptu et definitione constat, dominus est aliquid relativum, sicut pater, et magister; quare sicut nemo potest esse pater vel magister sui ipsius, ita nec potest esse sui ipsius dominus: nam dominus semper dicit superioritatem respectu illius cuius est dominus. unde nec Deus ipse potest esse dominus sui ipsius, quamvis possideat perfectissime seipsum. non potuit ergo homo fieri dominus sui ipsius, potest quidem esse dominus suarum operationum, et ideo potest vendere seipsum, et tunc dicitur improprie dare aleri dominium sui ipsius; sed revera non dat proprie dominium sui simpliciter sed solum in ordine ad aliquas suas operationes . . . solum ergo potest homo disponere de suis operationibus, quarum dominus est, non de seipso, vel, quod idem est, de vita sua, cuius dominus non est, nec esse potest»—J. de Lugo, op. cit., Disp. X, Sec. I, n. 9.

[27]Cf. ibid., n. 10 ss., where de Lugo refutes the objections made to his doctrine.

10

permission from God, because God, after all, possesses the most perfect dominion over life and man would act then as His instrument.[28] The theologians appreciated the value of this basic notion of dominion. It was quite logical then for them to take the next step and apply the distinction existing at the time in juridic terminology between dominion over the «substance» of a thing and dominion over its «usefulness». The first is known as a direct or radical dominion; the second, as an indirect or dominion of use.[29] With these terms then, the theologians explained the difference between God's status and man's status in regard to a man's human life. To God belongs the basic or radical dominion and He allows man an indirect dominion or possession of its usefulness. Regarding his human life, man has only the right to its proper use because God alone possesses the basic lordship over its substance.

It is in this manner that for centuries theologians have refuted the arguments in favor of suicide and proved its malice. The reasoning can be put in the form of traditional scholastic argumentation as follows:

Man in killing himself usurps the direct dominion over his life which belongs to God alone.
To usurp this dominion is a grave violation of a divine right.
Therefore, man in killing himself, violates in a serious way a divine right.

The proof then of the major is: the one having dominion over anything is the one for whom the usefulness of such a thing is primarily intended, so that he can dispose of it for his own benefit without fear of violating another man's prior rights. Man, however, has not been created primarily for his own convenience or utility, but rather, for the glory and worship of God. Thus, he can not dispose of himself without consideration of God's rights. Therefore, he is not his own master in regard to the basic rights over his life. The minor in the argumentation is clear enough and discussion concerns only the major.

Such is the argumentation that appear generally in the writing of the Catholic theologians and moral philosophers.[30] True, changes here and there

---

[28]Ibid., n. 10.
[29]Cf. F. Hürth—P. Abellán, *De Praeceptis* (Romae, Pontificia Universitas Gregoriana, 1948), p. 20, for a brief but precise explanation of these juridic terms.
[30]S. Alphonsus, *Theologia Moralis* (Romae, ex Typographia Vaticana, 1905), Lib. III, Tract. 4, Cap. 1, Dub. 1, n. 366; A. Lehmkuhl, *Theologia Moralis* (ed. 10; Friburgi Brisgoviae, Herder, 1902), I, pp. 346–347; H. Noldin—A. Schmitt, *Summa Theologiae Moralis* (ed. 27; Oeniponte/ Lipsiae, Rauch, 1940–41), II, p. 309; Aertnys-Damen, *Theologia Moralis* (ed. 16; Marietti, 1950), I, p. 458; L. Fanfani, *Manuale Theorico-Practicum Theologiae Moralis* (Romae, Libraria Ferrari,

in the presentation of the argument occur. The variation depends on the author. No change, however, is so singular as to warrant special mention here. These writers in their expression of the argument based on the divine dominion over human life obviously suppose the existence of God, creation and the end of man which is to be attained in the next life, as facts proved elsewhere.[31] They then proceed to set forth their argument. This procedure is, of course, legitimate enough. As a matter of fact, the suppositions are quite necessary if one is to capture the validity of the reasoning process.[32]

One frequently finds the argument from *charity* conjoined with the argument based on the exclusive dominion of God over human life. Man is bound to exercise the virtue of charity in regard to himself as he is in regard to others and this virtue he violates seriously by suicide.[33] However the argument based on the virtue of charity does not seem to find unconditioned favor because of what theologians feel is a lack of universality. For example, one might argue that a situation could arise in which a man would actually show more love for himself if he would kill himself, rather than live in the necessary proximate danger of sinning seriously. Thus the authors feel that the prohibition against suicide must be proved from some other source besides the virtue of charity alone.[34] Once suicide is proved illicit by another argument, e.g., the singular right which God has over human life, then, of course, it is true to say that man also sins against the love which he owes himself.[35]

An interesting treatment of this problem occurs in the writings of Father Vermeersch. His approach is slightly different. Vermeersch states the arguments based on the dominion of God and the charity due one's self. He then proceeds to show that suicide also offends against the virtue of piety towards

---

1950), II, p. 323; Regatillo-Zalba, op. cit., II, p. 258; V. Cathrein, *Philosophia Moralis* (ed. 20; Friburgi Brisg., Herder, 1955), p. 245; Schuster, *Philosophia Moralis* (Friburgi Brisgoviae, Herder, 1950), pp. 91–92; Costa-Rossetti, *Philosophia Moralis* (Oeniponte, Rauch, 1886), pp. 265 ss.; T. Meyer, *Institutiones Iuris Naturalis* (Fributgi Brisgoviae, Herder, 1900), II, p. 41; *Philosophiae Scholasticae Sunma* (Matriti, Biblioteca de Autores Cristanos, 1952), III, p. 553.

[31] Cf. Schuster, op. cit., p. 91.

[32] There are some who feel that there is apparent in the argument based on the dominion of God, an unwarranted influence of « juridism ». Cf. Bender, « Organorum humanorum transplantatio », *Angelicum*, XXI (1954), pp. 148–149. Of interest also is the contention of some that all the arguments against suicide are founded, in fact ultimately resolve themselves into the argument based on man's lack of perfect dominion over himself.

[33] Cf. Mt.: 22, 39; also Hürth-Abellán, *De Principiis* (Romae Pontificia Universitas Gregoriana, 1948), p. 276.

[34] Cf. Schuster, op. cit., p. 91.

[35] Cf. St. Thomas, op. cit., II: II, q. 64, art. 5.

one's self.[36] Vermeersch explains this by pointing out that when a man commits suicide, he removes the fundamental condition of all worship—his life. By so doing, he fails to acknowledge his essential dependence on God, the Creator, and thus refuses to recognize his obligation to revere in himself the image of God from Whom he has come and to Whom, alone, belongs the dominion over his life.[37]

By way of summary then, we may say the Catholic position in regard to suicide is that a man always sins seriously when he attempts to take his life on his own authority. This is so because suicide is a grave infraction of the natural law, the divine positive law, and the ecclesiastical law. The natural law is violated because man has only the right of using his life and never possesses a radical dominion over the substance of it. Hence, by suicide, he usurps a divine right. Suicide is prohibited also by the divine law in view of the fifth commandment,[38] the duty of loving one's self[39] and the open declaration in Scripture of God's dominion over life.[40] Finally, the ecclesiastical law forbids suicide and thus the perpetrator offends against Church law. Add to this the constant teachings of the ecclesiastical writers, theologians, and moralists and one understands plainly and appreciates fully the import of the teaching of the Church in this matter. Scripture,[41] Tradition, and the teaching Church all show the malice of suicide.

1.2 THE RESPONSIBILITY OF CONSERVING ONE'S HUMAN LIFE

A—Catholic teaching

Since man does not have perfect dominion over his life, but only a right to its use, which he receives from God, it follows that he is bound to take

---

[36]A. Vermeersch, *Theologiae Moralis Principia-Responsa-Consilia* (ed. 3; Roma, Pontificia Universitas Gregoriana, 1945), II, n. 296.

[37]Cf. A. Vermeersch, *Quaestiones de Virtutibus Religionis et Pietatis* (Brugis, Baeyaert, 1912), p. 205, n. 183 and p. 215, n. 190, for an added treatment of this argument.

[38]Exodus: 20, 13.

[39]Mt: 22, 39.

[40]Deuteronomy: 32, 39; Wisdom: 16, 13.

[41]History reveals instances in which saints and martyrs threw themselves into fire or undertook other fatal tortures. Because of this, an objection often arises against the Church's condemnation of suicide. Also, in the Old Testament, Samson (Judges: 17, 30) killed himself and yet St. Paul numbered him among the saints (Hebrews: 11, 32). The interpretation of these events can be found in de Lugo; op. cit., Disp. X, Sec. I, n. 15; Regatillo-Zalba, op. cit., II, p. 259. Cf. also

proper care of it. Since he does not own his life, he must conserve it until such time as is indicated by the rightful owner.

Man does have dominion over his actions and even a certain dominion over his life and members, but only such as allows him certain limited rights: «Furthermore private men have no dominion over the members of their body other than that which pertains to their natural ends . . .»[42]. Lacking therefore the perfect dominion, he not only must not destroy his life, but he must conserve it in a positive manner. He is not the lord of his life but only its custodian, and thus, he has the obligation and responsibility of caring for what has been entrusted to his charge. As the administrator of his life, he has the duty to take the steps necessary for its conservation. To him has been given life, not to be lost but to be conserved.

If however, man fails in this regard; if man decides to disregard his responsibility of administration and custody; if man does not conserve his life, he then violates the same law which forbids him to kill himself: «The same precept which prohibits suicide also prescribes by that very fact, the conservation of one's life, since not to conserve one's life and to commit suicide are virtually the same.»[43] Hence, there is no difficulty in recognizing the duty of conserving one's life as a rather obvious consequence of the doctrine that suicide is illicit. Also, from the realization that man is merely the custodian of his life, the inference is clear—namely, he must conserve it and care for it.

In the Decalogue, no one can find this specific command: Thou shalt conserve thy life. Yet, Sacred Scripture certainly extols the value of human life. God is the ultimate end of man and of his actions, so that in all his actions, he should direct himself to glorifying God and one day possessing Him.[44] Man accomplishes this end by the exercise of his powers and faculties. God has given certain natural gifts to man and, if he uses these properly, he will merit eternal salvation, thus giving glory to God and attaining the lasting possession of God.

Among these gifts of God, there is none more precious than life itself, for without life, there is no power or faculty or action. The first requirement,

---

S. Augustine, *De Civitate Dei,* Cap. 21; St. Thomas, op. cit., II:II, q. 64, art. 5, ad 4. Briefly, we may say that these authors interpret the actions of the saints and martyrs and usually explain them as having occurred due to an erroneous conscience or to a divine inspiration.

[42]«Ceterum, quod ipsi privati homines in sui corporis membra dominatum alium non habeant, quam quid ad eorum naturales fines pertineat . . .»—Pius XI. *Casti connubii,* D. 2246.

[43]«Idem praeceptum, quod prohibet sui occisionem, eo ipso praecipit etiam propriae vitae conservationem, cum virtualiter idem sit vitam non conservare et vitam sibi adimere».—Noldin-Schmitt, op. cit., II, p. 307.

[44]Regatillo-Zalba, op. cit., I, pp. 36–44.

therefore, for man in order that he may merit heaven is life here on earth. Then, as a true steward, he supervises these gifts of his Master until the Master demands an accounting.[45] His time of existence here on earth becomes for him a period of probation. The entire New Testament portrays life as the time in which man must use the God-given talents[46] with which he can save his soul. Life is a period of sowing good seed in preparation for the harvest.[47] It is during life that man has the opportunity of working in the vineyard of the Lord.[48] Thus he is able to store up treasures in heaven.[49]

If, therefore, the relation between man's life on earth and future happiness in heaven is so intimate, an appreciation of the value of his life immediately arises. Man then should guard it, protect it, care for it, and conserve it as he would any precious thing. Certainly, he should not injure it; much less, should he destroy it. However, since man in this present economy can not hold himself indifferent to his supernatural end which is obligatory,[50] and since this end is attained by the correct use of his powers and faculties here on earth, one can argue that, therefore, the use of these powers and faculties and the life which is their foundation is also obligatory, because he who is bound to an end is bound also to the means. Then, since the use of the means, which in this case have not been freely elected by man but assigned by God,[51] is obligatory, the conservation of them is also obligatory. This is true because the obligation to use a thing does not bind unless the thing exists. In this particular case, however, the thing concerned—his life and faculties—has been placed at man's disposal by a higher power precisely for that purpose— namely, use. Furthermore, it can be gathered from Sacred Scripture, as we saw above, that the time for meriting is not a period determined by the servant but rather, by the Master. Thus, the use of necessary means of meriting and their conservation is obligatory not merely for a stated time, but until such time as God demands a settling of man's eternal account. Hence, it is true to say that the responsibility which man has to conserve his life is evident also in Scripture.

From another point of view, Pope Leo XIII, in his Encyclical *Rerum Novarum,* expresses the necessity of conserving one's life. Writing about the nature of human work, the Pope remarks that work is not only something

---

[45]Luke: 16, 2.
[46]Mt: 25, 14.
[47]Mt: 13, 24 ss.
[48]Mt: 20, 1.
[49]Mt: 6, 20.
[50]Cf. Regatillo-Zalba, op. cit., I, pp. 45 ss.
[51]Cf. T. Meyer, op. cit., II, p. 48.

15

personal, but also something quite necessary because it is the way in which man can care for his human life. To take care of one's life, the Pontiff emphasizes, is a demand of the very nature of things with which it is necessary to comply.[52] The Holy Father says: «Indeed, to remain in life is a duty common to all—the non-fulfillment of which is a crime. Hence, the right of acquiring the goods by which life is sustained necessarily arises . . .».[53] The teaching of Leo XIII, therefore, declares openly that the right to work exists precisely because man has the duty to conserve his life which he accomplishes by means which his daily work provides.

In this matter, the doctrine of the Church and her theologians has been consistent and constant through the ages. This is not surprising because, first of all, the Church has always condemned suicide, as has been shown, and thus the logical concomitant, self-conservation, has been rather obvious. Secondly, because of the value of human life as a precious gift of God, and of its necessity for performing meritorious acts, the theologians have, as we shall see, constantly emphasized the responsibility of using the means of self-conservation. An understanding of creation, the value of man's body and soul, and his final end leaves room for no other doctrine in this regard.

Commonly, theologians are accustomed to use also the argument based on the virtue of charity.[54] Man is bound to love himself. Therefore, a fortiori, he must exercise charity in regard to his life and thus, he is bound to care for his life and conserve it as the means which serve for obtaining eternal salvation.[55] Most theologians, however, add this argument to the others by which they have already proved the necessity of self-conservation.[56]

St. Thomas employed the argument from charity when emphasizing the import of the natural attachment that all men have to life: «. . . it is by nature that everything loves itself so that everything conserves itself in being and resists, as far as it can, any corrupting influences. Therefore, he who kills himself, acts against a natural inclination and against the charity by which a man should love himself».[57] This excerpt from the *Summa Theologica* serves well

---

[52]Leo XIII, *Rerum Novarum*, D. 1938c.

[53]«Reapse manere in vita, commune singulis officium est, cui scelus est deesse. Hinc ius reperiendarum rerum, quibus vita sustentatur, necessario nascitur . . .»—loc. cit.

[54]Cf. St. Thomas, op. cit., II:II, 1. 25, art. 4–5.

[55]Cf. L. Fanfani, op. cit., II, p. 126.

[56]The theologians are somewhat reserved about this argument. They feel it is valid as far as it goes but that it is not sufficiently universal to prove by itself the necessity of self-conservation. This point has been mentioned already in the discussion on suicide, but it is worthwhile here to call attention to the treatment in Cathrein, op. cit., p. 247, n. 347.

[57]«. . . naturaliter quaelibet res seipsam amat: et ad hoc pertinet quod quaelibet res naturaliter conservat se in esse et corrumpentibus resistit quantum potest. Et ideo quod aliquis seipsum

16

as an introduction to the argument based on man's natural desire to live. St. Thomas recognized the instincts that man finds within himself. In his writings, therefore, he was quick to reveal their fuller meaning and implications. Certainly, the first instinct of man is the attachment to life and the desire to live. In fact, it is the first instinct of all living being. Quite properly, someone has defined life as «the internal power of development and of resistance to destruction».[58] Within himself, man senses a vigorous drive which urges him on to protect and perfect himself under all conditions, and to oppose all powers bent on his destruction. Deep within himself, he senses a passionate urge to live. Even in times of adversity, his basic concern is the protection of his well-being, and the fear of his own destruction initiates violent reactions throughout his whole human structure. His is an ardent love of life and a forceful instinct to live— and this he shares with every member of the human race.

There is no doubt that this basic instinct within man manifests the law of nature for him. Such a design of nature he must not only approve but effectively obey. Hence, he has the obligation to comply with nature and conserve his life in a positive manner. Not to do so constitutes a crime against nature, since he is acting against a natural inclination placed in him by the Author of nature itself.[59] One author phrases it this way: «It is *impossible that any appetite set up in us by nature should be directed to any other thing than the fuller being of the individual. It is impossible that it should aim at nothingness or at destruction*».[60] A simple glance at human life as it exists today in the world, and as it has existed since the beginning, reveals that what is said of the theory of this human desire to live and better one's self, has also worked out in practice. Man and woman unite to initiate the family by which they actually perfect their own personalities in addition to accomplishing other ends. The families have formed society, and all society is directed not only to the perpetuation and conservation of the human race, but also to its betterment and development by enabling man to accomplish in society what he could not do alone. Certainly, society is not bent on the destruction of the human race. Society represents the inner feelings of each individual of which it is comprised, and

---

occidat est contra inclinationem naturalem, et contra caritatem, qua quilibet debet seipsum diligere».—St. Thomas, op. cit., II:II, q. 64, art. 5, in corp.

[58]«Pouvoir interne de développement et de résistance à la destruction».—J. Leclercq, *Leçons de Droit Naturel* (Namur, Maison d'edition Ad. Wesmael-Charlier, 1937), IV, Les Droits et Devoirs Individuels, Première Partie, p. 14.

[59]Cf. R. P. Sertillanges, *La Philosophie Morale de Saint Thomas d'Aquin* (Paris, Aubier, editions Montaigne, 1946), p. 182.

[60]M. Cronin, *The Science of Ethics* (Dublin, Gill & Son, 1917), II, p. 53.

thus represents the individual's desire for life, development and perfection. If, at times, society fails in this regard, the reason does not lie in any basic drive or urge to self-destruction, but rather, in ignorance, blindness, bad will or in many of the other effects of sin. This is evident even in war itself. Although one segment of society does not hesitate to destroy another, yet each individual member of society fears self-destruction and aims at his own protection and conservation.

This theme runs through the works of St. Thomas, as these few examples, besides the one already quoted, demonstrate:

> It is natural for each individual to love his own life and things pertaining thereto, but in due measure: that they are loved not as if the end of life were rooted in them, but that they must be used in view of the ultimate end of life. Hence failure to love these things in due measure is contrary to the natural inclination, and consequently, a sin.[61]

> Love of self-preservation because of which the dangers of death are avoided, is much more connatural than any pleasures whatever of food or sex which are intended for the preservation of life. Hence, it is more difficult to conquer the fear of dangers of death, than the desire of pleasure in the matter of food and sex.[62]

> Particular nature is conservative of each individual as much as it can, hence it is beyond intention that it be deficient in conserving.[63]

> And according to this all corruption and defect is against nature because a power of this type intends its existence and the conservation of that of which it is.[64]

---

[61]«Inditum autem est unicuique naturaliter ut propriam vitam amet, et ea quae ad ipsam ordinantur, tamen debito modo: ut scilicet amentur huiusmodi non quasi finis constituatur in eis, sed secundum quod eis utendum est propter ultimum finem. unde quod aliquis deficiat a debito modo amoris ipsorum, est contra naturalem inclinationem: et per consequens est peccatum».—St. Thomas, op. cit., II:II, q. 126, art. 1.

[62]«. . . amor conservationis vitae, propter quam vitantur pericula mortis, est multo magis connaturalis quam quaecumque delectationes ciborum vel venereorum, quae ad conservationem vitae ordinantur. Et ideo difficilius est vincere timorem periculorum mortis quam concupiscentiam delectationum, quae est in cibis et veneres»—Ibid., q. 142, art. 3, ad 2.

[63]«Natura particularis est conservativa uniusquisque individui quantum potest: unde praeter intentionem eius est quod deficiat in conservando . . .»—S. Thomae Acquinatis, De Caelo et Mundo (Taurini, Marietti, 1952), Lib. II, Lec. 9.

[64]«Et secundum hanc, omnis corruptio et defectus est contra naturam . . . quia huiusmodi virtus intendit esse et. conservationem eius cuis est».—St. Thomas, I:II, q. 85, art. 6, in corp.

Finally:

> An act of this type, since one's intention is to conserve one's life, is not illicit because it is natural to everything to conserve itself in being in as much as it can . . . .[65]

These citations from the writings of St. Thomas emphasize not only the strength of his arguments in the particular matter he is treating but also, the fact that all men sense within themselves a drive urging them on to the conservation of their own lives. This tendency of nature is not passive. One could never call it mere wishful thinking. In point of fact, it is to a great degree the psychological basis for man's actions. He acts not only in order to live but also to satisfy the drive within himself to self-protection and development. One of the demands of nature then is the conservation of one's own life. Since, also, it is true that man is bound to live according to his nature, it is true to say that man is bound by the law of nature to conserve his own life.

This argument is based not on the presence or apparent absence of this natural inclination within a particular man. Rather, it is based on the presence of this inclination in an individual as is observed in the majority of mankind. The objection, therefore, that a man could easily fancy his self-development as existing in some form of suicide, in no way vitiates the argument. Reasoning in argumentation of this type should be grounded on the solid manifestations of the feelings and actions of mankind in general, not on the psychological quirks of any particular individual.

A review, therefore, of the foregoing discussions indicates that neither Scripture, the tradition of the teaching Church, nor the nature of man can be cited in support of an argument denying the obligation to conserve one's life. Indeed, the facts reveal the contrary. The reasons demonstrating the malice of suicide and the obligation of self-conservation are intimately related, and the common Catholic teaching has been consistent and constant in regard to both.

The teachings of Sacred Scripture and of the Church in this matter are merely authoritative restatements of what is already contained in the natural law[66]. Therefore, throughout this dissertation the malice of suicide is condemned as a grave infraction of the natural law and the obligation of self-

---

[65] « Actus igitur huiusmodi ex hoc quod intenditur conservatio propriae vitae, non habet rationem illiciti: cum hoc sit cuilibet naturale quod se conservet in esse quantum potest ».—Ibid., II:II, q. 64, art. 7, in corp.

[66] In this dissertation, the natural law is understood as the natural *moral* law, as distinct from the physical laws of nature.

conservation is urged as a positive precept of the natural law—the supposition being that the reader in both instances will advert to the fact that the natural law is the foundation for any teaching in these matters found in Scripture or the teaching of the Church. This applies also to man's natural inclination to conserve his life. Such an inclination manifests the content of the natural law for an individual in regard to the conservation of his life. The natural law in this matter, as in all others, is consonant with the very nature of man. Therefore, not to conserve one's life or, in effect, to commit suicide directly is entirely against nature and therefore intrinsically wrong.

B—Euthanasia and the precept of self-conservation

In the light of the foregoing arguments, a condemnation of euthanasia presents no problem. If euthanasia is inflicted without the consent of the patient, then it is intrinsically evil because it is murder. (The malice of homicide is treated elsewhere in the texts of Catholic Moral Theology.) If on the other hand, it is a form of voluntary euthanasia in which the person concerned gives permission on his own authority for his life to be taken, then it still remains intrinsically evil. The reason is a simple corollary to the discussions already made in this dissertation. Voluntary euthanasia is suicide and, as such, is a grave disregard of the obligation of self-conservation.

C—Epikeia and the precept of self-conservation

A question can easily arise which fittingly calls for attention here. Is it possible to apply epikeia to the natural law? More precisely, understanding epikeia as a correction of law made by a subject himself on the presumption that the legislator did not intend to include in a law his particular case,[67] is it possible to apply epikeia in the question of the demand of the natural law that a man must not commit suicide and that he must conserve his life?

We must reply that there can never be an application of epikeia to the natural law and therefore, not even in this case. In a thorough treatment of epikeia, L. Riley, in his doctoral dissertation, devotes an entire chapter to this subject.[68] In this chapter the author assigns the many reasons in support of this doctrine. First of all, since the acts prescribed by the natural law are intrinsically good, and those forbidden are intrinsically evil, any possible ex-

---

[67]L. Riley, *The History, Nature and Use of Epikeia in Moral Theology* (Washington, The Catholic University of America Press, 1948), p. 137.

[68]L. Riley, op. cit., pp. 258-291.

trinsic circumstances could never legitimately excuse an individual from positing the prescribed acts continuously or avoiding, as a rule, the prohibited actions.[69] Furthermore, presuming that the licit use of epikeia is conditioned on the existence of the fact that the law is deficient, there can be no licit application of epikeia in the question of the natural law because there can be no defect in the Legislator—God; the promulgator—right reason; or in the matter of the law because it is comprised of what is either intrinsically good or intrinsically evil.[70] Therefore, whether the precepts of the natural law are negative or affirmative, the conclusion is that the natural law never admits of epikeia. An example of a negative precept of the natural law is the prohibition of suicide; an affirmative precept would be the duty of self-conservation. The following lines from Riley's work, which are based on the teaching of Suarez, are of considerable interest:

For the negative precepts bind *semper* and *pro semper*, and hence the obligation can never cease. The affirmative precepts bind *semper* but not *pro semper*. Natural reason or positive law dictates when precisely they must be put into execution. Not to fulfill them *in actu secundo* when, in the judgment of natural reason such is not demanded, is certainly no example of *epikeia*—it is simply an instance of interpretation. on the other hand, there can be no licit use of *epikeia* when reason dictates that the affirmative precepts of the natural law must be put into action. For to allow *epikeia* in such an instance would be to permit an action admittedly contrary to right reason and ultimately to the Divine Essence.[71]

Hence since epikeia can never be licitly applied to the natural law,[72] the further deduction is true; namely, epikeia could never be employed by any individual on the grounds that his particular circumstances represent a case where the natural law would not require the fulfillment of the obligation of self-conservation.

---

[69]Ibid., p. 277.

[70]Ibid, pp. 280–282.

[71]L. Riley, op. cit., pp. 284–285.

[72]Further references to the question of epikeia and the natural law include: Aertnys-Damen, op. cit., I, p. 126, quaer. 3; Fanfani, op. cit., I. P. 197, dub II. Fanfani explains that the application of epikeia to the natural law is impossible because the natural law is founded in the very nature of man and comes from the supreme and most wise Legislator and thus, the law can not be deficient, neither can there be a particular case not foreseen by the omniscent Legislator.

D—Dispensation and the precept of self-conservation

A further question comes to mind. Is there such a thing as a dispensation from the natural law? Again, more precisely, can one obtain a dispensation from the obligation of conserving his life?

Dispensation is defined as the relaxation of a law in a particular case.[73] The natural law is by its very nature immutable and universal. Hence, there can be no dispensation from it. Since the natural law is immutable, it can not be either suspended or abrogated and since it is universal, it admits of no exception.[74] However, a certain type of mutability in the improper sense is admitted by some authors regarding the secondary precepts of the natural law.[75] They distinguish between the changing of a law and the changing of the matter of a law. Thus, a law properly could be called mutable if the obligation of the law ceases, while at the same time, the very same matter is involved. On the other hand, it would be called a mutable law in the improper sense if the obligation of the law ceases because the matter of the law has changed. The matter of the law here is understood as the item concerning which a law is formed and promulgated. Hence, these authors would say that regarding the secondary precepts, the natural law is mutable, in the improper sense, in a situation where the matter of the law has changed. Wherefore, a proper authority can dispense from the natural law in such a situation unless the law concerns a matter in itself everywhere and always intrinsically evil.

Others deny any type of mutation whatever in the natural law, as long as the demands of the law are expressed in complete and adequate terms with all the necessary restrictions, conditions, and determinations which would allow the applications of the law not only in general cases but also in particular and extraordinary cases.[76] Hence, these authors feel there is no possible dispensation from the natural law, because, as is known, the indispensability of the natural law derives from its immutability. Therefore, they would say that there is no dispensation from the natural law, even in the improper sense. Any cases which are brought forth as examples of a dispensation from the natural law merely manifest special conditions which do not permit the application of a principle of the natural law because it has been expressed in terms too general and indefinite.[77]

---

[73]*Code of Canon Law (1983)*, Canon 85.
[74]L. Fanfani, op. cit., I, p. 196.
[75]Cf. Noldin-Schmitt, op. cit., I, p. 123, n. 116; Aertny-Damen, op. cit., I, p. 125, n. 136; Lehmkuhl, op. cit., I, p. 122; Fanfani, op. cit., I, pp. 196–197.
[76]Regatillo-Zalba, op. cit., I, p. 354.
[77]Ibid., pp. 355–356.

Whatever else remains to be said of this dispute would not be to the point here. Perhaps, the whole matter represents merely an argument over words because all admit that the natural law in itself is immutable and admits of no dispensation in that sense.

Therefore, an individual can never receive a dispensation from the obligation of conserving his life. God could manifest His will and demand that a person give up his life by some form of non-conservation of self. This would not be a divine dispensation from the natural law. God has the dominion over life and He can cede this faculty to man, and thus the non-conservation of self or suicide would not be against the natural law since the individual would be acting, not on his own authority, but on God's. Killing is not against the natural law; it is killing without the proper authority that breaks the natural law. This authority, is not a dispensation; not a jurisdictional act whereby the natural law is relaxed in a particular case but rather, it is a divine permission to exercise a faculty which God ordinarily reserves to Himself. In passing, it should be noted that an individual must have positive evidence that this faculty has been granted him by God. Presumption, instigated by the onslaught of physical or psychological ills, is certainly no indication that God has given such a faculty.

E—Ignorance and the precept of self-conservation

Another interesting point is the possibility of invincible ignorance in this matter. In effect, the question is: can there be invincible ignorance of the natural law, or rather, is the natural law so well written and impressed in the hearts of men that it is quite inconceivable that a man could be invincibly ignorant of its demands. Certainly, one of the basic postulates of the natural law is the precept of self-conservation. This is grounded on a very natural inclination. It would seem, therefore, that no possibility of invincible ignorance in this matter could ever be present.

In point of fact, the history of the world and of different races testify that it has been with considerable difficulty that some peoples have arrived at the knowledge of even the most fundamental moral truths. It is also true that in the present condition of fallen nature, the promulgation of the natural law by the light of the human reason alone is sufficient physically for a man to know the content of the natural law. However, human reason alone is insufficient morally—hence the need of revelation. In fact divine revelation in this present economy is morally necessary in order that the natural law can be known with sufficient ease, certitude and completeness.[78]

---

[78]A.Vermeersch, *Theologiae Moralis Principia-Responsa-Consilia*, I, p. 127.

The common teaching holds that an individual enjoying the use of reason cannot be in ignorance of the first and most universal principles of the natural law.[79] Furthermore, the primary conclusions drawn from the most universal principles are also known and the individual can not be invincibly ignorant of these for any extended length of time, because the ordinary intellect can deduce these conclusions correctly with a minimum of effort. The foregoing, then, is the common teaching regarding the knowledge that a human being has of the natural law. However, it is necessary to admit that defects of education, past sins and evil habits, or false persuasions can be the cause of invincible ignorance for a time.[80]

Vincible ignorance, which is also culpable, obviously can be present, not because of a defect in the intellect but due to a bad will—with this point there is no argument.[81] Over and above this, there can also be a situation in which the intellect would draw the correct conclusion from a most universal principle but err in the application of the conclusion to a particular case.[82]

It is necessary, then, to admit theoretically first of all that cases of invincible ignorance of the natural law can occur and, therefore, the person concerned is free of the guilt of formal sin. The opposite opinion, once held by the Jansenists, was condemned by Pope Alexander VIII:

> Although there may be invincible ignorance of the law of nature, in the state of fallen nature, the one working in virtue of this ignorance is not excused from sin[83].

Secondly, one has to agree that an individual can err in good faith in the application of a natural law principle or deduction, and thus, also, be free of guilt.

Now to the case in point. The principle guiding an individual to the conservation of his life is self-evident. «Per se,» therefore, there can be no invincible ignorance in this regard. The drive leading a man forward to self-conservation finds its roots in the very nature of man. He can not be ignorant for any extended length of time of the obligation of self-conservation. However, the following would seem to be possibilities:

---

[79]Regatillo-Zalba, op. cit., I, p. 361, n. 344; Fanfani, op. cit., I, p. 198.

[80]Regatillo-Zalba, ibid., n. 345; Fanfani, ibid, p. 199.

[81]Noldin-Schmitt, op. cit., I, p. 122, n. 144.

[82]Regatillo-Zalba, op. cit., I, p. 362, footnote 48.

[83]«Tametsi detur ignorantia invincibilis iuris naturae, haec in statu naturae lapsae operantem ex ipsa non excusat a peccato formali».—D. 1292.

1. Theoretically, an individual, for a brief time, could be invincibly ignorant of the duty of self-conservation. Thus he would not be guilty of sin, if in that period of time, and acting in virtue of the invincible ignorance, he should take his life.

2. A situation can occur in which an individual would be vincibly and culpably ignorant of his obligation of self-conversation. Any action performed in virtue of this ignorance would, of course, be sinful.

3. An individual could fully realize his obligation to self-conservation, and admit its truth, but feel that his failure to satisfy the obligation would be licit because of some particular circumstances. A good example of this is euthanasia. The patient could falsely justify euthanasia because of the overwhelming pain he is suffering. The doctor could falsely justify his administrating of the euthanasia on the grounds of charity to the patient. This is ignorance not regarding the law itself, but, rather, in regard to the application of the law, and, thus, again an individual might escape formal sin.

> However it was conceded that per accidens the subject may conceive an action as justifiable in practical action surrounded with all its circumstances while fully admitting the general prohibition. This would hold in the present consideration. The aversion to the physical pain that causes men to subvert the value of life to the value of physical well-being is no doubt due to a long series of sins on the part of both individuals and society. However, as has been seen, ignorance which is a consequence of sin is not always culpable ignorance. If it is a result of previous sin, it is not culpable unless it had been foreseen. Though its admission constitutes an indictment of modern society, the possibility of invincible ignorance of the evil of euthanasia is to be admitted. The same principles can sometimes be applied to suicide[84].

One must enjoy the use of reason before the above-mentioned rules on ignorance of the natural law apply. This does not mean, of course, that those who have not as yet reached the use of reason and those who are insane are not bound by the natural law. Rather, the opposite obtains. These people, as all other human beings, by their very nature, are subject to the natural law and thus when they break this law, they sin—materially, however, and not formally.[85]

---

[84]S. Bertke, *The Possibility of Invincible Ignorance of the Natural Law* (Washington, The Catholic University Press, 1941), p. 103.

[85]Cf. Aertnys-Damen, op. cit., I, p. 124.

F—The principle of the double effect and the precept of self-conservation

The principle of the double effect also comes to mind and a question arises concerning it. Can the principle of the double effect be used in certain cases involving the dictate of the natural law requiring self-conservation? Is it licit to perform some action which will produce two effects—one of which will be an individual's won death? Up till now, therefore, the discussion has centered around the necessity of self-conservation and the malice of non-conservation of self by some form of direct suicide. Here, the question of indirect suicide comes into light.

Obviously, any form of non-conservation of self that happens without any intention at all on the part of the individual is without fault. It then is involuntary as, for example, in the case of an accidental suicide. However, in the case of an action which is entirely intended and willed, but which will produce two effects, one of which is good and the other evil, it would be licit to perform this action only if certain conditions are fulfilled. Edwin Healy, S. J. explains it this way:

> It is allowable to actuate a cause that will produce a good and bad effect, provided 1) the good effect and not the evil effect is *directly intended;* 2) the action itself is good, or at least, indifferent; 3) the good effect is not produced by *means* of the evil effect; and 4) there is a proportionate reason for permitting the foreseen evil effect to occur.[86]

Above all, it is necessary to underline the fact that, just as direct suicide performed on one's own authority is always illicit, so also, indirect suicide which is not accompanied by a proportionately grave reason is basically illicit. Indirect suicide is understood here as suicide eventuating from the performance or omission of an act on account of which death occurs. The moral difference in the two forms of suicide lies in the fact that indirect suicide can sometimes be licit if there is a proportionately grave reason on account of which the indirect suicide can be permitted.

Hence, the application of all the above principles to particular cases would show that the following solutions offered by the older moralists are valid. 1) A soldier may remain at his post even though he is morally certain that he will be killed.[87] 2) An individual in a ship-wreck may give his means of

---

[86]E. Healy, *Moral Guidance* (Chicago, Loyola University Press, 1942), p. 20.
[87]St. Alphonsus, op. cit., Lib. III, Tract. 4, Cap. 1, Dub. 1, n. 366.

safety to someone else, even though the loss of his own life may occur.[88] 3) One may minister to those infected with contagious fatal diseases even with great danger ot his own life.[89] 4) In the event of a fire, it is licit to jump from a high position with the intention of escaping the fire even though there is certain danger of death involved in such a high fall.[90] Likewise, a young woman could do the same in order to escape an attacker.[91] 5) Naval personnel could scuttle a ship at sea during war even with danger and possible death occurring to themselves, lest the enemy capture the ship and thus inflict heavy damage on their native land.[92] 6) It is also licit to fast and abstain, and inflict moderate injuries on one's body for the sake of penance, even though, unintentionally, one's span of life is considerably shortened.[93]

Certainly, these cases are not the only ones possible to mention. The principles involved are clear. With the examples that have been given, the distinction between direct and indirect non-conservation of self has been sufficiently outlined.

There is an interesting case, however, which is worthy of separate mention because there could be a serious temptation to solve the problem by means of the two-fold effect principle. This, however, would seem to be unlawful and not allowable. These days, an episode involving voluntary hungerstrike occasionally occurs. As a rule, it receives tremendous publicity in the ordinary daily journals. This is true especially when the ones involved undertake their hungerstrike in order to emphasize or solve some public issue. The fascinating story of the voluntary hungerstrike of the Lord-mayor of Cork, Ireland in 1920 is typical. This gentleman, in order to defend the autonomy of Ireland against England, had recourse to a voluntary hungerstrike and died on October 25, 1920 after a fast from food which lasted seventy-three days, twelve hours and forty minutes.[94]

It is quite simple to imagine that many, especially those emotionally connected with the situation, could fancy that some species of the principle of the double effect would justify the actual non-conservation of self on the part of the famous mayor of Cork. No doubt, there were several who felt at the time that the autonomy of the country, the striving after a great good, the interest in the common weal made his course of action licit.

---

[88]Loc. cit.
[89]Loc. cit.
[90]Ibid., n. 367.
[91]Loc. cit.
[92]Loc. cit.
[93]Ibid., n. 371. The foregoing examples are given also in St. Alphonsus, *Homo Apostolicus* (Torino, Marietti, 1848), Tract. VIII, Cap. 1, n. 1.
[94]Cf. editor's note, *La Documentation Catholique*, 30 oct. 1920, p. 333.

An examination of the case proves, of course, that only a valid application of the two-fold effect principle could justify the situation. Certainly, the bare action alone of the mayor was not allowable, because it was direct non-conservation of self. However, a thorough analysis revels that no application of the principle of the double effect would seem to be allowable here. The act of fasting is certainly good or, at least, indifferent. The good effect, namely, the recognition of Ireland's autonomy, was what was directly intended and certainly the bad effect was not the means by which the good effect would come. However it would seem that this particular hungerstrike was not allowable. Although the act of fasting in the beginning was good or, at least indifferent morally, the point eventually came when fasting ceased being a morally indifferent act. As the mayor's physical condition became worse, then fasting any longer became unlawful because of the grave injury to health and the danger of death involved. Furthermore, whether the action in itself were good or not, it certainly was an inefficacious means of obtaining the end in view. Thus, the mayor's action should be condemned also on the grounds of lacking a proportionately grave reason. It is difficult to agree that a voluntary hunger-strike on the part of the mayor of Cork would be a secure means, efficacious by its very nature, and the only means necessary and proportioned to the obtaining of national liberty and independence.[95]

This case is cited here to show, first of all, an example of an invalid application of the principle of the double effect, and also, to emphasize that even when suicide is not directly intended, a voluntary and direct abstinence from food, complete and lasting till death, even though performed because of high political or social motives, remains illicit nonetheless.[96] It can be said, in passing, that the mayor of Cork acted in good faith and thus was free from formal sin.

Thus far, the treatment of cases involving non-conservation of one's life has involved, first of all, direct suicide and this is always illicit. Secondly the possibilities of indirect suicide were mentioned together with stipulated reasons and conditions because of which the indirect suicide could be allowable. In the first of these cases, the non-conservation of self is said to be voluntary and thus, sinful. In the second, it is not voluntary but said to be permitted, and thus can, at times, be licit if certain conditions are verified. Thirdly, the case of the completely accidental, unforeseen non-conservation of self was mentioned. This is entirely involuntary, and therefore, free of any moral culpability. In all three of these cases, though, the common element is some

---

[95]*La Civiltà Cattolica*, IV (1920), pp. 530–531. Cf. also P. Gannon, «La Grève de la Faim», *La Documentation Catholique*, 30 cot., 1920, pp. 333–336; *L'Ami du Clergé*, 1920, pp. 529 ss.

[96]Cf. Aertnys-Damen, op. cit., I, p. 457, footnote 1.

positive action performed by the individual which directly or indirectly brings about his death. There is present, therefore, a cause which exerts a positive influence in the matter.

G—Moral impossibility and the precept of self-conservation

Now what about a mere omission of an action, when by this omission death of one's self occurs? Would it be illicit for an individual to omit an action when he foresees that he could perform the action and that should he choose not to, he will die? (Furthermore, the supposition in the case would be that he really would not intend to choose death, or else, of course, it would be suicide.)

In treating the famous Cork case, we mentioned actually a situation involving the omission of food. However, at the time, the point of main concern was an explanation of the conditions involved in the licit application of the two-fold effect principle. here our main concern is the direct treatment of the principles involved in the omission of an act. The reason for the separate mention of the moral principles involved in this question is the fact that they are of great importance in determining the obligation that an individual has of conserving his life in certain circumstances. We shall see the application of these principles more clearly as this dissertation progresses.

Three conditions are necessary in order that a person be charged with guilt in a situation which involves either the omission of an act in impeding evil, or the placing of an act which causes evil, even though the effects of evil are not intended. 1) In some manner, at least in a confused way, he must foresee the evil effect. 2) He must be able to prevent the evil either by acting or omitting an action. 3) He must be bound by some obligation to prevent the evil.[97]

In the case at hand, therefore, the supposition is that an individual can perform the action and that he foresees that if he does not, he will die; he does not, however, intend his death. Therefore, the response is that he is guilty of sin if he omits the conservation of his life, unless it should be in his case that he (this particular individual) is not bound to conserve his life. Yet, on the other hand, it is a dictate of the natural law that a person conserve his life.

When does the moral obligation of the natural law cease? The answer to this question is quite simple. The obligation imposed by the natural law never ceases. It binds every human being,— everywhere and always. However, it is possible that a human individual could be excused from the fulfillment of the natural law because of particular circumstances. One of the excusing causes is

---

[97]A. Lehmkuhl, op. cit., I, p. 20.

ignorance of the law. This has been treated earlier. Another, however, is inability to fulfill the law. This inability can be of a physical nature. Certainly, no one is bound morally to fulfill a law when he is physically unfit to do so. This is obvious in the question of the conservation of one's own life. Otherwise, an individual would be morally bound to the performance of the impossible and this is a patent contradiction.[98] On the other hand, the individual may be physically capable of fulfilling the law but unable to, here and now, because of some circumstance of fear, danger, or grave inconvenience which renders the observance of the law extremely difficult for him. It is then said to be morally impossible for him to fulfill the law. It is obvious that physical inability excuses from the observance of a precept of the natural law. Regarding moral inability, however, the following is to be noted. Theologians commonly distinguish between the affirmative and negative precepts of the natural law.[99] In the case of the negative precepts, it is necessary to emphasize that they are always binding even when their fulfillment involves a grave danger of death. This is so because these negative precepts forbid what is intrinsically evil and not even death itself would make it licit to perform evil. So, no grave inconvenience would produce a moral impossibility in this regard.

Where an affirmative precept is concerned, however, a moral inability would excuse from the fulfillment or observance of the precept. The reason is that these laws bind an individual *semper* but not *pro semper*, as the common dictum puts it. Whereas, in the case of negative precepts, the obligation is *semper* and *pro semper*.[100] It is a rational presumption then that since man is not always and everywhere, under every circumstance, bound to do something positively good, he would not be always and everywhere bound to fulfill an affirmative precept. Hence, a moral impossibility, while not freeing an individual from the basic obligation of the natural law, excuses him from the present observance of an affirmative precept of that law.[101]

One further point worthy of note is the fact that an instance of moral impossibility does not exist in a situation where the fulfillment of the law is intrinsically and radically accompanied by some considerable inconven-

---

[98]Cf. D. 804.

[99]Noldin-Schmitt, op. cit., I, p. 179, n. 177.

[100]Cf. L. Fanfani, op. cit., I, p. 184 and p. 272; also A. Lehmkuhl, op. cit., I, p. 108.

[101]There are occasions when an affirmative law binds even in the presence of moral impossibility: 1) if the violation of the law brings about common harm, 2) if the violation tends to the detriment of religion or hatred of God, 3) if the violation tends to the grave detriment of the spiritual condition of the individual concerned. Cf. A. Lehmkuhl, op. cit., I, pp. 108–109; Noldin-Schmitt, op. cit., I, p. 179, par. 177, n. 2.

ience.[102] This is a difficulty common to all men and thus would not generally constitute a moral impossibility for any one individual. So, for example, the ordinary individual usually could not excuse himself from the obligation of obtaining food on the grounds that working for the money to buy the food constitutes for him a moral impossibility. In the case, however, where working would entail a difficulty for him not commonly experienced by men in general, then a possible instance of moral inability to fulfill the law might exist.

Therefore, to summarize the above doctrine and apply it to the problem at hand: an individual is always bound by the affirmative precept of the natural law commanding him to conserve his life. However, the individual is licitly excused from the fulfillment of this precept by circumstances which constitute for him a moral impossibility not commonly experienced by men in general. How grave this difficulty has to be is the question which will occupy a great section of the remainder of this dissertation.

H—Ordinary and extraordinary means and the precept of self-conservation

The law that demands the conservation of one's own life, also commands that he employ the means necessary to conserve his life. Since, however, this law is an affirmative law and a licit application of the doctrine on moral impossibility may be made, theologians commonly divide the means of conserving life into two categories. The first includes those which are obligatory for everyone. The second is comprised of those means whose use would constitute a moral impossibility either for human beings in general or for one particular individual. The former they term *ordinary means;* the latter, *extraordinary means.* An individual must employ the ordinary means of conserving his life. *Per se,* he need not use the extraordinary means. *Per accidens,* however, someone might have the obligation of employing the means which are recognized as extraordinary for him and human beings in general.

In this chapter, we have investigated the basic obligation that binds each individual to conserve his life. We have seen also that because this precept is affirmative, the individual is held *per se* to employ only the ordinary means of conserving his life, *per accidens* the extraordinary means. In the next chapter, we shall review the teaching of Catholic theologians regarding the nature and use of these ordinary and extraordinary means of conserving life.

---

[102]A. Lehmkuhl, loc. cit.

31

CONCLUSIONS

1. God retains the radical possession of the rights over man's life. Man has full rights to the use of his life but to this only. Hence, any form of non-conservation of self, directly intended by an individual on his own authority, is illicit.

2. Likewise, man has the serious positive obligation of caring for his bodily life and health.

3. It is possible that an individual could be invincibly ignorant, for a time, of this obligation but certainly not for any extended length of time. However, it is possible that one might realize his obligation to conserve his life, but err in the practical application of the obligation to his status here and now.

4. There is no licit application of epikeia in this matter. Neither is a dispensation possible. However, an individual could receive the command from God to take his own life by some form of non-conservation of self. In such a case, the individual would then have permission to exercise a faculty ordinarily reserved as a divine prerogative.

5. The obligation to conserve one's life, being an affirmative precept of the natural law, does not require fulfillment under all circumstances. Hence a moral impossibility would excuse.

6. The means to fulfill this precept of self-conservation are obligatory. Those means binding everyone in common circumstances are ordinary means. Those means involving a moral impossibility are extraordinary means.

CHAPTER II
_____

Historical Report of the Opinions in Regard to the Ordinary and Extraordinary Means of Conserving Life

Inasmuch as the main object of this dissertation is an analysis of the Catholic teaching concerning the ordinary and extraordinary means of conserving life, it is fitting that, from the outset, a simple report of the traditional opinions on this subject be given. However, to conjoin an analysis with this report would be far too cumbersome. Hence, the reader will find that an attempt has been made to keep the commentary on the opinions cited here to a minimum. A more lengthy analysis will follow in the next chapter.

2.1 THE THIRTEENTH TO THE SIXTEENTH CENTURIES

Having in mind the basic duty which obliges an individual to conserve his life, as was seen in the preceding chapter, we will now find it rather interesting to follow the further development of this doctrine through the centuries. The present historical report commences with St. Thomas Acquinas. In point of fact, there was not much discussion of the problem of the ordinary and extraordinary means of conserving life in the writings of the theologians prior to the sixteenth century. However, in this report, we begin with St. Thomas because his treatment of the question of suicide in the Secunda Secundae, q. 64, art. 5 influenced later writers quite heavily. Furthermore, many of the commentators chose this article[103] and the one on mutilation (II: II, q. 65, art. 1)[104] as the place for their discussion of the ordinary and extraordinary means of conserving life. Citations have already been given from St. Thomas. The following one, however, is of interest:

> A man has the obligation to sustain his body, otherwise he would be a killer of himself . . . by precept, therefore, he is bound to nourish his body and likewise, we are bound to all the other items without which the body can not live.[105]

The theologians immediately succeeding St. Thomas were content merely to restate his arguments against suicide,[106] and one does not discover in their writings any lengthy speculation regarding the use of the ordinary and extraordinary means of conserving life.

2.2 THE SIXTEENTH CENTURY TO THE TIME OF CARDINAL DE LUGO

In the sixteenth century much discussion about the problem occurs. One of the notable theologians in this regard is *Vitoria*, O. P. († 1546). In his famous *Relectiones Theologiae*, there is much of considerable interest. This holds true of his commentary on the Secunda Secundae of St. Thomas also. First of all, in the *Relectio de Temperantia*, Vitoria treats many problems regarding one's

---

[103]Cf. *Somme Theologique*, op. cit., p. 149.

[104]For example, cf. D. Bañez, *Scholastica Commentaria in Partem Angelici Doctoris S. Thomae* (Duaci, 1614–1615), Tom. IV, Decisiones de Jure et Justitia, in II:II. q. 65, art. 1.

[105]«Praecipitur autem homini quod corpus suum sustentet, alias, enim est homicida sui ipsius . . . ex praecepto ergo tenetur homo corpus suum nutrire et similiter ad omnia sine quibus corpus non potest vivere, tenemur».—S. Thomas, *Super Epistolas S. Pauli* (Taurini-Romae, marietti, 1953), II Thess., Lec. 11, n. 77.

[106]Cf. e.g., S. Antonius, *Theologia Moralis* (Veronae, 1740), de Homicidio, tom. II, col. 861, lit. D.

life by means of food. He proves this obligation by arguments based on man's natural inclination to self-conservation, the love a man owes himself and the malice of suicide contained in the non-conservation of self. Therefore, if the conservation of self by food is an obligation, it would seem that a sick person who did not eat because of some disgust for food, would be guilty of mortal sin. Vitoria replies:

> Regarding the first argument to the contrary, . . . I would say secondly that if a sick man can take food or nourishment with some hope of life, he is held to take the food, as he would be held to give it to one who is sick. Thirdly, I would say that if the depression of spirit is so low and there is present such consternation in the appetitive power that only with the greatest of effort and as though by means of a certain torture, can the sick man take food, right away that is reckoned a certain impossibility, and therefore he is excused, at least from mortal sin, especially where there is little hope of life, or none at all. Responding by way of confirmation: first of all a similar case does not exist in reference to food and drugs. For, food is per se a means ordered to the life of the animal and it is natural, drugs are not: man is not held to employ all the possible means of conserving his life, but the means which are per se intended for that purpose . . . Thirdly, we say that if one were to have moral certitude that by means of a drug he would gain health, without the drug, however, he would die, he really does not seem to be excused from mortal sin: because if he did not give the drug to a sick neighbor, he would sin mortally, and medicine per se is intended also by nature for health, but since this rarely can be certain, therefore they are not to be condemned of mortal sin who have universally declared an abstinence from drugs, although this is not laudable because God created medicine because of its need, as Solomon says . . . [107]

---

[107]«Ad argumentum in contrarium, ad primum . . . Secundo dico quod si aegrotus potest sumere cibum, vel alimentum cum aliqua spe vitae, tenetur sumere cibum, sicut teneretur dare aegrotanti. Tertio dico, quod si animi dejectio tanta est et appetitivae virtutis tanta consternatio, ut non nisi per summum laborem et quasi cruciatum quendam, aegrotus possit sumere cibum, jam reputatur quaedam impossibilitas et ideo excusatur, saltem a mortali, maxime ubi est exigua spes vitae aut nulla. Ad confirmationem respondetur. Primo, quod non est simile de pharmaco et alimento. Alimentum enim per se medium ordinatum ad vitam animalis et naturale, non autem pharmacum: nec tenetur homo adhibere, omnia media possibilia ad conservandam vitam, sed media per se ad hoc ordinata . . . Tertio dicimus quod si quis haberet certitudinem moraliter, quod per pharmacum reciperet incolumitatem, sine pharmaco autem

Later on then, discussing the lawfulness of abstaining perpetually from a certain type of food, even in extreme necessity, Vitoria has this to say:

Finally, for a solution of the objections, it must be noted: it is one thing not to protect life and it is another to destroy it: for man is not always held to the first and it is enough that he perform that by which regularly a man can live: if a sick man could not have a drug except by giving over his whole means of subsistence, I do not think he would be bound to do so.[108]

Then he adds:

Second conclusion: One is not held to protect his life as much as he can by means of foods. This is clear because one is not held to use foods which are the best, the most delicate and most expensive, even though these foods are the most healthful, indeed this is blameworthy . . . Likewise, one is not held to live in the most healthful place, therefore neither must he use the most healthful food . . . .[109]

Again:

Third conclusion: If one uses foods which men commonly use and in the quantity which customarily suffices for the conservation of strength, even though from this his life is shortened, even notably and this is noticed, he would not sin . . . From this, the corollary follows that one is not held to use medicines to prolong his life even where the danger of death is probable, for example to

---

moreretur, noon videtur profecto excusari a mortali: quia si non daret pharmacum proximo sic aegrotanti, peccaret mortaliter et medicina per se etiam ordinata est ad salutem a natura, sed quia hoc xiv potest esse certum, ideo non sunt damnandi de mortali, qui in universum decreverunt abstinere a pharmacis, licet non sit laudabile, cum creaverit Deus medicinam propter necessitatem ut aid Salomon . . . »—F. a Victoria, Relec. de Temp., n. 1.

[108] «Pro solutione tandem argumentorum, notandum est: quod aliud est non protelare vitam, aliud est abrumpere: nam ad primum non semper tenetur homo et satis est, quod det operam, per quam homo regulariter potest vivere: nec puto, si aeger non posset habere pharmacum nisi daret totam substantiam suam, quod teneretur facere».—ibid., n. 9.

[109] «Secunda conclusio: non tenetur quis protelare vitam per alimenta quantum potest. Patet, quia non tenetur uti cibis optimis et delicatissimis et pretoisissimis etiamsi ea sint saluberrima, imo hoc est reprehensible, . . . Item non tentur vivere in loco saluberrimo, ergo nec uti cibo saluberrimo . . .»—ibid., n. 12.

take for some years a drug to avoid fevers or anything of this sort.[110]

Another pertinent passage comes from Vitoria's *Relectio de Homicidio.*

. . . One is not held, as I said, to employ all the means to conserve his life, but it is sufficient to employ the means which are of themselves intended for this purpose and congruent. Wherefore, in the case which has been posited, I believe that the individual is not held to give his whole inheritance to preserve his life, . . . From this also it is inferred that when one is sick without hope of life, granted that a certain precious drug could produce life for some hours or even days, he would not be held to buy it but it is sufficient to use common remedies, and he is considered as though dead.[111]

Vitoria uses the same reasoning in his commentary on St. Thomas.

. . . In the second place, I say that one is not held to lengthen his life because he is not held to use always the most delicate foods, that is, hens and chickens, even though he has the ability and the doctors say that if he eats in such a manner, he will live twenty years more, and even if he knew this for certain, he would not be obliged . . . So I say, thirdly, that it is licit to eat common and regular foods . . . Granted that the doctor advises him to eat chickens and partridges, he can eat eggs and other common items.[112]

---

[110]« Tertia conclusio—Si quis utatur alimentis, quibus homines communiter utuntur et in quantitate, quae solet sufficere ad valetudinem conservandam, dato quod ex hoc abbrevietur vita, etiam notabiliter et hoc percipiatur, non peccat . . . Ex quo sequitur corollarium, quod non tenetur quis uti medicinis, ad prolongandam vitam, etiam ubi esset probabile periculum mortis, puta quotannis sumere pharmacum ad vitandas febrew, vel aliquid huiusmodi».—loc. cit.

[111]« Non tenetur quis uti dixi, omnia media ponere ad servandum vitam, sed satis est ponere media ad hoc de se ordinata et congruentia. unde in casu posito credo quod non tenetur dare totum patrimonium pro vita servanda . . . Ex quo etiam infertur, quod cum aliquis sine spe vitae aegrotat, dato quod aliquo pharmaco pretioso posset producere vitam aliquot horas, aut etiam dies, non tenetur illud emere, sed satis erit uti remediis communibus et ille reputàtur quasi mortuus».—Relec. de Homicidio, n. 35.

[112]« Secundum dico non tenetur aliquis augere vitam quia non tenetur semper uti delicatissimis cibis, scilicet gallinis et pullis, etiamsi habeat facultatem et medici dicant quod si comedit ex illis vivet plus viginti annos et etiamsi hoc sciret pro certo, non tenetur . . . Et sic dico tertio, quod licet comedere cibos communes et regulares . . . Dato quod medicus consuleret illi comedere

Finally:

> Where, however, one were to live in a very strict and singular manner, for example, eating perpetually only bread and water so that he abbreviates his life, perhaps it would not be licit, or even to eat only once in the week would not be licit. But, this ought to happen in a manner common to good men so that it is beside one's intention that death follow and not by intention.[113]

Dominic Soto, O. P. († 1560), in his *Theologia Moralis* adheres to St. Thomas closely. Treating of suicide,[114] he explicitly repeats the arguments of the Angelic Doctor. Soto includes this treatment in his tract *De Justitia et Jure.* The next point for explanation is the problem of mutilation. Soto, in this particular question, treats not only the lawfulness and unlawfulness of mutilation, but touches also on the intriguing speculation of whether or not a person is ever bound to suffer a mutilation, and further, whether the individual could ever be forced to submit to a mutilation. In the course of his discussion, Soto writes:

> . . . a prelate indeed could force a subject, on account of a singular obedience promised to him, to take medicines which he can conveniently accept. But, really, no one can be forced to bear the tremendous pain in the amputation of a member or in an incision into the body: because no one is held to preserve his life with such torture. Neither is he thought to be the killer of himself.[115]

In his *De Justitia Commutativa, Molina* († 1600) gives a good treatment of the status of man as the custodian and guardian of his life and members. In

---

pullos et perdices, potest comedere ova et alia communia».—F. de Vitoria, *Comentarios a la Secunda Secundae de Santo Tomas,* in II:II, q. 147, art. 1.

[113] «Ubi tamen modo arctissimo et singulari quis viveret, puta non comendendo perpetuo nisi panem et aquam ut vitam abbreviaret, forte non liceret vel etiam semel tantum in hebdomada comedere non liceret. Sed debet hoc fieri modo communi hominum bonorum ut praeter intentionem mors sequatur, et non ex intentione».—ibid., q. 64, art. 5.

[114] D. Soto, *Theologia Moralis* (Lugduni, 1582), Tract. de Justitia et Jure, Lib. V, q. 1, art. 5.

[115] «. . . praelatus vero cogere posset subditum propter singularem obedientiam illi promissam, ut medicamina admittat quae commode recipere potest. At vero quod ingentissimum dolorem in amputatione membri aut corporis incisione ferat, profecto nemo cogi potest: quia nemo tenetur tanto cruciatu vitam servare. neque ille censendus est sui homicida».—D. Soto, *Theologia Moralis,* Tract. de Justitia et Jure, Lib. V, q. 2, art. 1.

the course of this treatment he describes the necessity «per accidens» of using the extraordinary means of conserving life. The section has these words:

> Fourth conclusion. Because man has been constituted the custodian and administrator of his own life and members, when he is unwilling, no one can cut a member from him for the sake of curing him or apply any other medicinal remedy to him . . . [116]

Soon again then, he says:

> The conclusion proposed, therefore, is understood only when it is not entirely certain that the remedy will be of profit for avoiding the grave harm of a neighbor: or when the remedy is such that because of too intense a pain or another legitimate reason, he is not obliged to undergo that which he needs in order to conserve his life or member.[117]

In this particular subject, namely, the necessity of using the ordinary means of conserving life and the lawfulness of shunning the extraordinary means, the teaching of Vitoria had tremendous influence.[118] Many of the authors used his speculation as the foundation for their own thinking in the matter. Others were quite content with repeating verbatim his doctrine. An example of this latter approach is found in the writing of *Gregory Sayrus* († 1602). His famous *Clavis Regia Casuum Conscientiae* contains in the ninth chapter of the seventh book much of what has already been cited from Vitoria. For instance, in the question of the lawfulness of abstinence from food, and penances administered to the body, when such procedures injure one's health or shorten one's life, Sayrus uses the very arguments and words of Vitoria. Thus, one finds that he emphasizes that an individual is not bound to prolong

---

[116]«Quarta conclusio. Quia homo custos et administrator est constitutus suae propriae vitae ac membrorum, nullus ipso renuente, potest secare ab eo membrum gratia curationis, aut medicamentum aliud ei applicare . . .»—L. Molina, *De Justitia,* Tom. IV, Tract. III, disp. I, col. 514.

[117]«Conclusio ergo proposita solum intelligitur, quando certum omnino non est remedium profuturum ad grave malum proximi, vitandum: aut quando remedium est tale quod propter nimium dolorem, vel alia legitima causa, non tenetur is sub reatu lethalis culpae illud subire, qui eo indiget ad vitam aud membrum conservandum».—loc. cit.

[118]The influence of Vitoria is recognized not only in regard to this problem, but also in regard to many other aspects of Moral Theology. "Vitoria fama celebratus ob suas Relectiones, in quibus, derelinquens sententias Lombardi, felici innovatione a posteris imitanda sollerter Summam Aquintis commentatus est, cum applicationibus ad quaestiones novas sui temporis . . . " Regatillo-Zalba, *op. cit.,* vol. I, p. 25.

his life,[119] nor is one held to use the very best and more delicate foods.[120] However, Sayrus adds to the expression «common foods» the notion of their being produced naturally.

> No one in order to prolong his life is bound to use the best and more delicate foods, even though he can, but the common ones, naturally produced.[121]

Later then, he expresses in his own words an idea also found in Vitoria.

> For although a man is held not to cut off his life, he is not held, however, to seek all the means, even licit ones in order to make his life longer. This is manifest because, granted that an individual should know for certain that in India or in another city, even nearby, the air is more healthful and milder and that there he would live longer than in his native land or in his own city, he is not bound, however, to seek all the means, even licit and exquisite ones in order to make his life longer.[122]

Then again Sayrus repeats the teaching of Vitoria cited earlier in this chapter regarding the use of medicine,[123] after which one reads: «. . . not all means must be furnished for the sake of conserving life, but those only which for this purpose are necessary and congruous.»[124] Finally, Sayrus reaches the problem of mutilation and answers the question whether or not, when a sick person is unwilling, he may be forced as a citizen by the state, as a son by his father or as a subject by a prelate to submit to the mutilation of one of his members. Sayrus shows himself indebted to Soto in his answer. His general response is in the affirmative if the person is necessary for the common good.

---

[119]G. Sayrus, *Clavis Regia Casuum Conscientiae* (Venetiis, 1625), Lib. VII, cap. IX, n. 28.

[120]*Loc. cit.*

[121]"Nemo ad vitam prolongandam, cibis optimis et delicatioribus uti tenetur, etiamsi possit, sed communibus naturaliter productis." G. Sayrus, *Clavis Regia Casuum Conscientiae.* Lib. VII, Cap. IX, n. 28.

[122]«Quamvis enim teneatur homo non abrumpere vitam non tenetur tamen omnia media etiam licita et exquisita quaerere, ut longiorem vitam faciat. Id quod manifeste patet, quia dato, quod aliquis certo sciat, quod in India aut in alia civitate etiam propinqua salubrior et clementior aura sit et quod ibi diutius viveret, quam in patria, aut propria civitate, non tenetur tamen omnia media etiam licita et exquisita quaerere ut longiorem vitam faciat».—loc. cit.

[123]*Loc. cit.*

[124]". . . non enim vitae conservandae gratia omnia media adhibenda sunt, sed illa tantum, quae ad hoc sunt necessaria et congrua." *Ibid.,* n. 29.

If the mutilation, however, is necessary only for the particular good and health of the sick individual, then he can not be forced. To this he adds:

> . . . furthermore, since by the natural law each one is bound to employ for the conservation of his body those licit means which he can conveniently undertake, the individual undoubtedly would sin who, when there is not question of great pain, would permit himself to die when he could take care of the health of his body. To this, however, that he suffer the very intense pain of the amputation of a member or of an incision into his body, neither a prelate can oblige his subject, nor a father his son.—The reason is both because the sick individual is not held to conserve the life of his body with such great pain and torture and because superiors can not prescribe all things licit and honest but those only which are moderate.[125]

Before leaving the teachings of Sayrus, it is well to point out that what was said earlier regarding the fact that he in many points merely repeats the writings of other authors, in no way diminishes the value of his work. All through this report the reader will see evidence of the effect that one writer has had on another. To cite, however the same doctrine as each author comes into focus is not just simple repetition, but rather it is an attempt to show the constant tradition that has existed in this matter. Sayrus, for example, perhaps has added very little original thought to this subject. His work is of tremendous importance, nonetheless, because it mirrors the opinions prevalent in his age regarding the necessity of using the means of conserving one's life. Such will be the case also as the different authors come up for review.

Among the commentators on the writings of St. Thomas, one of the most famous is *Dominic Banez* († 1604). Writing about St. Thomas' article on mutilation, Banez treats the question of whether or not the state can force a citizen to undergo an amputation.[126] After this problem, he then places the query

---

[125]«. . . ac proinde cum unisquisque jure naturali media licita, quae commode sumi possunt ad sui corporis conservationem ponere tenetur, peccaret sine dubio, qui absque magno dolore, cum possit saluti corporis succurrere, se mori permitteret. Ad hoc tamen, ut ingentissimum dolorem in membri amputatione, vel corporis incisione ferret nec subditum praelatus, nec pater filium, obligare potest. Ratio est tum quia nec infirmus tenetur cum tanto dolore et cruciatu vitam corporis conservare . . . Tum quia superiores non possunt omnia licita et honesta praecipere sed ea tantum quae moderata sunt».—Ibid., n. 38.

[126]D. Banez, op. cit., in II:II, q. 65, art. 1.

before himself:« . . . is the man himself bound to suffer the amputation of a member in order to save his life?»[127] In response, he writes:

It seems as though the answer is yes: because he is held to conserve his life through means which are ordered for this purpose and proportioned: but the cutting off of a member is a means proportioned to conserving life; therefore, he is bound to suffer the amputation. In answer here is the first conclusion. He is not bound absolutely speaking. The reason is that, although a man is held to conserve his own life, he is not bound to extraordinary means but to common food and clothing, to common medicines, to a certain common and ordinary pain: not, however, to a certain extraordinary and horrible pain, nor to expenses which are extraordinary in proportion to the status of this man. So that if, for example, it were certain that a common citizen would gain health if he spent three thousand ducats for a certain medicine, he would not be held to spend them. Thus, the argument is clear, for although that means is proportioned according to right reason and from the consequence is licit, it is, however, extraordinary.[128]

Sanchez († 1610) has substantially the same doctrine. This teaching is found in his famous *Consilia seu opuscula moralia.* Two of the more pertinent passages are the following.

One must suppose that it is one thing not to prolong life and it is another to shorten life. Let the first conclusion be; no one is held to prolong life, indeed neither is he held to conserve it by using the best and most delicate foods, rather this is reprehensi-

---

[127]« . . . an ipsemet homo teneatur pati abscissionem membri propter sevandam vitam?»—Loc. cit.

[128]« Et videretur quod sic: quia tenetur servare vitam per media ordinata et proportionata: sed abscissio membri est medium proportionatum ad servandam vitam, ergo tenetur pati abscissionem. Respondetur et sit prima conclusio. Quod non tenetur absolute loquendo. Et ratio est quia quamvis homo teneatur conservare vitam propriam, non tenetur per media extraordinaria, sed per victum et vestitum communem, per medicinas communes, per dolorem quendam communem et ordinarium: non tamen per quendam dolorem extraordinarium et horribilem, neque etiam per sumpus extraordinarios, secundum proportionem status ipsius hominis. Ut, si v.g. communem civem salutem consequuturum esset certum, si insumeret tria millia ducatorum in quadam medicina, ille non tenetur insumere. Per hoc patet ad argumentum, nam quamvis illud medium sit proportionatum secundum rectam rationem et ex consequenti licitum, est tamen extraordinarium».—D. Banez, in II:II, q. 65, art. 1.

ble. This is proved by reason of the fact that one is not bound to live in the most healthful place but can dwell in a region which is harmful due to the cold or heat neither is he held to seek out the most exquisite medicinal remedies etc., therefore. Likewise, he is not bound to abstain from wine in order to live longer . . . Hence the first inference that if one uses foods which men commonly use and in the quantity which customarily is sufficient for conserving strength, although he realizes due to this he will shorten his life considerably, he does not sin. Secondly, it is inferred that one is not obliged to use medicines to prolong life even where there would be the probable danger of death, such as taking a drug for many years to avoid fevers etc. The second conclusion; one is held however, while sick, to consult doctors and use healthful foods.[129]

Further on then, he writes:

It is licit to fast and abstain even from common foods, not only in regard to the plurality of meals but also, in regard to the quantity as long as the food necessary for the nourishment and conservation of the individual is taken . . . This is proved by reason of the fact that this is not to intend to abbreviate life or kill one's self but it is only to use means directed by nature for sustenance and not to prolong life, to which no one is bound, as I said.[130]

---

[129]« Supponendum est aliud esse non prolongare vitam et aliud abbreviare vitam. Sit prima conclusio. nullus tenetur prolongare vitam, immo nec illam conservare utendo optimis et delicatissimis alimentis, immo hoc est reprehensible. probatur quia non tenetur quis vivere in loco saluberrimo sed potest habitare in regione nociva ratione frigoris vel caloris: nec tenetur exquirere exquisitissima medicamenta etc., ergo. Item, non tenetur abstinere a vino ut diutius vivat . . . Hinc infertur primo, quod si quis utitur alimentis, quibus homines communiter utunter et in quantiate, quae solet sat esse ad valetundinem conservandam, licet percipiat, ex hoc abbreviare vitam notabiliter, non peccat. Secundum infertur, quod non tenetur quis uti medicinis ad prolongandam vitam etiam ubi esset periculum probabile mortis, ut quotannis sumere pharmacum ad vitandas febres etc. Secunda conclusio, tenetur tamen quis dum morbo laborat, consulere, medicos et uti cibis salutaribus». Sanchez, *Consilia,* Tom. II, Lib. V, Cap. 1, dub. 33.

[130]« Licitum est jejunare et abstinere etiam a communibus cibus, non tantum, quo ad pluralitatem comestionum sed etiam quantum ad quantitatem, dummodo sumatur cibus necessarius ad alimentum et conservationem individiu . . . Probatur, quia hoc non est intendere abbreviare vitam, seu occidere se, sed tantum est uti mediis ordinatis a natura ad sustentationem et non prolongare vitam, ad quod nullus tenetur ut dixi».—loc. cit.

Francis Suarez († 1617) has a very interesting article which treats of the necessity that a man has of guarding his life. The question proposed is whether a man is bound to think of himself rather than his neighbor when a situation of danger to his own temporal goods arises.[131] Naturally, his life comes into question here. A good deal of the discussion would not be to the point just now, but there are a few passages which are of interest and which will prove helpful later on.

> The reason is that although a man may never kill himself, he is not bound, however, to conserve his life always and by every means, even by taking less account of the life of a neighbor, especially a friend or father . . . .[132]

Again he writes:

> . . . without mortal sin one, even in extreme necessity, may take less account of himself in order to assist any other neighbor, even a stranger, in similar necessity. By the way of conclusion, it must be noted that we are speaking with only the consideration of charity in mind; for it is otherwise, if the obligation of another virtue comes into question, as for instance justice or piety, as if he is the father of a family who is bound to make provisions, and conserve himself for his sons and family . . . .[133]

Another interesting sentence is, «. . . since mutilation in a principal member is almost equivalent to death, for this reason a man is not bound to undergo it in order to save his life.»[134]

Straight away, one can recognize that a problem that perplexed the moralists of this age was the doubt about whether anyone could be forced to

---

[131]F. Suarez, *Opera Omnia* (Paris, ed. Berton, Vives, 1858), Tom. XII, disp. 9, sect. 3.

[132]« Ratio est quia licet homo nunquam possit se occidere, non tamen semper, et omni medio, et ratione tenetur servare vitam, etiam postponendo vitam proximi, praecipue amici, vel patris . . . »—F. Suarez, op. cit., Tom. XII, Tract. III, Disp. 9, Sect. 3, conclu. 3.

[133]« . . . potest quis sine peccato mortali in necessitate etiam extrema se postponere, ut simili necessitati cujusvis alterius proximi etiam extranei subveniat. Advertendum pro conclusione est, nos loqui considerata propria sola ratione charitatis; nam secus est si intercedat obligatio alterius virtutis, ut justitiae, vel pietatis, ut si sit paterfamilias, qui ex officio tenetur providere, et se conservare pro filiis et familia . . . »—ibid., conclu. 4.

[134]"et quia mutilatio in membro principali quasi aequiparatur morti; unde non tenetur homo illam pati ut vitam servet." *Ibid.*, concl. 5.

44

submit to an amputation in order to save his life. Interesting speculation arose around this problem, and in it, the writers have left indirectly, if not directly, their teaching on the ordinary and extraordinary means of conserving one's life. A good example of these is *Lessius* († 1623).

> . . . notice that a man is bound to permit a member to be cut from him, if the doctors judge this necessary and he will not have to suffer great pains . . . The reason is that he is bound to help his endangered life by ordinary means which are not extremely difficult. If however, tremendous tortures have to be suffered, he is not held to permit this nor can he be forced to this. The reason is because no one is obliged to conserve his life through such torture with an uncertain result . . . .[135]

Lessius makes two exceptions however. The first is the individual who is necessary for the common good. This person is bound to conserve his life even if an amputation is necessary, and it is the opinion of Lessius that he can be forced to submit to it by the State. The second exception involves the religious who is entirely under the power of his Superior. However, even Lessius doubts if this second exception is valid because he does not feel that a Superior could licitly command under obedience such heroic an undertaking.[136]

When discussing the problem of impure touches and glances, Lessius brings up the question of whether or not a virgin, in order to conserve her life, is bound to undergo treatment from a male doctor in the more private parts of her body, when such treatment would be a cause of intense embarrassment and shame. He replies:

> . . . women, especially virgins, are not bound to accept from men medical treatment of this type in the more secret parts . . . The reason is because no one is held to accept a cure which he abhors no less than the disease itself or death: but many modest virgins prefer to tolerate a disease or death rather than to be

---

[135]«. . . adverte hominem teneri permittere sibi membrum secari, si medici id judicent necessarium, nec magni dolores sint preferendi . . . Ratio est quia tenetur vitae suae periclitanti, emdiis ordinariis non admodum difficilibus opitulari. Si tamen ingentes essent cruciatus tolerandi, non tenetur permittere, neque etiam potest ad hoc cogi. Ratio est quia non tenetur quisquam cum tanto cruciatu vitam incerto eventu conservare».—L. Lessius, *De Justitia et Jure,* Lib. II, Cap. 9, dub. 14, n. 96.

[136]Loc. cit.

touched by men. Furthermore, no one is obliged to accept that to which is conjoined the danger of an evil motion or carnal pleasure; indeed it pertains to the heroic grade of chastity to prefer death rather than permit in one's self evil imaginations or any sense of evil desires.[137]

Martin Bonacina († 1631) also writes concerning the necessity of submitting to an amputation.

It is licit to amputate a member or a part of a member from one's self when such an amputation is necessary for the health of the whole body. Indeed, in such an event, there is an obligation of amputating if in the judgment of the doctor the pains are slight. The reason is that a man is bound to help his endangered life by ordinary remedies which are not too difficult; when therefore, a certain member is injurious to the whole body, the law of nature dictates that it be cut off in order that we may help our life.[138]

Similarly, *Paul Laymann* († 1635):

The second resolution is that we are not obliged for the most part to free our life from a disease or extrinsic violence by a means which is very difficult or not customary; v.g., by cutting off the feet, or by using very precious medications. The reason is that the precept of preserving life is affirmative, not obliging in all times and in every way.[139]

---

[137]«. . . mulieres, praesertim virgines, non teneri huiusmodi genus medicandi in locis secretioribus a viris admittere . . . Ratio est, quia nemo tenetur admittere curationem, a qua non minus abhorret quam ab ipso morbo, vel morte: at multae virgines pudicae malunt tolerare morbum, vel mortem quam a viris contingi. Deinde nemo tenetur admittere id, cui conjunctum est periculum turpis motus, aut delectationis carnalis: imo ad heroicum castitatis gradum pertinet malle, mori quam permittere in se turpes imagines aut sensum ullum libidinis».—Ibid., Lib. IV, Cap. 3, dub. 8, n. 60.

[138]«Licitum est sibi amputare membrum, vel membri partem, quando illius amputatio necessaria est ad salutem totius corporis. Imo, in tali eventu extat obligatio amputandi si dolores sint exigui, ita judicante medico. Ratio est quia homo tenetur vitae suae periclitanti opitulari remediis ordinariis nonn valde difficilibus, quando igitur membrum aliquod est toti corpori perniciosum jus naturae dictat abscindendum esse, ut bitae opitulemus . . .»—M. Bonacina, *Moralis Theologica,* Tom. II, Disp. 2, Quaest. Ultim., Sect. 1, Punct. 6, n. 2.

[139]«Resolvitur secundo: Quod propriam vitam a morbo vel exstrinseca violentia plerumque liberare non tenemur per medium valde difficile et insolitum; v.g. pedum sectione, medicamentis

In the *De justitia et Jure of Gabriel of St. Vincent,* the same doctrine is found.

In the seventh place, you ask whether one is obliged to yield to a doctor or surgeon who judges that it is necessary for the conservation of the whole life that a leg or arm or other member be amputated? The response is affirmative when this can happen without great pain; the reason is that no one is held to take care of his life by extremely troublesome means nor by extremely torturous ones as neither by extremely costly means. Hence, I said that a certain nun was not obliged to reveal to a surgeon a disease which she had in the more secret parts of her body, because of the excessive modesty ("verecundia") which appeared to her to be more serious than death itself.[140]

2.3 FROM THE TIME OF CARDINAL DE LUGO TO THE NINETEENTH CENTURY

The first section of *Cardinal De Lugo's* († 1660) tenth disputation in his *De justitia ct jure* has for its title: « Whether it is licit for a man to kill or mutilate himself. »[141] Throughout this section the Cardinal treats the many problems that concern suicide, mutilation and the conservation of one's life. In the first chapter we have made mention of De Lugo's approach to the question of suicide. Here what is of interest is his treatment of the obligation that an individual has to conserve his own life and the necessity of using the means thereto. In the course of this section, De Lugo discusses a good number of particular cases. His solutions enable one to gather his teaching on the obligation of using the ordinary means of conserving life and the lawfulness of not employing the extraordinary means.

---

pretiosissimis. Ratio est: quod praeceptum servandi vitam affirmativum sit, non omni tempore ac modo obligans».—P. Laymann, *Theologica Moralis,* Lib. III, Tract. 3, p. 3, cap. 1, n. 4.

[140]«Quaeres 7 an teneatur quis parere medico, vel chirurgo judicanti necessarium esse pro totius vitae conservatione, quod crus, vel brachium, aut aliud membrum amputetur? Resp. affirmative, quando id fieri potest sine magno dolore, ratio est, quia nullus tenetur tueri vitam per media valde laboriosa, nec valde cruciativa, sicut neque per media vlde pretoisa. hinc dixi non fuisse obligatam quandam monilemostendere chirurgo quendam morbum, quem habebat in partibus secretioribus ratione maximae verecundiae quae sibi gravior apparebat quam esset moris ipsa».—Gabrielis a S. Vincentio, *De Justitia et Jure,* Disp. 6, de restitutione, q. 6, n. 86.

[141]"Utrum liceat homini seipsum interficere, vel mutilare." J. De Lugo, *op. cit.,* Disp. 10, Sect. 1.

In number twenty-one the Cardinal reviews the malice of mutilation. Just as a man does not possess full dominion over his life, so also he lacks complete power over his members. Therefore any mutilation that is not justified by the necessity of his body's health is illicit. Here too, he explains what he understands by mutilation: to take away a member from one's self.[142] Since the necessity of mutilation for the conservation of life can render the mutilation licit, is it ever obligatory to suffer it? (Here again is evidence of the traditional approach. First an author will treat of suicide and the necessity of self-conservation. Then almost automatically, the next question is mutilation and the conditions which make it not only licit but obligatory.) De Lugo answers that an individual is obliged to permit a mutilation as a means of cure when the doctors judge this necessary and when it can be performed without intense pain. If, on the other hand, the mutilation is accompanied by very intense pain, then of course, it ceases to be obligatory because it becomes an extraordinary means of conserving life.

> . . . he must permit this cure when the doctors judge it necessary, and when it can happen without intense pain; not, if it is accompanied by very bitter pain; because a man is not bound to employ extraordinary and difficult means to conserve his life.[143]

Therefore, De Lugo exempts an individual from employing the extraordinary means of conserving his life. However, it could happen that some individual because of certain circumstances would be bound to employ the extraordinary means. For instance, in De Lugo's own words, this would apply to one « whose life is very necessary for the public good. »[144]

It has been seen even thus far, that a discussion of mutilation among the authors of this age usually included some speculation on whether a religious, or for that matter, any person could be forced by the proper authority to submit to a mutilation in order to conserve his life. De Lugo mentions it too. He mentions the religious who is bound by a vow to obey his Superior. Now, supposing that an amputation of some limb is necessary for the health of that religious and his Superior orders him to undergo it, must he do so? De Lugo cites the fact that some hold that the religious is bound to submit, even in this

---

[142]« membrum aliquod sibi auferre ».—Ibid., n.21.

[143]« . . . debere eam curationem permittere, quando medici necessarium judicarent, et absque intenso dolore fieri posset; secus si acerbissimo dolore fieret; quia non tenetur homo media extraordinaria et difficillima adhibere ad vitae conservationem . . . »—J. De Lugo, *De Justitia et Jure*, Disp. 10, Sect. I, n. 21.

[144]« . . . cuius vita bono publico sit valde necessaria." *Loc. cit.*

case, to the will of his Superior. However, the Cardinal judges that the opposite opinion is more probable:

> Some except also the religious obliged to obey his Superior who commands that he undergo the necessary amputation of a limb. Others, and more probably, deny this because such difficult things seem beyond the items of the rule in which religious are bound to obey.[145]

Then De Lugo interjects a thought of great importance. He states that this religious however, would be held to undergo the amputation if he were necessary to the State or the Community,—to which he adds: «and the remedy were entirely secure and certain».[146] Notice that this last element was mentioned also by Lessius when he taught that «no one is obliged to conserve his life under such torture with an uncertain result».[147] Even Vitoria, much earlier, had insinuated the same when he demanded that there be a hope of life which rightly interpreted, would seem to mean a hope of recovery.[148]

In succeeding numbers, De Lugo treats different problems regarding the unlawfulness of certain types of mutilation and suicide.[149] Not all of this is to the point here. However, in number twenty-eight, he outlines the distinction between the positive and negative influences that an individual can have on his own death.[150] There are two ways in which a man sins against the obligation of conserving his life. The first is in a positive way by performing something that will bring on death. The second is in a negative manner; that is, by not fleeing the danger of death when this can be accomplished easily:

> . . . note that a man sins against the obligation of conserving his life, first in a positive way, by doing something that is inductive of death, as for example, to pierce one's self with a sword, to cast

---

[145]«Aliqui excipiunt etiam religiosum, qui obedire debet praelato praecipienti, quod eismodi membri sectionem necessariam sustineat. Alii probabilius id negant, quia res adeo difficiles videntur esse extra res contentas in regula, in quibus religiosi obedire tenentur».—loc. cit.

[146]«. . . nisi religiosus necessarius esset reipublicae, vel communitati, et remedium esset omnino securum et certum.—Loc. cit.

[147]«. . . non tenetur quisquam cum tanto cruciatu vitam incerto eventu conservare».—Lessius, op. cit., Lib. II, Cap. 9, cub. 14, n. 96.

[148]«. . . si aegrotus potest sumere cibum vel alimentum cum aliqua spe vitae, tenetur summere cibum . . .»—Vitoria, Relectio de Temp, n. 1.

[149]J. De Lugo, op. cit., nn. 22-27.

[150]Ibid., n. 28 has this title in the edition cited, «Alius est concursus positivus ad propriam mortem, alius negativus.»

one's self into a fire or a river etc. Secondly, in a negative manner, by not fleeing the dangers of death, as when seeing a raging lion coming to devour him, an individual wills to wait unmoved although he could turn away and flee; or when seeing a fire already approaching him, he does not will to move from his place but awaits the flames . . . [151]

De Lugo admits that in this latter situation a man can not be said to bring about his death in a positive manner; that is, by exerting some positive influence himself. Nonetheless, because the individual does not flee the cause of death when this is possible «in an ordinary and easy way»,[152] his behavior is «against the common obligation of caring for one's own life».[153]

Now, in which category should the individual be placed who abstains from food necessary to sustain his life? De Lugo answers that «to abstain from food necessary for the sustenance of life when a person can sustain his life by ordinary means, would pertain to the first genus».[154] Hence, for De Lugo, the refusal to employ the ordinary means (in this case, food) when this can be accomplished easily and in a normal manner is equivalent to performing an act which has a positive influence in bringing about one's own death.

Another important distinction is next outlined by De Lugo. He points out that danger of death can come from two different types of causes. The first is a natural and purely necessary cause; for example, a flood or a fire. Danger of death arising from such a cause, one must attempt to escape. It would not be lawful to await its eventual destructive force. The second is a free cause; for example, the situation in which one knows that an individual is intent on killing him. In this case the person concerned would not always be bound to flee but for a proportionately grave reason could await possible death. In other words, the obligation of fleeing the danger is greater in the first instance:

---

[151]«. . . adverte, dupliciter posse hominem pecare contra obligationem conservandi vitam, primo positive aliquid faciendo inductivum mortis, ut si ferro se percutiat, si in ignem se conjiciat vel in flumen, etc. Secundo negative, hoc est, non figiendo pericula mortis, ut si videns leonem furiosum ad ipsum devorandum venire, et potens facile decinare et fugere, velit immobilis expectare: vel si videns incendium jam ad ipsum appropinquare, nolit locl moveri, sed flammam expectare . . .»—ibid., n. 28.

[152]«. . . ipsum tamen non fugere et declinare modo ordinario et facili mortem advenientem . . .»—Loc. cit.

[153]« . . est contra obligationem communem tuendi propriam vitam».—Loc. cit.

[154]«Ad hoc autem primum genus pertineret abstinere a cibo necessario ad vitam sustentandam quando facile potest mediis ordinariis illam sustentare».—Loc. cit.

Again it seems that a distinction has to be made concerning this obligation of conserving life. For, sometimes the danger comes from natural and purely necessary causes; sometimes from free causes. In the first case the obligation is greater: v.g., if a flood from a river or sea, or a fire approaches you, you can now await it but you must flee lest it encompass you . . . In the second case however, there is not so great an obligation: v.g., if you know that someone is seeking to kill you . . . you are not held always to flee, but for a grave reason you can patiently await the death inflicted or to be inflicted by another.[155]

De Lugo offers a reason for his reply. In the first case, the natural and necessary cause is determined in itself and does not operate with any indifference. Therefore, the one who wills the necessary cause would seem to will its effect also. Such being the case, a man could really be called the author of his own death since he wills the set of causes from which death necessarily arises. Certainly, he does not will to impede it when he easily could. The second case is different because there is a question of a free cause. Since an effect follows a free cause contingently and not of necessity, it is not necessarily true that a person who would not flee such a cause would will its effect. Rather, he only permits this effect, if it should occur. In such a case, he would not be the author of his own death:

The point of difference in the two cases seems to be that in the first case, he who wills the necessary cause, seems to will the effect since a natural and necessary cause is determined in itself and does not operate with indifference: therefore, a man seems to be the author of his death when he wills the complexity of causes from which death arises; or certainly, he does not will to impede it when he easily could. In the second case however, since a free cause intervenes from which an effect follows contingently, it is not necessary that he will the effect when he does not flee this cause,

[155] « Rursus circa hanc obligationem conservandi vitam distinguendum videtur. Aliquando enim periculum provenit ex causis naturalibus et mere necessariis: aliquando vero ex causis liberis. in primo casu obligatio est major: si v.g. inundatio fluminis vel maris, aut incendium ad te appropinquat, non potes illud expectare, sed debes fugere ne te comprehendat . . . In secundo autem casu non est tanta obligatio v.g. si scis aliquem te ad necem quaerere . . . non teneris semper fugere, sed potes ex causa gravi patienter mortem ab alio illatam vel inferendam expectare ».—ibid., n. 29.

but he holds himself permissive in relation to it . . . Hence, the man is not the author of his death . . . .[156]

The point of main concern in the foregoing discussion is the emphasis which De Lugo places on the necessity of conserving one's life. It will also prove helpful later on to have the clear distinction between natural and free causes in mind. So often in the disputations in theology, confusion arises because of the lack of clear-cut distinctions. This is true also in the matter of ordinary and extraordinary means.

For De Lugo then, the necessity of conserving one's life by ordinary means is beyond dispute. Not to use the ordinary means is the same as to inflict death on one's self.

> I said, however, that a man must guard his life by ordinary means against dangers and death coming from natural causes . . . because the one who neglects the ordinary means seems to neglect his life and therefore to act negligently in the administration of it, and he who does not employ the ordinary means which nature has provided for the ordinary conservation of life is considered morally to will his death . . . [157]

Such is not the case however, with the extraordinary means of conserving life. In this paragraph, De Lugo gives a minor discussion on the nature of extraordinary means and the reason why they are not obligatory. However brief this discussion is, his teaching is of great importance and assistance to one trying to determine the nature of the extraordinary means of conserving life. First of all, De Lugo rules out the necessity of any extraordinary diligence in accomplishing the conservation of life. For him, there is a clear distinction between the blameworthy neglect of one's life and the necessary

---

[156]«Ratio differentia inter utrumque casum haec videtur esse, quod in primo casu, qui vult causam necessariam, videtur velle effectum ipsum, cum causa naturalis et necessaria determinata sit ex se, et non operetur cum indifferentia: quare tunc homo videtur auctor esse suae mortis, cum velit eam complexionem causarum, exqua necessario mors oritur, vel certe non vult illam impedire, cum facile possit. In secundo autem casu, cum interveniat causa libera, ex qua contingenter sequitur effectur, non est necesse quod velit affectum qui non fugit illam causam, sed solum permissive se habet respectu illius . . . Unde homo tunc non est auctor suae mortis . . . »—loc. cit.

[157]«Dixi tamen, contra pericula, et mortem ex causis naturalibus provenientem debere hominem *mediis ordinariis*, vitam tueri . . . quia qui media ordinaria negligit, videtur negligere vitam, atque ideo negligentem se in ejus gubernatione gerere, et moraliter censetur velle mortem, qui mediis ordinariis non utitur, quae natura providit ad ordinariam vitae conservationem . . . »—loc. cit.

care of it by very extraordinary means. The reason which De Lugo gives is that the «bonum» of a man's life is not so tremendously important that it demands conservation by all possible means. Perhaps this statement may appear a bit shocking at first. Rightly interpreted however, its meaning is clear. The affirmative precept of the natural law obliging conservation of one's life does not bind in the presence of a proportionately grave difficulty. Not every possible means must be employed but only those which ordinary diligence requires. If in using ordinary means death occurs, his death nevertheless can not be imputed to the individual as morally culpable:

> . . . he is not held to the extraordinary and difficult means . . . the 'bonum' of his life is not of such great moment, however, that its conservation must be effected with extraordinary diligence: it is one thing not to neglect and rashly throw it away, to which a man is bound: it is another however, to seek after it and retain it by exquisite means as it is escaping away from him, to which he is not held; neither is he on that account considered morally to will or seek his death.[158]

De Lugo applies the principle again and says that in a situation where life is being taken away by another man, «you are not held to the ordinary means of fleeing death, except per accidens in a particular case on account of the inconveniences which will follow from your death».[159] The reason is that as far as the individual is concerned, he is conserving his life and the responsibility for death lies with the other person.[160]

A teaching of momentous importance is found under number thirty in De Lugo's treatment of ordinary and extraordinary means. He supposes a situation in which a person is condemned to death by fire. While surrounded by the flames, he notices that he has sufficient water to extinguish some of the fire but not all of it. Must he use this water? De Lugo says no, and gives his reason:

---

[158]«. . . nec etiam tunc tenetur ad media extraordinaria et difficilia . . . non tamen est tanti momenti hoc vitae bonum ut extraordinaria diligentia procuranda sit ejus conservatio: aliud est eam non negligere et temere projicere, ad quod homo tenetur: aliud vero est eam quaerer et fugientem ex se retinere mediis exquisitis, ad quod non tenetur, nec ideo censetur moraliter mortem velle aut quarerere».—loc. cit.

[159]" . . . nec ad ordinaria media teneris ut mortem fugias, nisi per accidens in aliquo casu propter inconvenientia quae ex tua morte sequuntur . . . " Loc. cit.

[160]" . . . quia tunc jam quantam ex te est, vitam conservas, nec ex te provenit ejus amissio, sed ex alio quod tibi non imputatur, sed illi." Loc. cit.

. . . if a man condemned to fire, while he is surrounded by the flames, were to have at hand water with which he could extinguish the fire and prolong his life, while at the same time other wood is being carried forward and burned, he would not be held to use this means to conserve his life for such a brief time because the obligation of conserving life by ordinary means is not an obligation of using means for such a brief conservation—which is morally considered nothing at all . . . .[161]

However, if he could put the fire out once and for all, and thus escape death, it would seem that the use of the water would be obligatory because then his death could not be considered as coming absolutely from an extrinsic source «since there would be left to him the free ability of defending himself from the fire by ordinary means . . .».[162] In other words, here again the element of benefit is introduced. The means and remedies employed, even though in themselves common and ordinary, must offer some hope of benefit or help to the conservation of life before they become obligatory. Furthermore, this benefit must be of some considerable duration—in other words, proportionate. Otherwise, if the profit from using these means is only brief, then for De Lugo, it must be considered of no value morally and thus not obligatory. «Parum pro nihilo reputatur».

De Lugo also treats the opinion already reviewed here that a man is not bound to effect a prolongation of his life by using choice and delicate foods. In similar fashion, neither is he bound to abstain from wine in order to live longer. He expresses it as follows:

Whence, much less is a man bound to effect a lengthening of his life by choice and delicate foods, for just as one is not held to abstain from wine in order to live longer, so neither is he bound to drink wine for the same purpose: because just as a man is not bound to seek a more healthful and wholesome locality and air in

---

[161]«. . . si enim quis ad ignem damnatus, dum jam flamma circumdatus est haberet ad manum aquam, qua posset ignem extinguere et vitam protrahere, quamdiu alia ligna afferuntur et accenduntur; non ideo teneretur ei medio uti, ut vitam illo brevi tempore conservaret: quia obligatio conservandi vitam per media ordinaria, non est obligation utendi mediis ad illam brevem conservationem quae moraliter pro nihilo reputatur . . .»—ibid., n. 30.

[162]". . . cum relinqueretur ei facultas libera defendendi se ab igne per media ordinaria . . . " *Loc cit.*

order to prolong his life, so neither is he held to eat better or more healthful food.[163]

The reader has taken note without doubt, that the theologians cited thus far, when discussing ordinary means, have constantly referred to a comparison with the manner in which men «commonly» live. An interesting application of this principle occurs in De Lugo. He repeats the difference between bringing about one's own death in a positive manner and omitting the use of certain means of conserving life. The first is never licit; the second can be licit in certain circumstances. In harmony with this principle therefore, «according to the common opinion of the Doctors, there is no obligation of using choice and costly medicine to avoid death».[164] This omission does not imply a direct killing of one's self but rather, the person concerned permits his death and rests content with using only the ordinary and common means by which men commonly live.[165] Hence, the person does not positively influence his death, but dies on account of old-age or the weakness of his own life.[166] With this in mind therefore, we may conclude that a religious novice would not be bound to return to the world to eat better and seek other conveniences for the sake of his health when those in religion do not commonly live in that manner.[167] Here is the interesting application made by De Lugo because he is obviously taking the measure of comparison from the surroundings which are required by the individual's state in life. Hence, although strictly speaking given the common food for common men living in the world may be an ordinary means for them, nevertheless, it remains extraordinary for the religious who in his cloister would not ordinarily eat in the manner ordinary or customary in the world.

---

[163]«Unde multo minus tenetur homo vitae elongationem procurare cibis exquisitis et delicatis, sicut enim non tenetur quis abstinere a vino, ut longius vivat, sic nec vinum libere ad eundem finem: quia sicut non tenetur homo salubriorem locum, et aerem quaerere ad vitam prolongandam, sic nec meliorem et salubriorem victum sumere.»—ibid., n. 32.

[164]«. . . juxta communem doctorum sentintiam, non est obligatio utendi medicina exquisita et pretiosa ad vitandum mortem . . .»—Ibid., n. 36.

[165]«. . . haec enim omittere non est se occidere, sed permittere mortem ex se obvenientem, et relinquere se ordinariis et communibus mediis, quibus alii homines communiter vivunt . . .»—Loc. cit.

[166]«. . . neque enim hic se occidit, sed moritur prpter aegritudinem, vel infirmitatem suae naturae . . .»—Loc. cit.

[167]«Cur ergo novitus tenebitur sub peccato redire in saeculum, ut quaerat delicias, delicatos cibos, et luxum, nec satisfaciet utendo victu, et mediis quibus alii communiter in religione utuntur et vitam conservant?»—Loc. cit.

The foregoing report on the teaching of De Lugo reveals his strict adherence to the traditional doctrine in these matters. Likewise, it shows the clever and precise explanations and applications of the principles involved which the Cardinal makes—all of which will be of assistance further on in this dissertation.

It is the same doctrine that is given by *Anthony Diana* († 1663). Citing Vitoria he admits that a sick person for whose health there is no hope, can refuse to buy a costly drug that will prolong his life for some days, even though he is able to buy it.[168] Diana also follows previous teaching in he matter of mutilation. Even though an amputation is necessary for the health of the individual, he need not feel obliged to suffer it when it is accompanied by intense pain and torture.[169] Actually Diana is more forthright than his predecessors when he includes in this exception the religious bound by obedience. He says categorically that the religious is not bound to the amputation and can not be forced to it, «even if . . . the Superior commands this (surgery) to him».[170]

Each theologian makes a contribution in his writings. Many in the matter of the ordinary an extraordinary means of conserving life, have perhaps served only to reflect the teachings prevalent in their age. Others carry on the existing tradition and add a different approach or solve a different case. Some perhaps even point out a new problem. Others relate the old teaching in a more precise manner.

Tournely in his *Theologia Moralis* reiterates much of what went before him. For instance, he excludes the necessity of using very costly medications which would consume a considerable amount of one's resources. Neither is it obligatory to undergo very intense pain such as in the amputation of feet or arms.[171] Tournely not only excludes the necessity of using these means but he also assigns the reason: «Means of this type are morally impossible».[172]

---

[168] «Et idem Victoria ait, licet aegrotus, di cuius salute desperature, posset aliquot dies pharmaco protrahere vitam, non teneri illud emere . . . »—A. Diana, *Coordinatus,* per R. P. Mrtinum de Alcolea (Lugduni, 1667) Tom. VIII, Tract. V, Resol. 53., (ex Diana, p. 5, tr. 4, res. 33).

[169] « . . . hominem teneri permittere sibi membrum secari, si medici id judicent necessarium, nec magni dolores sint perferendi, si tamen ingentes essent cruciatus tolerandi . . . non tenetur permittere, neque potest ad hoc cogi . . . »—Ibid., Res. 57.

[170] « . . . etiam si Religiosus et Superior id ei praeciperet».—Loc. cit.

[171] «Sic non habetur ut homicida sui, qui abstinet a pretiosissimis medicamentis, in quibus profundi deberent opes patrimonii; item qui non vult gravissimos cruciatus pedum v.g. vel brachiorum sectionem pati, ut vitam diutius protrahat . . . »—H. Tournely, *Theologica Moralis* (Venetiis, 1756), Tom. III, Tract. de Decalogo, cap. 2, de Quinto Praec., Art. I, conc. 2.

[172] « . . . cum huiusmodi media moraliter impossibilia sint».—Loc. cit.

Interestingly enough, this author next discusses the person who does not agree to suffer even moderate pain in order to conserve his life. Can he be forced to submit to an amputation if it involves only moderate pain? Tournely's answer is that this individual can be forced by those who are entrusted with his care, or even by someone acting in virtue of a mandate from such persons. Tournely is hesitant about enlarging the circle of those who have the authority to command such a procedure.[173] However, what is of importance is the fact that Tournely recognizes and teaches that moderate pain does not constitute moral impossibility and hence, generally speaking, does not make a means extraordinary.

The Carmelite Fathers of Salamanca, known as the *Salmanticenses,* have this precise wording of the doctrine on the ordinary and extraordinary means of conserving life:

> . . . also, in order to conserve his life, one is not bound to use all possible remedies, even extraordinary ones, really choice medicines, costly foods, a transfer to more healthful territory, so that he will live longer: he is not held to give over all his wealth in order to avoid death which is threatened by another person, whether justly or unjustly: neither is a sick individual in desperate condition bound to employ very costly remedies, even though he should know that with these remedies his life would be extended for some hours, or days or even years.[174]

The intense pains of amputation excuse a person from the obligation of employing such a remedy for the further conservation of his life. In this, the Salmanticenses adhere to previous teachings. Likewise, they make only one exception and state that a person who is necessary for the common good should submit to such a procedure in order to save his life. Furthermore, the

---

[173] « Sed quid si homo ne moderatos quidem dolores pati velit, ut vitam servet, poteritne invitus abscindi? Poterit ab iis aut de mandato eorum, qui curam ejus gerunt, ut pater, tutor, Superior, et similes: an autem et ab aliis mutilari possit, non ita constat ». —Loc. cit.

[174] « Nec etiam tenetur aliquis ad conservandam vitam ut omnibus possibilbus remediis, etiam extraordinariis, nimirum exquisitis medicinis, cibis pretiosis, ire ad terras salubriores ad amplius vivendum: nec dare omnes suas divitias pro evitanda morte juste vel injuste ab alio minata: nec tenetur infirmus desperatus uti remediis pretiosissimis, tametsi cum illis sciret vitam per aliquas horas, vel dies, vel etiam annos fore extendendam . . . » —Salmanticenses, *Cursees Theologia Moralis,* Tom III, Tract. XIII, de restit., Cap. II, Punct. 2, Sect. 2, n. 26.

proper authority can command him to submit.[175] However, they add «if the remedy is entirely certain for the conservation of his life».[176] No one, ordinarily then, is bound to permit an amputation «because, as the Roman said, the opening up of whose leg caused him intense pain, health is not worth such pain,—for no one is held to conserve his life by extraordinary and horrible means».[177]

The doctrine on the ordinary and extraordinary means of conserving life as found in the *Medulla Theologiae Moralis* of H. Busenbaum is merely a collection of all that has been reported here so far. It is known that the first edition of *St. Alphonsus' Moral Theology* in 1748 actually was the *Medulla Theologiae Moralis* of Busenbaum to which Alphonsus added certain notes.[178] Even in succeeding editions, Busenbaum's *Medulla* was the basis for Alphonsus' noted work. Especially, in the matter of the ordinary and extraordinary means of conserving life, this is true. Hence it seems well to treat merely the writings of both these authors together.

In point of fact, nothing new is added by either of these authors in this matter. However, for future reference, it will be profitable here to outline the elements and conditions which these authors feel render a means of conserving life extraordinary. First of all, there is no obligation of using any costly and uncommon medicine.[179] There is no need of changing one's place of residence in order to get a more healthful climate outside one's native land.[180] No one is held to employ extraordinary and very difficult means such as an amputation of a leg in order to conserve his life.[181] True, the obligation of taking an expensive medicine does not exist but if it is an ordinary medica-

---

[175]«. . . nec tenetur infirmus eam patio ob conservationem vitae nec posset hoc Respublica, aut Praelatus illis praecipere, nisi esset persona multum necessaria bono communi . . .»—Ibid., Punct. 3, n. 50.

[176]«. . . si remedium esset omnino certum ad illius vitae conservationem».—Loc. cit.

[177]«. . . quia, ut dicebat ille Romanus, cui crus cum ingenti dolore aperiebatur; 'non est tanto dolore digna salus'—non enim quis tenetur per media extraordinaria, et horrenda vitam conservare . . .»—Loc. cit.

[178]Cf. S. Alphonus, *Theologia Moralis,* praefatio editoris, for historical study on the editions of St. Alphonsus' Theologia Moralis and the influence that hte *Medulla* of Busienbaum exerted on St. Alphonsus.

[179]«Ideoque non teneri . . . nec aliquem alium uti pretiosa et exquisita medicina ad mortem vitandam . . .»—H. Busenbaum, *Medulla theologiae moralis* (Romae, 1757), Lib. III, Tract. IV, de Quinto-Sexto Praecepto, cap. 1, n. 371; S. Alphonsus, *Theologia Moralis,* Lib. III, Tract. IV, cap. 1, n. 371.

[180]«. . . nec secularem, relicto domicilio, quaerere salubriorem aerem extra patriam . . .»—Busenbaum, loc. cit.; S. Alphonsus, loc. cit.

[181]«. . . non teneri quemquam mediis extraordinariis, et nimis duris, v. gr. abscissione crucis, etc. vitam conservare . . .»—Busenbaum, ibid., n. 372; S. Alphonsus, ibid., n. 372.

tion, one would be bound to employ this means of conserving his life provided that some hope of future health could be foreseen.[182] The abhorrence that a sick woman, particularly a maiden, might have for medical treatment by a male doctor or surgeon would seem to be sufficient, ordinarily speaking, to excuse her from this treatment.[183] However, if the services of a woman doctor or surgeon are available, certainly this treatment would be obligatory.[184]

As can be seen, both Busenbaum and Alphonsus adhered strictly to the traditional teaching on this subject. No doubt, it has become obvious to the reader by now that the moralists at this period are merely repeating the very same phrases and examples which their predecessors used. Perhaps the reason is that at this time there were other, more important, problems confronting the moral theologians. Perhaps also, the reason is that progress in the medical field had not actually reached such a degree as to initiate any speculation on whether a particular remedy should be considered obligatory or not. Evidently an amputation, at this period in history, was the perfect example of a terrible torture which no one ordinarily could be held to undergo. When, evidently, an interpretation of the obligations imposed by religious obedience presented a problem in this matter, the theologians solved it. Had doctors and other scientists created doubts or difficulties by advancing new and secure methods of heath and cure, no doubt these very moralists would have settled them, as they did in so many other instances. The absence of speculation therefore seems due to the fact that difficulties in the matter were not presented to the moralists, rather than to any want of appreciation of the problem itself.

Anthony de Escobar († 1669) took from Vitoria much of his teaching on the necessity of using the ordinary means of conserving life. He uses Vitoria's example of the man who, according to the judgment of a doctor, would be able to prolong his life ten years if he would drink wine. Escobar with Vitoria answers that this individual «can nevertheless abstain from the wine.»[185]

---

[182]«. . . infirmum in periculo mortis, si sit spes salutis non posse medicamina respuere».—Busenbaum, loc. cit.; S. Alphonsus, loc.cit.

[183]«Non videtur tamen virgo aegrotans (per se loquendo) teneri subire manus medici vel chirurgi quando id ei gravissimum est, et magis quam mortem ipsam horret».—Busenbaum, loc. cit., S. Alphonsus, loc. cit.

[184]«Posset tamen virgo permittere tangi; immo teneretur sinere, ut ab alia femina curetur . . .»—S. Alphonsus, loc. cit.

[185]«. . . posse nihilominus a vino abstinere».—A. de Escobar, *Universae Theologiae Moralis, Receptiores absque Lite Senteniae nec-non Controversae Disquisitiones* (Lugduni, 1663), IV, Lib. 32, Sect. **, Cap. V, Prob. XXIV, n. 128.

This very same doctrine is taught by *Thomas Tamburini* († 1675) in his *Explicatio Decalogi.*[186] This author also lists great pain as a cause excusing a man from undergoing an amputation because «charity in regard to your own life is not demanded with such great inconveniences.»[187] For that very reason, medication that can be obtained only at a high price is not obligatory.[188] Interestingly enough, Tamburini is quite realistic in his treatment of the necessity of undergoing an amputation. As has just been said, he teaches that it is not obligatory, but he takes notes of the fact that many previous authors have excepted the individual who is necessary for the common good. Then Tamburini adds that this «at least practically, does not apply because ordinarily you can prudently consider that when you die, another just as capable will take your place.»[189]

The necessity of suffering a surgical intervention in order to conserve one's life is also excluded by *Holzmann*. For this author also, the obligation of conserving one's life does not require the use of extraordinary and very difficult means. Since a surgical section would involve pain and be in fact extraordinary, it can not be said to be obligatory.[190]

Sporer in his *Theologia Moralis* has the following very concise treatment. It is worthy of quote, since he gives in this excerpt most of the conditions which the moralists of his time considered as the identification marks of extraordinary means:

> It is for this reason that they sin mortally who have a gravely dangerous or deadly disease and are not willing to employ the ordinary and conveniently procurable remedies, and thus having neglected these remedies, permit their death when it can be very conveniently and reasonably impeded; for, since we are not the

---

[186]«. . . qui te non obligat ad utendum vino, vel carnibus; etiamsi Medicus dicat te victurum cum illis amplius decem annis quam si utaris aqua et piscabus . . .»—T. Tamburini, *Explicatio Decalogi* (Venetiis, 1719), Lib. Vi, Cap. II, Sect. II, n. 11.

[187]«. . . cum tanto incommodo non urget charitas in tuam ipsammet vitam».—Ibid., Sect. III, n. 3.

[188]«Nam propter eandem rationem modo diximus, non obligari nos medicamentis magno pretio conquisitis et extraordinariis vitam annosque protrahere».—Loc. cit.

[189]«. . . saltem practice non urget, quia regulariter potes prodenter existimare, tibi morienti alterum non minus aptum successurum».—Loc. cit.

[190]«Ratio est quia nemo per se loquendo, tenetur suam vitam conservare per media extraordinaria et admodum difficulia; cum non sit tanto digna dolore salus, juxta commune adagium: sed sectio est medium extraordinarium et admodum difficile—ergo.»—A. Holzmann, *Theologia Moralis* (Benevento, 1743), Vol. I, Pars II, Tract. II, Disp. V, Cap. III, Cas. II.

masters of our lives, but the guardians only, we are bound to conserve our life only by means which are ordinary and per se directed to the conservation of life; not, in like manner, by means which are extraordinary, unusual and very difficult either because of suffering v.g., in the amputation of a member, arm or leg, or because of price v.g., a medicine which is too expensive considering one's position . . . The reason is because the precept of conserving life is affirmative, and therefore does not bind pro semper but only at certain times and in a certain manner.[191]

Among the conditions which could render a means extraordinary, there are three that *Reiffenstuel* († 1703) seems to emphasize. He gives a very precise discussion of the matter in his *Theologia Moralis*.[192] First of all, no one is obliged to conserve his life except by means which are ordinary, considering his position or status. Secondly, there must be a considerable hope of recovery from the illness by using these means. Thirdly, Reiffensteul requires that the individual be able to employ the means without tremendous difficulty. All three of these conditions must be fulfilled simultaneously in the same individual, otherwise the means is an extraordinary means of conserving life. These three conditions are not listed numerically in Reiffensteul, as they have been here. Rather, they have been gathered from the elements included in a difficulty which he presents and answers in the negative:

> . . . no one is bound to conserve his life except by means which are ordinary in respect to his status . . . Do not say: if no one is bound to conserve his life, except by ordinary means, then a sick man without being accused of indirectly killing himself, can in good conscience refuse medicines when in danger of death even though these medicines are not too costly and furthermore, even

---

[191]«Quando nimirum commode et rationabiliter impediri potest: qua ratione peccant mortaliter, qui in gravi periculoso aut lethali morbo nolunt adhibere remedia ordinaria, et commodo parabilia, iisque neglectis mortem permittunt; cum enim non simus domini sed custodes tantum vitae nostrae, tenemur vitam nostram conservare mediis ordinariis, et per se ordinatis ad vitam conservandam tantum; non item mediis extraordinariis insolitis, multumque difficilibus, aut ob cruciatum, v.g. abscissione membri, brachii, vel tibiae aut ob pretium v.g. medicina nimium sumptuosa comparatione sui status: . . . Ratio est quia praeceptum servandi vitam affirmativum est, ideoque non pro semper sed certo tantum tempore et modo obligat».—P. Sporer, *Theologia Moralis,* Tom. I, Tract. V, Cap. III, SEct. I, n. 13.

[192]A. Reiffenstuel, *Theologia Moralis* (Mutinae, 1740), Tract. IX, Distinc. III, Quaes II, n. 14.

though there would be a great hope of recovery if he took the medicines, which he could do without tremendous difficulty.[193]

Reiffenstuel, quite significantly, finds no trouble in stating that the sick individual in the circumstances just outlined must accept the medicines because they are ordinary means of conserving his life and therefore obligatory.[194]

In his treatment of this problem, La Croix († 1714) repeats much of what was written by the moralists before him. This is especially true since this author is basing his work on that of Busenbaum. La Croix acknowledges his debt to such authors as Vitoria, Lessius, De Lugo, Laymann etc.[195] For example, he mentions costly and choice medicines and voluntary exile from one's native land as examples of means which are not of obligation. One of the conditions that this moralist also requires before any means can be termed ordinary is the hope of deriving some good from the use of a remedy.

In a sort of postscript to this whole discussion, La Croix has some speculation on just how great the obligation of conserving or prolonging one's life can be said to be.[196] First of all, he indicates that the obligation of prolonging one's own life is not the same as the obligation of conserving it. The reason is that « the prolongation of life implies a singular assiduity to which we are not held, whereas the non-abbreviation or the conservation of life implies only a common diligence to which we are obliged . . . . »[197]

Later on, La Croix cites a dispute regarding the necessity of undergoing a surgical section or amputation of a leg when one foresees that the neglect of such a procedure could result in his death. As to the obligation entailed, he writes: « some say yes because you are not the master of your life; others say

---

[193]« . . . quia nemo tenetur suam vitam servare nisi mediis respectu sui status ordinariis . . . non dicas: Si nemo tenetur suam vitam servare, nisi mediis ordinariis, tunc aegrotus, quin dicatur se ipsum indirecte occidere, potest bona conscientia respuere medicinas in periculo mortis, quamvis illae medicinae non sint nimium pretiosae et caeteroquin foret magna spes reconvalescentiae, si easdem, quas asque ingenti difficultate posset, etiam summeret ».—A. Reiffenstuel, *Theologia Moralis,* Tract. IX, Distinc. III, Quaest. II, n. 14.

[194]« Respond. enim negando illatum et eiusdem suppositum, quasi nimurum medicinae respectu status infirmorum essent quid extraordinarium: etenim hae, praesertim non ninmis pretiosae . . . non sunt extraordinaria sed potius ordinaria remedia ».—Loc. cit.

[195]Cf. C. La Croix, *Theologia Moralis* (Ravennae, 1761), Vol. I, Lib. III, Pars I, Tract. IV, Cap. I, dub. I.

[196]Ibid., addenda.

[197]« Ratio est *vitam prolongare* importat singulare studium, ad quod non tenemur, e contra *non abbreviare et conservare* importat commune tantum stadium ad quod tenemur. »—Ibid., n. 3.

no because no one is held to employ extraordinary and very difficult means to conserve his life. »[198]

Finally, it is well to note that this moralist considers the notion of incertitude when determining a means as ordinary or extraordinary. Giving reference to Vitoria, La Croix says a man is not held to conserve his life by medicines because it is uncertain whether the effects of the medicine will be good or bad. Actually we do not know whether medicines will prolong one's life or shorten it.[199]

Roncaglia's († 1737) teaching follows the general outline of that of his predecessors. Ordinary means are obligatory, and extraordinary means are not usually of obligation. An individual can not be said to be negligent in caring for his life if he employs the ordinary means. This is true because one could never be called negligent in this mode of acting « if he uses all those means which ordinarily are in use in any project to be undertaken. »[200] However, one would not be obliged to use means which are very costly, very painful or means which cause great shame.[201]

This theologian agrees with the moralists before him that an amputation of a diseased member of the body would not usually be obligatory if it involves tremendous suffering. However, his teaching is not quite so unconditional in this matter as was the case with earlier authors. Regularly, the moralists cite an amputation as an example of extraordinary means. Roncaglia agrees with this if unbearable pain accompanies the cutting away of a limb. Whenever, however, « from the amputation, future pains of notable proportion will not arise but only moderate pains, then one is bound to suffer the abscission; for everyone is held to conserve his life by ordinary means and it is an ordinary means to suffer something to conserve this same life. »[202]

Naturally enough, Roncaglia excludes the necessity of undergoing tremendous torments in order to conserve one's life. It is significant, however, that he is willing to distinguish surgical procedures into the type involving extraordinary pain and difficulty and the type involving only a moderate pain. All previous theologians have recognized the distinction in theory. The

---

[198]« . . . aliqui affirmant quia non es dominus vitae tuae; alii negant quia nemo tenetur media extraordinaria et valde difficilia adhibere ad conservandam vitam . . .»—Ibid., n. 16.

[199]Cfr. ibid., n. 6.

[200]« . . . si utatur iis omnibus, quae ordinarie sunt in usu in aliqua re peragenda . . .»—C. Roncaglia, *Theologia Moralis* (Lucae, 1730), Vol. I, Tract. XI, Cap. I, Q. III

[201]« . . . non vero extraordinariis et valde pretoisis sicut etiam valde doloriferis, seu magnam afferentibus erubescentiam».—Loc. cit.

[202]« . . . ex abscissione non sint futuri dolores ingentes, sed moderati, tunc tenetur mediis ordinariis vitam conservare et medium ordinarium est aliquid pati pro eadem vita conservanda».—Ibid., Q. IV.

application of it, however, to a surgical section or abscission is noteworthy and important. Roncaglia also underlines the necessity of suffering a moderate difficulty for the conservation of one's life. This too is of considerable import. Pain of itself does not render a means extraordinary. It must be a pain that will involve intense torment in such a way as to constitute a certain impossibility or unproportionate difficulty. All this was recognized by previous moralists, but it certainly is stated more precisely in Roncaglia.

In discussing the question whether a sick man is bound to take means to gain his health again, *Mazzotta* († 1746) gives certain elements that would render a means extraordinary and thus not obligatory. First of all, if there is no hope of recovery, a means need not be employed. Secondly, great horror or torment or extraordinary expenditure of money would excuse an individual from employing these means. The reason is that duty requires only ordinary diligence and expense. The use of extraordinary means is considered to involve some sort of impossibility. This teaching is found in his *Theologia Moralis.* [203]

The traditional doctrine is also taught by *Benjamin Elbel* († 1756) in his work on Moral Theology.[204] Likewise, *Billuart* († 1757) states that « they are guilty who, while they are sick, refuse common remedies which will certainly or more probably be of benefit and not harmful, if from the lack of these death results. »[205] On the other hand, remedies which are unusual, very difficult or very expensive considering the person's status are not of obligation because we are held to conserve our life only by ordinary means. Furthermore, « God does not command that we be solicitous of a longer life. »[206]

Vincent Patuzzi († 1769) agrees in general with the teaching of his predecessors in the matter of the ordinary and extraordinary means of conserving

---

[203]« . . . hinc tenetur cibum vel medicamentum sumere etc. si inde affulgeat spes vitae. Caeterum, si non possit ea sumere sine magna consternatione, cruciatu etc. non peccat, quia tunc reputatur impossibilitas quaedam. item nec peccat, qui, etiamsi possit, non facit expensas extraordinarias pro medicis, medicamentis, etc. etiamsi prudenter timeatur mors; quia sufficit adhibere expensas et diligentiam ordinariam. »—N. Mazzotta, *Theologia Moralis* (Venetiis, 1760), Tom. I, Tract. II, Disp. II, Quaest. I, Cap. I.

[204]Cf. B. Elbel, *Theologia Moralis per modum Conferentiarum*, ed. I Bierbaum (Paderbornae, 1891–1892), II, n. 25 and n. 27, and particularly « . . . etiamsi quilibet teneatur conservare vitam suam mediis ordinariis secundum dicta, nullus tamen (per se, nisi scilicet bonum publicum, charitas erga Deum aut proximum aluid suadeat) teneatur in hunc finem uti mediis nimis difficilibus vel medicamentis extraordinariis seu etiam nimis sumptuosis ».—Ibid., n. 28.

[205]« Rei sunt qui dum aegrotant recusant remedia communia, certo seu probabilius profutura et non nocitura, si ex earum defectu mors sequatur ».—C. Billuart, *Summa S. Thomae* (Parisiis, 1852), Tom. VI, Dissert. X, Art. III, Consect. n. 3.

[206]« . . . neque jubet Deus ut de vita longiore ita simul solliciti ».—Loc. cit.

life. He holds that a sick person would not be bound to employ the extraordinary means. As examples of extraordinary means, he gives the abscission of a member, choice and more costly medicines, a long journey or absence from one's native land undertaken for the sake of a better climate, and finally grave expense.[207] The reason assigned by Patuzzi is that most of the remedies involve a difficulty which is too burdensome and even produce harm. Furthermore, their results are uncertain and very often useless.[208] Even if, however, one would have a morally certain hope that the recovery of health would eventuate from the use of these means, an individual would not have to use them because the law of charity and the natural law do not demand that one employs such extraordinary, harsh and violent remedies in order to conserve his life.[209] The question is impractical anyway, according to Patuzzi, because people usually sin by being too solicitous of conserving their lives rather than the other way around.[210]

However, there is one notable departure from tradition in the writings of Patuzzi. He holds a stricter view regarding the maiden's obligation to accept treatment from a surgeon even at the price of great embarrassment and shame. Actually, it is not surprising to find that in this matter, one of his views is stricter than that of other moralists because Patuzzi has somewhat of a reputation for being rigorous in his opinions.[211] It will be well though, to quote the passage in question because it reveals a different approach, an approach which Patuzzi borrowed from Franzoja:[212]

I agree, however with Franzoja when he teaches well that it is not licit for a girl to refuse the healing hand of a surgeon and thus undergo death, because her shame or foolishness deem it something most grave and even more painful than death; since this is

---

[207]«Non tenetur infirmus saluti suae providere extraordinariis remediis, puta abscissione membri, exquisitis et pretioribus medicinis, longa a patria peregrinatione et absentia ob aeris mutationem, vel gravioribus expensis».—V. Patuzzi, *Ethica Christiana sive Theologia Moralis* (Bassani, 1770), Tom. III, Tract. V, Pars V, Cap. X, Consect. sept.

[208]«. . . quia haec remedia plurimum incommodi et damni afferunt, graviora et incerta sunt ac plerumque inutilia . . .»—Loc. cit.

[209]«non ergo legem naturae et caritatis violabit qui recto fine justaque de causa remediis extraordinariis, acerbioribus et violentis vitam conservare recusarent».—Loc. cit.

[210]Cf. loc. cit.

[211]Lehmkuhl says of him, «. . . in re morali rigidus, S. Alphonsi adversarius erat quem scriptis impugnativ—Op. cit., II, p. 838.

[212]Regarding Franzoja, Lehmkuhl writes «paravit editionem theolgiae Lacroix et Zaccariae *cum notis* in quibus rigidissimum se ostendit».—Ibid., p. 831.

not in itself troublesome, harsh or difficult, but arises only from the imprudent and inane idea of the patient which she ought to subject to the law of charity and the law of nature; especially since the doctor's hand is not an extraordinary remedy but a common one, in itself simple and easily procurable; furthermore, one which by the law of nature and charity should be employed when necessity demands it.[213]

2.4 THE NINETEENTH CENTURY TILL THE PRESENT TIME

After St. Alphonsus and in the nineteenth century, the characteristics of the treatments given this problem of the ordinary and extraordinary means of conserving life were fairly well standardized. St. Alphonsus had emerged as a recognized authority and leader in the field of Moral Theology. What he had learned from the previous theologians was now to be passed down by the authors who followed him. This is particularly true regarding the problem of the ordinary and extraordinary means of conserving life. Here and there different speculation is discovered, but for the most part, the authors are content to paraphrase Alphonsus.

For example, writing his Moral Theology according to the teaching of St. Alphonsus, *Scavini* says:

But one is not held to the extraordinary (means), namely when the remedy is very hard; or very repugnant to modesty: unless his life is entirely connected with the common good. Hence, one is not held to conserve his life by the amputation of a leg or another operation of the same genus which involves pains

---

[213]«Assentior tamen Franzojae optime docenti, non licere puellae recusare medicam Chirurgi manum ac proinde mortem subire, quia eius sive verecundiae, sive imbecillitati id gravissimum et etiam ipsa morte acerbius videtur cum hoc non in se molestum, asperum, arduumque sit, sed ex sola patientis imprudenti et inani apprehensione oritur, quam legi caritatis et naturae subjicere debet; praesertim cum medica manus non extraordinarium remedium sit, sed commune & in se facile ac obvium; proinde necessitate urgente lege naturae et caritatis adhibendum».—V. Partuzzi, *Ethica Christiana sive Theologia Moralis,* Tom. III, Tract. V, Pars V, Cap. X, Consect. sept.

entirely too intense since this is beyond human endurance. In this case, the common estimation of men, he is thought only to permit his death for a just cause.[214]

Another author of great importance is *John Gury*. Gury mentions in his *Compendium Theologiae Moralis* that severe pain[215] would render a means extraordinary and as an example, he cites the amputation of a leg or arm, or an incision into the abdomen. Another element influencing the determination of means as ordinary or extraordinary is the question of expense in relation to the individual's status.[216] This author also holds the opinion that a maiden is excused from submitting to the treatment of a male doctor when her modesty causes her to fear this more than death itself.[217]

The teaching of Gury in the matter of the ordinary and extraordinary means of conserving life has been repeated substantially and most often verbatim by the authors who have produced editions of his work on Moral Theology.[218] However, there is a discussion in the Ballerini-Palmieri edition which is of considerable interest and significance. Relating the traditional teaching that intense pain would render a means extraordinary, and thus, such operations as an amputation or incision into the abdomen would not be of obligation, the writer then goes on to speculate a bit. If by some artificial means, it would be possible to induce sleep and thus relieve the pain, would the individual be bound to accept this type of sleep and submit to the operation. The answer is «as long as such inducing of sleep is a dangerous thing, certainly it is an extraordinary means: really, the very loss for some time of the use of

---

[214]« Sed non tenetur ad extraordinaria, nempe quoties remedium durissimum est; vel pudori valde repugnans: nisi ejus vita bono communi sit omnino conducens. hinc non tenetur quis abscissione cruris, vel alia ejusdem generis operatione dolores nimis atroces afferente, vitam sibi servare; cum id sit extra communes vires positum. Eo in casu in communi aestimatione censetur justa de causa mortem tantummodo permittere».—P. Scavini, *Theologia Moralis*, II, n. 649.

[215]«. . . remediis extraordinariis, quaeque maximum dolorem afferant . . .»—J. Gury, *Compendium Theologiae Moralis* (ed. 17; Romae, 1866), I, n. 391.

[216]Ordinary means «. . . nec sumptus pro varia cuiusque conditione ingentes exposcunt . . .»—Loc. cit.

[217]« Non tenetur virgo operationem pati per manus medici, licet eius vita periclitetur, quando ea in re verecundia aequare potest aut etiam superare malum, quod morte pertimescitur».—Loc. cit.

[218]Cf. J. Gury-A. Ballerini—D. Palmieri, *Compendium Theologiae Moralis* (ed. 14; Romae, 1907), I, nn. 389–391; J. Ferreres, *Compendium Theologia Moralis* (ed. 16; Subirana, Barcinonae, 1940), I, n. 489; T. Jorio, *Theologia Moralis* (ed. 4; Neapoli, D'Auria, 1954), II, n. 165.

reason and the mastery of his acts, such as occurs in this hypothesis seems an extraordinary thing. »[219]

It is very interesting to note this discussion because it does not occur in the edition of Gury's *Compendium Theologiae Moralis* which was published with the help of Ballerini in 1866, the last year of Gury's life, and yet a somewhat similar discussion is found in the *Opus Theologieum Morale of Ballerini*, published posthumously by Palmieri. In a footnote in this latter work, the following is found:

> Theologians speak of the very bitter pains which an amputation produces. What if there is no pain because the senses have been put to sleep? Would it not be that the grave disadvantage of living with a mutilated body would just as readily excuse a sick man from undergoing the abscission as would the very harsh pains which last only a short while. This I leave for the learned to decide.[220]

In this period one begins to find reference to the new discovery of anaesthesia. Anaesthesia had been somewhat known. As regards its medical use, for all practical purposes, it was first successfully demonstrated in Boston, Massachusetts in 1846.[221] The growing use of anaesthesia did not have any world-shaking effect on the writings of the moralists. After a while, they began to acknowledge its advent and use but they commented on it in terms which are obviously reserved and hesitant. The constant tradition of many years among so many great theologians had forced the moralists of this age to proceed carefully when faced with the numerous advances being made in the medical field.

In the two excerpts already cited, it can be seen that although there is recognition of the existence of anaesthesia, doubt remains as to its safety. Furthermore, even supposing that the use of anaesthesia will be successful,

---

[219]«Quamdiu talis immissio soporis sit res periculosa, certe este medium extra-ordinarium: verum vel ipsa amissio per aliquod tempus, usus rationis et dominii suorum actuum, qualis in hac hypothesi occurrit, res extraordinaria videtur».—Gury-Ballerini-Palmieri, op. cit., n. 391.

[220]"Theologi de acerbissimis doloribus, quos gignit amputatio, loquuntur. Quid, si nullus sit dolor propter sopitos sensus? Nonne grave imcommodum ducendi vitam cum corpore mutilato, tantumdem valet ad excusandum aegrum, ne abscissionem subeat, ac valent acerbissimi dolores brevi desituri? Id relinquo doctis definiendum." A. ballerini, *Opus Theologicum Morale in* Basenbaum medullam (absolvit et edidit D. Palmieri, Prati, 1899), II, p. 645, n. 868, footnote "b".

[221]Cf. D. Guthrie, *A History of Medicine* (London, Nelson & Sons, 1947). The History of Anaesthesia, pp. 301–306.

the added difficulty of the temporary loss of the use of reason is mentioned. In the *Opus Theologicum Morale,* no doubt is left regarding the hesitancy insinuated there, even though it is disguised in question form. To submit to an amputation, whether it be performed painlessly or not, is too much to expect of any man and therefore such surgery should not be classed as an ordinary means.[222] Except for this treatment, the work of Ballerini-Palmieri follows the traditional outline and in fact, represents substantially the teaching of Busenbaum.

Dr. Capellmann, in his famous *Medicina Pastoralis,* has a section entitled «De Operationibus Vitae Periculum Afferentibus.»[223] In this section, he discusses the lawfulness of dangerous operations, and also, mentions the obligation of conserving one's life by these operations. He recalls the traditional teaching in the matter; namely, that the actual danger of surgical intervention renders these means extraordinary and therefore not obligatory. His source is St. Alphonsus. To this Capellmann replies:

> In this matter, I think one should note however, that this opinion seems perhaps less appropriate because of the present standing of medicine and surgery, since difficult operations are performed now in circumstances entirely different and for the most part with greater success than before.[224]

Here full recognition of the progress of medical science is noted and Capellmann is trying to apply the principles of Moral Theology to changed conditions. Immediately then, he cites Gury and Scavini to show that the traditional teaching is that the excessive pain involved in a surgical operation renders such a means of conserving one's life extraordinary. Again Capellmann wonders whether anaesthesia might put a different light on the subject. He asks:

> Does this resolve of probably escaping death, which otherwise would be certain, through an operation not painful in itself, exceed the ordinary strength of men? It is sufficiently known even to the unskilled man that when chloroform is used, an operation can

---

[222]Ballerini-Palmieri, loc. cit.

[223]Cf. C. Capellmann, *Medicina Pastoralis* (ed. 13; Aquisgrana, 1901), pp. 24 ss.

[224]«Qua in re advertendum tamen esse puto, hanc sententiam pro praesenti medicinae et chirurgiae ststu ideirco forte jam minus convenientem videri, quia operationes difficiles nunc circumstantiis plane mutatis ac plerumque meliori successu peraguntur quam antea».—Ibid., p. 25.

be performed without pain and it can do much to lessen the anxiety and fear of a more difficult operation.[225]

Anticipating then an objection that even though anaesthesia lessens, even eliminates pain during the operation, nonetheless there will be pain after the anaesthesia loses its effect. Capellmann answers that the post-operative pains generally are not as intense as those during the operation and for the most part are less than the pains arising from the disease which makes the operation necessary in the first place and which the individual will still have to suffer if he does not submit to the operation.[226] The deformity left by an operation is not as cogent an excuse these days from undergoing the operation as in earlier times because now technical remedies for the loss of a member are more advanced and offer a means of substitution.[227] However, as advanced as Capellmann was in his thinking, he still was quite hesitant about being dogmatic in this matter—perhaps because of the long tradition to the contrary—and he ends the discussion with these words: « Therefore it seems that the opinion of theologians published up to now on this subject either could be or perhaps should be moderated. Certainly, however, I by no means intend to pass judgment on the matter. »[228] The fact remains however, that Capellmann was very impressed with the new use of anaesthesia and for him, at least, the whole moral aspect of surgical interventions had changed.[229] The next change that he could envision was the new application of the standard moral principles to the situation brought about by medical progress.

Lehmkuhl discusses the problem of the ordinary and extraordinary means of conserving life. This moralist mentions the traditional teaching in the matter and includes all the elements of extraordinary means which had been given by the preceding theologians. He cites the example of an amputation

---

[225]« Haeccine *voluntas,* cum aliqua probabilitate mortem certam operatione in se minime dolorosa effugiendi, communes hominum vires superat? Adhibito chloroformio operationem sine dolore perfici posse, etiam imperito jam satis compertum est, multumque valet ad demineundam anxietatem timoremque operationis difficilioris ».—Ibid., p. 26.

[226]Cf. loc. cit.

[227]« Etiam huic malo ars technica huius aetatis valde emendata levamen, atque saepius verum remedium praebet ».—Loc. cit.

[228]« Quapropter sententia theologorum de hac re hucusque vulgata videtur vel posse vel forte debere temperari. Equidem tamen rem diiudicare minime intendo ».—Loc.c it.

[229]« Nunc vero quomodo mutata sunt omnia! En Aegrotum prorsus tranquillum sopore chloroformii, carentem dolore, libero voluntatis exercitio atque renisu. Perfecta cum quiete operatio firmiter ac diligenter perfici potest, aegrotus autem expergefactus, quum dolor pro rerum circumstantiis sit exiguus, non laborat nisi ex effectibus soporis chloroformii raro molestioribus. Quod sane miseris aegrotis magni est momenti magnumque beneficium ».—Ibid., p. 41.

and recalls that the common teaching is that such an operation is not obligatory. Lehmkuhl admits that this teaching does not now enjoy the same favor with doctors and men of medicine as it once did, precisely because anaesthesia can eliminate much of the pain previously connected with the procedure. However, Lehmkuhl insists that it is still not of obligation because, even if the element of pain be removed, the horror which would cause one to refuse the operation, would still excuse from sin.

> . . . even now, I think scarcely is a mortal sin committed by the one who, terrified of an amputation, refuses to submit to it . . . one should not omit the fact that not the torments alone, which partly can be deadened now, but also great horror can be the reason why it would be licit to refuse a great operation—I am not speaking now v.g. of cutting off a finger and its joint.[230]

It is the opinion of Lehmkuhl, therefore, that the advent of anaesthesia has not eliminated all the elements of extraordinary means and therefore one should proceed carefully before imposing under moral obligation a procedure which under one aspect or another has enjoyed considerable progress, even success, in the medical field.

The writings of *Cardinal Vives* and *Canon Pighi* adhere closely to tradition. These authors list as examples of extraordinary means, the amputation of a leg and the surgical operation which appears to a virgin more terrifying than death itself.[231]

Waffelaert follows De Lugo quite closely in his treatment of the ordinary and extraordinary means of conserving life.[232] The ordinary means are of obligation and the extraordinary means are not. What are the ordinary means? Waffelaert replies that «they do not consist 'in individisili' but must be determined from the various considerations indicated in the proposition

---

[230]«. . . mortale peccatum etiam nunc vix committi puto ab eo, qui amputationem multum horrens eam pati detrectet . . . tamen omitti non debet, non cruciatus solos, qui ex parte sopiri nunc possunt, sed etiam horrorem magnum pro ratione haberi posse, cur magna operationem— non enim loquor v. g. de digito ejusque articulo abscindendo—detrectari liceat».—Op. cit., I, p. 345.

[231]Cf. J. Vives, *Compendium Theologiae Moralis* (ed. 9; Romae, Pustet, 1909), n. 308; J. Pighi, *Cursus Theologiae Moralis* (Veronae, 1901), III, n. 180. Cf. also in this matter: C. Marc-F. X. Gestermann, *Institutiones Morales Alphonsianae*, recog. a J. Raus (ed. 18; Lugduni, 1927), I, n. 754; J. Aertnys-C. Damen, *Theologia Moralis* (ed. 16; Marietti, 1950), I, n. 566.

[232]Cf. G. Waffelaert, *De Virtutibus Cardinalibus* (Brugis, Beyaert-Storie, 1886), Vol. II, De Justitia, nn. 39 ss.

and finally, the matter must be settled in a determined event from moral judgment.»[233]

Bucceroni says that extraordinary means lie outside the limits of common endurance.[234] Therefore, a sick person must take only ordinary medications and need not spend great sums of money or employ unusual remedies.[235] Likewise, *A. Vander Heeren* writes that an individual is bound «to make use of all the ordinary means which are indicated in the usual course of things . . .».[236]However, one is not bound «to employ remedies which, considering one's condition, are regarded as extraordinary and involving extraordinary expenditure . . .»[237]

Vermeersch does not depart from tradition either. He is content with mentioning the usual examples of extraordinary means.[238] This is, in general, true also of *Joseph Ubach,* although he is inclined to go a bit further. For example, Ubach[239] lists vehement pain, danger of death, extraordinary expenditure of money and great fear as elements which make a surgical operation an extraordinary means. Pain, he says, is generally removed by anaesthesia; extraordinary cost is often absent because a surgical operation is usually performed in a public hospital. Fear frequently is not present and if it should be, one should try to eliminate it, if it is irrational. However, if considerable fear of the operation remains, then this would be a legitimate excuse from undergoing it. Ubach, when treating danger of death, however, is quite reserved. Much has been said, he feels, to extoll the progress made in the medical field but he emphasizes that one must never forget that an element of danger still exists and this can render such an operation extraordinary, and thus, not obligatory. He then makes the statement that «since some one of these reasons is not usually lacking, ordinarily a major surgical operation is not obligatory.»[240]

---

[233]«. . . media illa ordinaria non consistant in individibili, sed ex variis considerationibus in propositione indicatis sint dimetienda et denique tandem ex morali judicio sit in determinato eventu res absolvenda».—Ibid., n. 43.

[234]« Et sane media extraordinaria extra communes vires posita sunt . . .»—J. Bucceroni, *Institutiones Theologiae Moralis* (ed. 6; Romae, 1914–1915), I, n. 715.

[235]Ibid., n. 716.

[236]A. Vander Heeren, «Suicide», *The Catholic Encyclopedia* (New York, Appleton Co., 1912), XIV, p. 327. Cf. also *Dictionnaire de Théologie Catholique* (Letouzey et Ané, 1941), Tom. 14, col. 2748.

[237]A. Vander Heeren, loc. cit.

[238]Cf. A. Vermeersch, *Theologia Moralis,* II, n. 300.

[239]Cf. J. Ubach, *Theologia Moralis* (Bonis Auris, Sociedad San Miguel, 1935), I, n. 488.

[240]«Quare, cum aliqua ex his causis conseuverit non deesse, ordinarie magna operatio chirurgica non est obligatoria . . .»—Loc. cit.

The treatment found in *Noldin-Schmitt*[241] is quite good. It is precise and to the point. After stating that extraordinary means are not usually of obligation, these authors then note that extraordinary means should be determined from the common estimate of men. Those who are gravely sick and refuse to employ the services of a doctor and abide by his advice, when this can be done easily and when there is hope of recovery, are guilty of sin. Any remedy however, that is very costly considering one's status, or very painful and thus difficult is not obligatory. Since a remedy that is very costly is not of obligation, would a rich man be bound to employ this remedy even though he can afford to pay for it? Noldin-Schmitt answer that not even a rich man would be bound to employ the services of very skilled doctors or to leave his home in order to seek a better climate. This is true because « all these means are extraordinary. »[242] Hence, it can be seen that these authors feel that there is a definite limit beyond which a remedy should be considered extraordinary, absolutely speaking.[243]

Regarding major surgical operations or a major amputation, Noldin-Schmitt are rather definite.[244] They recognize that the older moralists excused an individual from submitting to these operations. However, since many of the elements on which these moralists based their reasoning have now been eliminated, it seems as though such operations should be called obligatory. Anaesthesia has removed pain. Operations now enjoy much greater success and artificial substitutes for natural limbs have been perfected. Two conditions however are posited by these authors before such an operation can be called obligatory. First there must be a great probability that certain danger of death will be avoided. Secondly, there should not be any intense subjective horror of the operation present.[245]

A somewhat similar treatment of surgical operations is found in *Genicot-Salsmans*.[246] They state that even when a major surgical operation can be performed without tremendous pain or great danger, it would be difficult to say that *per se* such an operation is obligatory even when vehement subjective

---

[241]Cf. Noldin-Schmitt, op. cit., II, pp. 307–308.

[242]« . . . quia haec omnia extraordinaria sunt ».—Ibid., p. 308.

[243]Cf. E. Healy, op. cit., p. 162. In an example, Father Healy suggests $2,000 as an absolute norm—an amount that even a rich man would not be obliged to spend. Extraordinary means for this author, are those means which « exceed the normal strength of men in general. » Cf. also Genicot-Salsmans, *Institutiones Theologiae Moralis* (ed. 17; Bruxelles, L'Edition Universelle, 1951), I, n. 364, where one reads: « . . . vim pecuniae ingentem expendere, nemo, etiam ditissimus, tenetur, etiamsi aliter vitam protrahere nequeat. ».

[244]Noldin-Schmitt, loc. cit.

[245]Loc. cit.

[246]Cf. Genicot-Salsmans, op. cit., n. 364.

horror is present. Certainly this horror would produce an extraordinary difficulty.[247] Furthermore, they feel that often a prudent doubt remains especially in regard to the enduring success of major operations. These authors do suggest, however, that an individual should rid himself of any exaggerated fear of operations and generally speaking, consent to them when it is necessary for the conservation of his life.[248]

Merkelbach excuses a man from employing «extraordinary, choice, unusual, more costly and very difficult means,»[249] in order to recover his health. These, he says, are not obligatory because the law demanding one to «protract»[250] his life does not oblige him at the cost of «such great trouble.»[251] Today, however, the author notes, many operations which in days gone by were quite difficult and dangerous, are now performed very easily and safely. Therefore, it can be said that «they have now become ordinary means.»[252]

In treating this very point, *Fanfani* uses the same words as Merkelbach except that he concludes this way «therefore operations of this type can not always be called extraordinary means.»[253] It is interesting to note this because the very same idea is expressed in just slightly different terms; different enough however, to make one realize that Fanfani is a bit more hesitant about stating categorically that a modern surgical operation is now an ordinary means.

In his *Moral and Pastoral Theology*, *Henry Davis* is content to say that a man must preserve his life by the use of ordinary means. He is not bound however, to employ «extraordinary expensive methods, nor methods that would inflict on him almost intolerable pain or shame.»[254]

Bert Cunningham, in his doctoral dissertation, *The Morality of Organic Transplantation*, says: «Man's custody of his own body demands that he conserve his life by every reasonable means, for that is in agreement with his position as custodian of the life given to him by God . . .»[255]

---

[247]Loc. cit.

[248]Loc. cit.

[249]«. . . media extraordinaria, exquisita, inusitata, pretiosiora, valde difficilia . . .»—B. Merkelbach, *Summa Theologiae Moralis* (Parisiis, Desclée, 1935), II, n. 353.

[250]«protrahendi»—loc. cit.

[251]«cum tanto incommodo»—loc. cit.

[252]«. . . ac ita jam facta sunt media ordinaria».—Loc. cit.

[253]«. . . ideoque huiusmodi operationes nequeunt semper dici media extraordinaria».—Fanfani, op. cit., II, n. 225, dubium I. Cf. also Fanfani's other references to ordinary and extraordinary means.—Ibid., nn. 88 and 169.

[254]H. Davis, *Moral and Pastoral Theology* (ed. 3; London, Sheed and Ward. 1938), II, p. 141.

[255]B. Cunningham, *The Morality of Organic Transplantation* (Washington, Catholic University Press, 1944), pp. 95-96.

M. Zalba requires a man to use only congruous and common means and ordinary diligence.[256] There is no obligation to use extraordinary means or extraordinary diligence except per accidens.[257] In applying the principle, Zalba feels that one would not be bound «to undergo a very dangerous operation or a very troublesome convalescence.»[258] Neither is a person bound to suffer the extraordinary pain of a surgical operation «if however, this case ever occurs supposing modern methods.»[259] It is interesting to take cognizance of the fact that Zalba recognizes that a period of recovery can be very harsh and thus be an extraordinary means. His opinion about the moral obligations involved in modern operations is guarded, as the reader can see. Perhaps, he does not want to state definitively that many major operations today are ordinary means, as Merkelbach did.

In the latest edition of *Lanza-Palazzini's Theologia Moralis,* one reads that «what at another time was held to be an extraordinary means, today on account of the progress of science, perhaps has become ordinary.»[260] What means are extraordinary? This should be decided in individual cases. However, it must be kept in mind that in ordinary circumstances, no one is obliged to undergo a «grave inconvenience» to conserve his life.[261]

The shorter manuals of Moral Theology are in great measure synopses of the teaching already recorded here as regards the doctrine on the ordinary and extraordinary means of conserving life. *Tanquerey* mentions that one need not prolong his life with great inconvenience.[262] Neither is an individual bound to undergo a dangerous or very painful or greatly displeasing operation.[263] *Arregui* gives the same doctrine.[264]

---

[256]«. . . media congrua; sed per se solum communia . . . et per ordinariam diligentiam . . .»—Regatillo-Zalba, op. cit., II, n. 254.

[257]«. . . per accidens tamen potest aliquis teneri ad media extraordinaria applicanda vel ad extraordinariam diligentiam adhibendam . . .»—Loc. cit.

[258]«. . . neque operationi valde periculosae vel convalescentiae molestissimae se submittere . . .»—Ibid., n. 254, aplicatio 3.

[259]«. . . si tamen casus iste eveniat unquam suppositis mediis hodiernis . . .»—Loc. cit.

[260]«. . . quod alias ut medium extraordinarium habebatur, hodie, ob scientiae progressum, forte ordinarium factum est».—A. Lanza-P. Palazzini, *Theologia Moralis* (Taurini-Romae, Marietti, 1955), II, n. 125.

[261]«. . . obligatio subeundi grave incommodum ad ipsum servandum non probatur».—Loc. cit.

[262]«. . . lex enim diu vitam protrahendi non obligat cum tanto incommodo».—A. Tanquerey, *Synopsis Theologiae Moralis et Pastoralis* (Parisiis, Desclée & Socii, 1953), III, p. 248.

[263]«. . . nec quisquam obligatur periculosam aut valde dolorosam vel maxime displicentem operationem subire . . .»—Loc. cit.

[264]«. . . non autem necessario mediis extraordinariis, sc. pro sua condicione valde sumptuosis, vel dolore aut pudore nimis arduis».—A. Arregui, *Summarium Theologiae moralis* (ed. 18; Bilbao, 1948), n. 234.

However, *Jone-Adelman* are inclined to be a little more specific. They exempt even wealthy people from the necessity of going to a far-distant place or health resort. Even the wealthy would not be obliged to summon the best known physicians. It is the opinion of these authors also that no one is gravely obliged to undergo a major surgical operation except per accidens and even then, the success of the operation must be morally certain.[265]

One of the few modern theologians to afford any special treatment of the problem of the ordinary and extraordinary means of conserving life is *Gerald Kelly*, S. J. His writings will be seen more closely in succeeding chapters of this dissertation. Suffice it to say now that these writings are of definite importance because of the author's experience and skill in treating medico-moral problems, and secondly, because of his realization of the practical import of the problem of the ordinary and extraordinary means of conserving life in modern medical procedure.[266]

This chapter has included the opinions of the most noteworthy moral theologians regarding the means of conserving life. It is with this teaching in mind that in the next chapter an attempt will be made to study more closely the nature of the ordinary and extraordinary means. In this way, it is hoped that the entire study will be based on traditional teaching. While it is true that theologians of past ages perhaps never imagined the almost miraculous progress of medical science which is so well known today, nonetheless, they left behind them the basic principles whereby even the moral problems of modern day medicine can be solved correctly.

---

[265]Cf. H. Jone-U. Adelman, *Moral Theology* (Westminister, Newman Press, 1948), n. 210.

[266]Cf. G. Kelly, «The Duty of Using Artificial Means of Preserving Life», *Theological Studies*, XI (1950), pp. 203-220; «The Duty to Preserve Life», ibid., XII (1951), pp. 550-556; *MEdico-Moral Problems* (St. Louis, The Catholic Hospital Association of the U. S. and Canada, 1954), V. pp. 6-15. Another treatment of considerable import, which has been published is J. Paquin, *Morale et Medicine* (Montreal, L'Immaculée-Conception, 1955), pp. 398-403.

CHAPTER III

The Nature of the Ordinary and Extraordinary Means of Conserving Life and the Moral Obligation of Using These Means

In the previous chapters, we have presented a discussion of the basic duty of conserving one's life and a report of the opinions of the most noteworthy moral theolgians in regard to the ordinary and extraordinary means of conserving life.

The nature of the ordinary and extraordinary means of conserving life, and the moral obligation of using these means are the subjects of the present chapter. In determining the nature of these means, of necessity we shall see more closely the opinions already presented in Chapter Two. An analysis of the writings of the theologians will give the elements by which we can determine more precisely the nature of the ordinary and extraordinary means of conserving life. These theologians, as a rule, did not define the terms ordinary and extraordinary means of conserving life, but they did describe them and they did underline the elements which constitute these means.

Once we have determined the nature of the ordinary and extraordinary means of conserving life, we shall discuss in the second section of this chapter the moral obligation of using them and the extent to which this obligation binds.

3.1 THE NATURE OF THE ORDINARY AND EXTRAORDINARY MEANS OF CONSERVING LIFE

In this section, we intend to gather from the writings of the moralists the elements which they consider essential to the concept of the ordinary and extraodinary means of conserving life. We shall then study the implications in these elements and thus be able to determine the nature of ordinary and extraordinary means. However, prior to this, it will be profitable to discuss some preliminary notions.

A.
PRELIMINARY NOTIONS

1) Natural and Artificial Means of Conserving Life

One of the first distinctions which we find made in this matter by the moralists is the one in which the natural means of conserving life are distinguished from the artificial means. In this present discussion, we are using the word *artificial* to designate a means which is devised and made by man for the conservation of his life. A *natural means* is a means which nature itself provides for the conservation of man's life. The older moralists used the term *natural means*. They did not, however, use the term *artificial means* but usually they described an artificial means in a negative way by pointing out that such a means is not a natural means. We have seen this already in the writings of Vitoria: « . . . a similar case does not exist between food and drugs. For food is per se a means ordered to the life of the animal and it is natural, drugs are not . . . »[267] Vitoria wants to emphasize that a man is not obliged to use every

---

[267]« . . . quod non est simile de pharmaco et alimento. Alimentum enim per se est medium ordinatum ad vitam animalis et naturale, non autem pharmacum . . . »—F. A Victoria, O.P., Relectio IX, de Temp., n. 1.

possible means of conserving his life but that, basically, his obligation begins only with those means that are natural and intended by nature for the conservation of man's life: « . . . man is not held to employ all the possible means of conserving his life, but the means which are per se intended for that purpose . . . »[268] Fundamentally, there is a clear distinction in the mind of Vitoria between natural means of conserving life and artificial means. It would seem, also, that he would say that natural means are obligatory and artificial means are not obligatory. In any event, he definitely assigns a stricter moral obligation of employing natural means than of employing artificial means of conserving life.

Reading further on in this same section of Vitoria's writings, we note an apparent contradiction to what has just been stated. Vitoria proposes the situation in which a person would have moral certitude that if he should take a certain medicine, he would regain his health; if he refuses to take the medicine, he will die. Is he obliged to take the medicine? Vitoria seems to reply that he is bound to use the medicine, and that if he does not take it, «he really does not seem to be excused from mortal sin . . . ».[269] The reasons for this answer are first of all, that this same person would be required to give the medicine to a sick neighbor, otherwise he would be guilty of sin. Secondly, Vitoria says « . . . medicine per se also is intended by nature for health . . . ».[270]

Hence, we see that Vitoria apparently is saying that drugs and medicines are not obligatory because they are not natural means intended by nature for the conservation of man's life and saying also in the same section that drugs and medicines are per se intended by nature for health and are obligatory. There is no doubt that an apparent contradiction exists. However, it would seem that a correct understanding of Vitoria's words can come only from an understanding of the entire context. Recall that he said that the case existing between food and drugs is not a similar one. This is true. Food is primarily intended by nature for the basic sustenance of animal life. Food for man is basically and fundamentally necessary from the very beginning of his temporal existence. It is basically required by his human life and nature intends food for this purpose. That is why man has the right to grow food and kill animals. Furthermore, because it is a law of nature that man sustain himself by food, it is a duty for man to nourish himself by food. In the case of drugs and medicines, the same is not true. Drugs and medicines are intended per se

---

[268]« . . . nec tenetur homo adhibere omnia media possibilia ad conservandam vitam. sed media per se ad hoc ordinata».—loc. cit.

[269]« . . . non videtur profecto excusari a mortali . . . »—loc. cit.

[270]« . . . medicina per se etiam ordinata est ad salutem a natura . . . »—loc. cit.

by nature to help man conserve his life. However, this is by way of exception. Drugs and medicines are not the basic way by which man is to nourish his life. They are intended by nature to aid man in the conservation of his life when he is sick or in pain or unable to sustain himself by natural means. These artificial means are not natural means but they are intended by nature to help man protect, sustain and conserve his life. If man were never to be sick, he would never need medicines. If he is sick, however, it is quite *natural* for him to make use of *artificial* means of *conserving* his life.

Vitoria is correct therefore, in making a clear distinction between natural means of conserving life and artificial means of conserving life. He is also correct when he explains that natural means, such as food, are intended per se by nature for the conservation of man's life, whereas artificial means are intended per se by nature for this same purpose but as a means of supplementing the natural means when this becomes necessary.

In regard to the obligation of using natural means of conserving life, Vitoria clearly states that the natural means are obligatory. With regard to the obligation of employing the artificial means of conserving life, his teaching again appears contradictory. In one place he seems to say that artificial means are not obligatory; in another place, he clearly states that there is a moral obligation to employ them when necessary for the conservation of one's life. In this particular matter also, an understanding of what Vitoria means to imply will render his actual words more understandable.

Vitoria's statement that an artificial means is per se intended by nature for the health of a person is quite understandable. It is also clear that Vitoria makes the use of artificial means a matter of obligation when the physical condition of the individual requires it. We must recall however that Vitoria is positing a condition in this matter. He states in his proposed case that the individual concerned has moral certitude that a medicine will bring him health. Further on in the same discussion, he actually admits that the possession beforehand of moral certitude of benefit deriving from the use of medicines is not obligatory. His words are: « . . . but since this rarely can be certain, therefore they are not to be condemned with mortal sin who have declared universally an abstinence from drugs . . . ».[271]

We can see, therefore, that the teaching of Vitoria in this matter is that medicines and drugs—in fact artificial means in general—are intended by nature to supplement the natural means of conserving life. They are intended to help man to conserve his life when the use of merely natural means, such as food, sunshine, rest etc. are not sufficient because of the individual's physi-

---

[271]« . . . sed quia hoc vix potest esse certum, ideo non sunt damnandi de mortali, qui in universum decreverunt abstinere a pharmacis . . . ».—loc. cit.

cal condition. As such, therefore, the artificial means are obligatory. However, in Vitoria's time, the development and progress of medical helps to conserving life had not reached the point where their use would give any sure hope of benefit. One could not have moral certitude of benefit. Hence, Vitoria is quite logical and quite correct in not demanding a person under obligation to use these artificial means.

To summarize Vitoria's teaching in this matter, we may say that natural means of conserving life are per se intended by nature as the means whereby man is to conserve his life and ordinarily these are strictly obligatory. Furthermore, artificial means of conserving life are per se intended by nature as a means whereby man can supplement the natural means of conserving life when these natural means are lacking or insufficient etc. Ordinarily, these artificial means are obligatory too if they can be obtained and used conveniently and with some certitude of benefit.

Sayrus makes the very same distinction. In fact, it is interesting to note that he uses Vitoria's very words in this section.[272] Actually, all he has done has been to repeat verbatim Vitoria's argument. One notion however, is his own. He adds the term «naturally produced» to the expression, «common foods»: « . . . no one in order to prolong his life is bound to use the best and more delicate foods, even though he be able; he need use only the common ones, naturally produced».[273] Here again, the same reasoning that motivated Vitoria in this matter is apparent in the writings of Sayrus. Basically, he feels that only what is a natural means of conserving life is obligatory. He repeats the case, which was proposed by Vitoria, about the necessary use of medicine, and we can see that Sayrus also is influenced by the condition of the medical science of his day. One can not be sure of success in the use of medicines, therefore, they can hardly be called obligatory. However, the use of these medicines would be obligatory if one could be sure that they would benefit him.

Sanchez also says that one would not be bound to use medicines to prolong his life, such as taking a drug for many years to avoid fevers.[274] He also uses the expression: «means directed by nature for sustenance.[275] It would seem that Sanchez does not oblige a person to make use of a drug for many

---

[272]Sayrus, op. cit., Lib. VII, Cap. IX, n. 28.

[273]« . . . nemo ad vitam prolongandam, cibis optimis et delicatioribus uti tenetur, etiamsi possit, sed communibus naturaliter productis».—loc. cit.

[274]« . . . non tenetur quis uti medicinis ad prolongandam vitam . . . ut quotannis sumere pharmacum ad vitandas febres etc.»—Sanchez, op. cit., Tom. II, Lib. V, Cap. I, dub. 33.

[275]« . . . mediis ordinatis a natura ad sustentationem . . .».—ibid., n. 11.

years in order to avoid a fever not because the use of a drug could never be obligatory but because the use of a drug *for many years* is not obligatory.

When one reads the writings of these older moralists in the whole context, one understands rather easily why they are eager on the one hand to term medicines a means of conserving life directly intended by nature for the purpose of conserving life, and therefore obligatory when necessary, and why then, on the other hand, these same authors seem willing to contradict themselves. As the success of medicine became more certain, the authors wrote differently. For example, Tamburini writes that one is bound to use only «ordinary foods per se intended to conserve life».[276] Then he says in the same section that one is not obliged to take very costly and extraordinary medicines «since it is sufficient to use common medicines».[277] Here we can see clearly that while the term *per se intended* is used for ordinary foods and these are obligatory, yet in the same section Tamburini calls common medicines obligatory. In the writings of the previous authors there is hesitancy about stating any obligation even in regard to the use of common medicines. Hence, we can appreciate that the moral teaching of the older moralists in this matter is quite solid even though in their writings they would seem to confuse principle and practice. *In principle,* artificial means of conserving life are obligatory; but for these authors, *in practice,* these means are not obligatory because of some circumstance which eliminates the duty of using them. For example, the medicines are too costly or they do not provide any serious hope of benefit. This seems to be the reason why in one and the same context an author will require the use of artificial means, and then say that these means are not of obligation.

Actually what these older moralists were saying can be well explained by the terms ordinary and extraordinary means of conserving life. When these moralists were living, artificial means of conserving life were extraordinary means because they were too costly or did not offer any hope of benefit. When, however, medicines became useful and offered some hope of success, these means became ordinary means and the moralists then called them obligatory. It does not seem, therefore, that the writings of the older moralists provide any argument for the opinion that artificial means of conserving life are never obligatory. When one understands the meaning in these writings, he will see that these moralists in principle do oblige a person to make use of artificial means of conserving life when these means are truly ordinary means. They seem to make the distinction between natural and artificial

---

[276]«. . . non tenetur quis uti cibis nisi ordinariis per se ordinatis ad vitam conservandam . . .».—Tamburini, op. cit., Lib. VI, Cap. II, Sect. II, n. 11.

[277]«. . . cum satis sit medicinis uti communibus».—loc. cit.

means because natural means generally were ordinary means and thus obligatory, whereas artificial means in this period of history were usually for one reason or another extraordinary means.

God intends the development of science for the good of man. When science can provide a means of conserving man's life which can be a supplement to a natural means, then this artificial means would seem to be obligatory. It is true, however, that whereas natural means in general are ordinary means, artificial means of conserving life can quite often be extraordinary means and thus not obligatory. When artificial means are ordinary means, then they are obligatory. We will see more closely, as this chapter progresses, the conditions required in determining a means as ordinary or extraordinary. The object of this discussion so far has been to show that the terms *artificial means* and *extraordinary means* are not coextensive. An artificial means can be an ordinary means of conserving life.

As a final point, we may point out that an artificial means of conserving life can be either a cure for a disease, such as a medicine, or it can be a means of supplanting a natural means of sustaining life, such as intravenous feeding. This distinction would not seem to change either in theory or in practice the teaching mentioned here. If the artificial means, whether a cure or a substitution for a natural means of conserving life, is an ordinary means it is obligatory. It is for this reason that in mentioning the artificial means, we have referred to them as means of supplementing the natural means of conserving life, intending thereby to include in the term artificial means both the means of curing a disease and means which supplant a natural function.

2) Ordinary means of conserving life and Ordinary medical procedures

The distinction existing between the expressions *ordinary means of conserving life* and *ordinary medical procedures* is a very interesting and important one. It is particularly important in any practical question concerning the duty of employing an artificial means, because there is danger of confusing the terms. In point of fact, an ordinary medical procedure is not necessarily an ordinary means of conserving life. What is an ordinary treatment in medical procedure can easily be a means of conserving life which the moralist will not term either ordinary or obligatory.[278] The moralists of past ages had no need of

---

[278] « La difficulté consiste a préciser le sens de ces deux expressions: remèdes ou traitements ordinaires, remèdes ou traitements extraordinaires. Le language médical appellera traitements ordinaires ceux qui sont habituellement employés pour telle ou telle maladie; mais, au point de vue theologique, de tels traitements peuvent parfois ??etre extraordinaires ».—Paquin, op. cit., p. 398.

making this distinction because most medical and surgical procedures were admittedly extraordinary means. Today, however, men are more conscious of the wonders of medical progress and they are more accustomed to employing medical and surgical remedies. Therefore, it is easy to imagine that what is surely ordinary as a medical procedure might appear ordinary also as a morally obligatory means of conserving life. However, such a case is not necessarily true. For example, a surgical intervention is an ordinary medical procedure today in case of acute appendicitis. It probably is also morally an ordinary means of conserving life in most instances. However, for some individuals, it still could be an extraordinary means due to some unusual set of circumstances. Thus it would not be obligatory. The expense involved in the operation or the lack of proper medical and surgical facilities could easily render the operation an extraordinary means for a particular individual. It is true that usually an extraordinary medical procedure will also be an extraordinary means of conserving life. However, it is well to understand from the beginning of this discussion that an ordinary medical remedy is not necessarily an obligatory ordinary means of conserving life.

B.
THE ELEMENTS INVOLVED IN THE TERMS ORDINARY AND EXTRAORDINARY MEANS OF CONSERVING LIFE

We have noted above that this study of the nature of the ordinary means of conserving life will be founded on the elements derived from an analysis of the writings of the moral theologians. This will be true also of the study of the nature of the extraordinary means of conserving life, which will be found in a succeeding section of this chapter.

In order that the elements involved in these terms may be seen more clearly, a list of moral theologians and the elements which they include in their discussions of the means of conserving life can be consulted in the preceding outline. [The letter « X » signifies that the appropriate element was mentioned by the author under whose name the letter « X » occurs.] This outline is by no means exhaustive, but it is representative and can be of assistance in appreciating the frequency with which some elements are mentioned in the theological discussions of the ordinary and extraordinary means of conserving life. There are other elements mentioned by the moralists which have not been cited in this outline because they have not been common to many authors. Where, however, there is need of mentioning such elements, proper citation will be made in the text itself. It is also well to note that in this outline the terms have been kept in Latin. Usually this exact expression is common to all the designated authors. Occasionally, however, an author may have used a different expression or a different language to connote the same idea. He is marked, nontheless, as having used the more common phrase.

The reader will note that we are going to discuss separately the nature of the ordinary means of conserving life and the nature of the extraordinary means. Although this method is not common in the treatises found in the Moral Theology books, we feel that to separate the two discussions will emphasize more the difference involved in the two terms.

1) The nature of the ordinary means of conserving life
a) Spes salutis

It is clear from the writings of the moralists that a means of conserving life must offer some *hope of a beneficial result* before such a means can be termed ordinary and obligatory. Vitoria speaks of the obligation that a sick man has to take food or nourishment if he can take it« . . . with a certain hope of life . . . »[279] Further on in the same writing, he says that a man who has moral certitude that he can regain his health by the use of a drug is bound to use the drug.[280] After Vitoria, this notion of a hope of benefit in the question of the ordinary means of conserving life was repeated by many moral theologians.

The teaching that an ordinary means of conserving life must offer a hope of benefit is certainly in harmony with common sense. It would be unreasonable to bind an individual with a moral obligation of employing a remedy or cure which offers no hope of benefit. All theologians agree to this, although not all moralists actually mention it in their discussions of the ordinary and extraordinary means of conserving life. No one, however, writes in opposition to this teaching.

The question of more practical import is how much hope of benefit must a means offer before it can be called an ordinary means. We have mentioned in Chapter Two the case cited by De Lugo, in which a man is condemned to death by fire.[281] Surrounded by flames, the man notices that he has sufficient water to extinguish some of the fire, but not all of it. De Lugo notes that the man concerned is not morally obligated to use the water because he can not extinguish the flames once and for all, and thus escape death. If he could extinguish the fire, he would be obliged to do so. However, he is not obliged

---

[279]« . . . cum aliqua spe vitae . . . »—a Victoria, Relectio de Temp., n. 1.
[280]Loc. cit.
[281]De Lugo, op. cit., De Justitia et Jure, Disp. X, Sect. I, N. 30.

ORDINARY MEANS

		Vitoria	Soto	Molina	Sayrus	Banez	Sanchez	Lessius	Bonacina	Laymann	Gabr. a S.V.	De Lugo	Diana	Tournely	Salmantic.	Busenbaum	Escobar	Tamburini	Holzmann	Sporer	Reiffenstuel	La Croix	Roncaglia
(1)	Spes Salutis	x		x	x						x				x	x					x	x	
(2)	Media communia	x		x	x	x					x							x			x		x
(3)	Sec. Proportionem status				x									x	x								
(4)	Non difficilia							x	x	x	x		x						x	x	x	x	
(5)	Facilia																						

ENGLISH Translations: (1) Hope of benefit (4) Means which are not too difficult
(2) Means commonly used (5) Reasonably simple means
(3) Current status factor

EXTRAORDINARY MEANS

		Vitoria	Soto	Molina	Sayrus	Banez	Sanchez	Lessius	Bonacina	Laymann	Gabr. a S.V.	De Lugo	Diana	Tournely	Salmantic.	Busenbaum	Escobar	Tamburini	Holzmann	Sporer	Reiffenstuel	La Croix	Roncaglia
(1)	Quaedam impossibilitas	x			x									x									
(2)	Summus labor	x			x												x						
(3)	Nimis dura														x						x	x	
(4)	Quidam cruciatus	x	x		x		x				x		x	x						x			
(5)	Sumptus extraord.	x				x									x	x			x	x			
(6)	Media pretiosa	x			x					x	x	x	x	x	x						x	x	x
(7)	Ingens dolor		x	x	x	x		x	x			x	x	x	x				x	x			x
(8)	Vehemens horror				x										x	x	x						x
(9)	Media exquisita				x		x					x			x	x						x	

ENGLISH Translations: (1) A certain impossibility factor (6) High priced means
(2) Greatest effort required (7) Excessive pain factor
(3) Excessive hardship factor (8) Intense fear/repugnance
(4) A certain excruciating pain (9) Very best means
(5) Extraordinary expenditure

1	2	3	4	5	6	7	Author
×			×		×		Mazzotta
		×					Elbel
	×						Billuart
	×	×		×	×		Patuzzi
×			×				S. Alphon.
×	×		×				Scavini
	×	×					Gury
×	×		×				Ballerini-P.
	×						Pighi
×		×	×				Lehmkuhl
×	×		×	×			Marc-Gest.
							Waffelaert
×		×	×				Bucceroni
	×	×					Ferreres
	×	×					Vander Heer.
×	×	×					Genicot-Sal.
×	×	×					Noldin Schm.
		×		×			Aertnys-Dam.
×	×	×		×			Vermeersch
×	×	×					Ubach
×		×	×		×		Merkelbach
	×	×					Davis
							Jone-Adelm.
	×						Zalba
×	×	×		×			Kelly
×	×						Paquin

1	2	3	4	Author
		×		Mazzotta
×	×			Elbel
×	×	×	×	Billuart
×		×		Patuzzi
		×		S. Alphon.
				Scavini
	×			Gury
		×		Ballerini-P.
				Pighi
×	×			Lehmkuhl
				Marc-Gest.
×	×		×	Waffelaert
		×	×	Bucceroni
	×			Ferreres
	×			Vander Heer.
×	×			Genicot-Sal.
×	×	×	×	Noldin Schm.
×	×			Aertnys-Dam.
				Vermeersch
				Ubach
×		×		Merkelbach
				Davis
		×		Jone-Adelm.
×	×			Zalba
×		×		Kelly
×		×		Paquin

merely to postpone his death by extinguishing part of the fire. In other words, the element of benefit is introduced. The means and remedies employed, even though in themselves common means, must offer some hope of benefit or help to the conservation of life before they become obligatory ordinary means. The benefit to be derived from the use of these means must be worthwhile. It must be worthwhile in quality and duration. Furthermore, it must be worthwhile in consideration of the effort expended in using the means. In a word, the use of a means must offer a *proportionate* hope of benefit or else it is not an ordinary means.

Hence, we can see that a means of conserving life, even though it be a very common remedy, can not be termed an ordinary means if it offers little or no hope of benefit. The fact that a means very definitely gives hope of some benefit but not a hope of proportionate benefit in no way changes the case. A hope of little benefit is to be considered morally as nothing. De Lugo phrases this doctrine in the following manner: « . . . the obligation of conserving life by ordinary means is not an obligation of using these means for such a brief conservation—which is morally considered as nothing at all . . . »[282]

De Lugo clearly states that any means which is to be employed for the conservation of one's life must give definite hope of being proportionately useful and beneficial before it can be called obligatory. It is noteworthy also that De Lugo applies this doctrine even to the taking of food[283] which is a purely natural means of conserving life. In other words, for De Lugo, any means whether natural or artificial, must give proportionate hope of success and benefit, otherwise it is not an ordinary means and thus not obligatory. G. Kelly, S. J. commenting on these words of De Lugo writes: « It may be that the principle, *parum pro nihilo reputatur,* is really contained in the preceding principle, *nemo ad inutile tenetur.* Yet there seems to be a slight difference. Furthermore, De Lugo applies his principle even to the taking of food, which is a purely natural means of preserving life, whereas the other authors were speaking only of remedies for illness. »[284]

Closely allied to this notion of proportionate hope of benefit is the element of danger which many recent authors mention in connection with their discussion of modern remedies and treatments. The earlier moralists were cognizant of the same element of danger and that is why they spoke so clearly

---

[282]« . . . obligatio conservandi vitam per media ordinaria, non est obligatio utendi mediis ad illam brevem conservationem, quae moraliter pro nihilo reputatur . . . ».—loc. cit.

[283]Loc. cit.

[284]Kelly, « The Duty of Using Artificial Means of Preserving Life », p. 208.

on the notion of proportionate benefit. In other words, a remedy or treatment must give definite and proportionate hope of success. If a procedure does not offer this proportionate hope of success it is clearly not an ordinary means. It is true that as medical science has progressed, many surgical operations and medical treatments that were dangerous and offered no proportionate hope of success, today have been perfected. Since they are not usually dangerous now, and do give hope of success and benefit, they have become ordinary means, at least in regard to the element of success and benefit.

If a medical procedure involves risk or danger and does not at the same time offer proportionate hope of success, the procedure is not morally obligatory. This teaching is an application of the principle *nemo ad inutile tenetur.* Oftentimes even though medical science has technically perfected a treatment or surgical procedure, the hope of success and benefit does not outweigh the risk involved. Hence, even though there be hope of benefit, it is not a hope of sufficient proportion to make a procedure obligatory. In an article reprinted in the *Linacre Quarterly* in November, 1955, Raber Taylor speaks of risks involved in some modern treatments.[285] He relates the case of a man who has a swollen hand. The case was diagnosed as Dupuytren's contracture and the doctor recommended corrective surgery without disclosing, however, to the patient the considerable risk involved. Actually, the operation was unsuccessful. Taylor says: «The operation was skillfully performed, but failed to achieve the expected result. The patient was left with greater disability than he had originally.»[286] The author relates this incident in order to note that the doctor in question was legally prosecuted in the civil courts for his failure to disclose properly to the patient the risk involved in the recommended surgery before obtaining the patient's consent. Furthermore, he writes: «The skillful performance of the operation did not, ruled the Supreme Court, excuse the doctor who had breached his duty to make a full disclosure of the surgical risk . . . »[287]

What is of interest in this case is the fact that even the civil laws recognize the element of danger and risk in many modern medical techniques. Hence they protect the patient's right to know this fact before any consent is given. How much more important it is, therefore, for the moralists to take cognizance of the possible risk or danger involved in a means of conserving life prior to imposing it as an obligatory ordinary means. If a procedure, whether

---

[285]R. Taylor, «Consent for Treatment», *The Linacre Quarterly*, Nov., 1955, pp. 131–135, (reprinted from *The Rocky Mountain Medical Journal*, May, 1955).
[286]Ibid., p. 133.
[287]Loc. cit.

medical or not, does not offer proportionate hope of success and benefit in the conservation of one's life, it is hardly an ordinary means.

Absolute and relative norms in determining the ordinary and extraordinary means of conserving life

Another point to understand clearly is the fact that in determining whether a means offers proportionate hope of success and benefit, one must consider some relative factors. It is hardly possible to establish categorically that a particular means of conserving life will always offer proportionate benefit under all circumstances and to all people. In other words, it is difficult to establish an absolute norm when determining the required hope of success and benefit in any procedure designed to conserve life. In point of fact, it is difficult to apply an absolute norm to any of the elements of ordinary means. Therefore it is well to call attention to that fact here.

It does seem that an absolute norm can be established regarding clearly extraordinary means. Certainly, there are means of conserving life that are not binding morally to anyone. We have already referred to the suggestion of E. Healy, S. J. that $2,000 is an amount that no one, even a rich man, is bound to expend for the sake of conserving his life.[288] It would be difficult to dispute the fact that an absolute norm exists in regard to extraordinary means and we shall see this more closely in the discussion of moral impossibility in the next section of this chapter. Suffice it to say now that since an extraordinary means is one that exceeds the strength of men in general, any means that exceeds the strength of men in general is obviously not binding on any man and therefore, is an extraordinary means absolutely speaking.

The question of an absolute norm in regard to ordinary means, however, is more intricate. It does not seem that one can successfully establish such a norm because even the older moralists[289] teach that such a purely ordinary and common means of conserving life as food, admits of relative inconvenience and difficulty. Furthermore, they point out that this very common means, food, sometimes can offer no proportionate hope of success relative to a particular individual.

There are many factors in this notion of relativity. For example, the age of an individual can be a determining factor. The person's physical and psychological condition enters the question. His financial status also can weigh heavily in determining a means as ordinary or extraordinary for him. This

---

288Healy, op. cit., p. 162.

289Cf. e. g., a Victoria, Relectio de Temp., n. 1; De Lugo, op. cit., De Justitia et Jure, Disp. X, Sect. I, n. 30.

doctrine on the relative nature of ordinary means should be kept in mind, therefore, in regard to all the elements involved in ordinary means, not only in regard to the hope of proportionate success and benefit.

There is one last point in this connection which is worthy of mention. We have stated that it seems difficult to establish the presence of an absolute norm in regard to ordinary means. We are not denying thereby that there are many means of conserving life which are certainly common means or remedies and which usually do not exceed the strength of men in general. It would be allowable, therefore, to make a *general* norm in regard to these means, by which they are characterized as ordinary for most men. To make this norm absolute, however, it is to imply that these means are obligatory for all men because ordinary means are obligatory means. It is in this sense that we say that it seems difficult to establish a norm which would be absolute in determining the nature of ordinary means.

Hope of success and benefit and the relative norm

An application of the relative norm can be made in reference to the element of proportionate hope of success and benefit. G. Kelly, S. J.[290] uses the example of the use of oxygen in tiding a patient over a pneumonia crisis. The oxygen is easy to obtain and easy to use and generally is quite inexpensive for short periods of use. If the patient overcomes the pneumonia crisis, he usually will recover from his illness. Fr. Kelly writes: «I would say that under these conditions the patient is obliged to use the oxygen if there is any solid hope of getting through the crisis.»[291] This author then remarks that any change in either the cost or use of the oxygen which would make its use more difficult, would also effect the need of an increase of hope of recovery as a basis for obligation.[292] There is therefore a definite relation between the notion of proportionate hope of benefit and the nature of ordinary means. The more a means involves difficulty, the more definite must be the hope of proportionate success and benefit. Kelly suggests this principle and is seems quite valid: « . . . a remedy, which includes rather great difficulty, though not moral impossibility, is hardly obligatory unless the hope of success is more probable, whereas a remedy which is easily obtained and used seems obligatory as long as it offers any solid probability of success. »[293] This seems to be a precise interpretation of the notion, proportionate hope of success and benefit.

---

[290]Kelly, «The Duty of Using Artificial Means of Preserving Life», —p. 214.
[291]Loc. cit.
[292]Loc. cit.
[293]Ibid., pp. 214–215.

In summary, therefore, we may say that the notion of proportionate hope of success and benefit is an essential part of the nature of ordinary means. Without this hope of benefit, a means is hardly an ordinary means and therefore it is not obligatory. In determining the presence of this hope of success and benefit, one must consider not only the nature of the particular remedy or means involved, but also the relative condition of the person who is to use this means. Then, and then only, can the moral obligation of using such a means be properly determined.

b) Media Communia

The next element that is frequently mentioned in referring to ordinary means of conserving life is the notion of being *common*. We have seen this in the writings of Vitoria: « . . . foods which men commonly use and in the quantity which customarily suffices for the conservation of strength . . . »[294] Sayrus also refers to the need of employing only the means in common use.[295] We not the same in the writings of Sanchez.[296] In similar manner, De Lugo writes that a man would be guilty of suicide not only if he were to kill himself with a sword, but also if he did not conserve his life by common means.[297]

Although the moralists use many expressions to describe the nature of ordinary means, the notion of being common seems to be basic. Even when the expression «common» is not used, it is presumed, and from the whole context, the reader is aware of the presumption. For the moralists, the duty of conserving one's life does not demand a diligence or a solicitude that exceeds the usual care that most men normally give their lives. Any means of conserving life that is not the normal or usual course of action adopted by men in general is out of the ordinary—extraordinary—and therefore per se not obligatory. Recall Vander Heeren's phrase that an individual is only bound «to make use of all the ordinary means which are indicated in the usual course of things . . . »[298]

Common diligence, therefore, requires the use of common means only. The ordinary conservation of one's life does not imply the singular assiduity

---

[294]« . . . alimentis, quibus homines communiter utuntur et in quantitate quae solet sufficere ad valetudinem conservandam . . . »—a Victoria, Relectio de Temp., n. 12. Cf. Also Vitoria, Comentarios a la Secundae, q. 147, art. 1.

[295]Sayrus, op. cit., Lib. VII, Cap. IX, n. 28.

[296]Sanchez, op. cit., Tom. II, Lib. V, Cap. I, dub. 33.

[297]« . . . non solum dicitur se interimere homo, quando ferro se occidit, sed etiam quando mediis communibus vitam non Conservat . . . »—De Lugo, op. cit., De Justitia et Jure, Disp. X, Sect. I, n. 27.

[298]A. Vander Heeren, «Suicide», *Catholic Encyclopedia*, XIV, p. 327.

involved in prolonging life by unusual and uncommon means. In determining, however, whether or not a means is common, it is necessary, of course, to consider the relative factors involved. For this reason, the moralists frequently mention in their writings the next element of ordinary means, viz., secundum proportionem status.

c) Secundum proportionem status

The element of comparison with one's social position or particular status in life is frequently mentioned by the moralists not only in connection with the notion of common means but also with the notion of the cost involved in using a certain means of conserving life. De Lugo calls attention to it relative to common means.[299] Banez mentions it in connection with cost.[300] Very often however, the notion of one's status is introduced into the very concept of ordinary means. Reiffenstuel, for example, uses such a method.[301]

De Lugo's example of the comparison with one's status is very interesting and helps to accentuate the principle involved.[302] He notes that Vitoria had taught long before that one who cares for his life by means which other men commonly use certainly is satisfying the obligation of caring for his life. De Lugo then applies this same principle to the religious novice who is advised to return to the world in order to obtain food and surroundings which are more healthful for him. The supposition is that ordinary life in religion is having an ill effect on the novice's life and health. De Lugo prefers to ignore the fact that the novice can licitly be given permission to return to the world. That fact is obvious for De Lugo, but beside the point. The question is whether the novice has the *obligation to return* to the world in order to conserve his life. In other words, must the religious novice who is in ill health exchange the ordinary life of religion for the ordinary life of the world in order to conserve his health? Does the duty of self-conservation require that such a novice relinquish the life men commonly live in the monastery for the life that men commonly live in the world? Is the accent, therefore, only on the expression «common,» or must consideration also be given to the particular status that a man has in life?

De Lugo replies that the obligation of conserving one's life and health does not require the novice to return to the world. This author indicates that the novice satisfies his obligation by using food and means which *other men in*

---

[299]De Lugo, op. cit., De Justitia et Jure, Disp. X, Sect. I, n. 36.

[300]Banez, op. cit., in II: II, q. 65, art. 1.

[301]Reiffenstuel, op. cit., Tract. IX, Distinc. III, Quaes. II, n. 14.

[302]De Lugo, op. cit., De Justitia et Jure, Disp. X, Sect. I, n. 36.

religion commonly use to conserve their lives.[303] As a matter of fact, further on, De Lugo completely denies any moral obligation in this regard, which binds the novice to leave the monastery.[304]

We have cited this case to emphasize De Lugo's teaching that very often one must take into consideration an individual's particular status before a means can be properly determined as ordinary for him. Furthermore, this principle applies not only to the determination of ordinary means in general but actually each element of ordinary means must be considered in the light of one's conditions or status. The elements of extraordinary means also are subject to a comparison with one's status in life and this must be kept in mind too.

It may appear that this element of comparison with one's status is merely the relative norm that we mentioned earlier. The notion of comparison with one's status is contained in that relative norm. Our treatment of it here, however, is no mere repetition of what we have already said. When the author's refer to a comparison with one's status they seem to be implying a relation with one's social or financial condition. Hence, they speak in terms of means being common or ordinary with respect to one's status. They also mention that a means must not be too costly in consideration of an individual's position. The relative norm, however, which we discussed before, is broader than that. It considers not only the financial or social position of an individual but also his physical condition. The relative norm clearly encompasses also the psychological outlook that an individual possesses in regard to the use of a particular means of conserving life. Our task here has been to discuss the elements which the moralists mention and in the light of the discussions which they give. That is the reason that we have allotted separate treatment to the element of comparison with one's status.

d) Media non difficilia

Many of the moralists show a very definite preference for describing in a negative way the ordinary means of conserving life. They seem to reason that if the elements which make a means extraordinary can be shown to be lacking in a certain means, then the means is clearly an ordinary means of conserving life. Since the difficulty involved in an extraordinary means is usually easier to describe, they seem content to show what an extraordinary means is, and

---

[303] «Cur ergo novitius . . . nec satisfaciet utendo victu, et mediis quibus alii communiter in religione utuntur et vitam conservant?»—loc. cit.

[304] «Propter haec itaque existimavi, medicorum illud consilium de obligatione novitii rejiciendum omnino esse . . .».—loc. cit.

then say that an ordinary means is one which does not entail such difficulty. Hence, we note that very often in their writings, they use the phrase *media non difficilia.*

Not all authors refrain from a positive expression in this regard. Soto notes that a « . . . prelate could indeed force a subject, on account of a singular obedience promised to him, to take medicines which he can conveniently accept. »[305] Sayrus too remarks that « . . . by the natural law each one is bound to employ for the conservation of his body those licit means which he can conveniently undertake . . . ».[306]

More often however, the authors prefer to say that one is bound to employ only the means which are not too difficult. For example, Lessius teaches that a man is held to care for his health by ordinary means «which are not extremely difficult. »[307] Bonacina uses practically the same words.[308] Laymann also excludes means which are very difficult.[309]

Does any amount of difficulty at all cause a means to be extraordinary? It is essential to the nature of an ordinary means that the means be entirely free of difficulty? From a study of the writings of the moral theologians, one can not help but realize that these authors certainly require an *excessive* difficulty before terming a means *extraordinary.* They clearly state however, that a *moderate* difficulty does not constitute an extraordinary means. Furthermore, from a study of their writings, one can not say that the moralists teach that the terms «difficulty» and «ordinary means» are mutually exclusive.

In order to make their teaching clearer, the moralists usually give examples of the elements which they are discussing. When the notion of excessive difficulty is treated, very often the authors use the example of an amputation. These authors consider an amputation an example of excessive difficulty which all will recognize and appreciate. We shall mention the example of an amputation again when we treat the nature of extraordinary means. Here, however, it is worthwhile to call attention to the teaching of Roncaglia in regard to amputation. Roncaglia mentions an amputation as an extraordi-

---

[305]« . . . praelatus vero cogere posset subditum propter singularem obedientiam illi promissam, ut medicamina admittat quae commode recipere potest».—Soto, op. cit., Lib. V, Quaes. II, art. 5.

[306]« . . . jure naturali media licita, quae commode sumi possunt ad sui corporis conservationem ponere tenetur . . . ».—Sayrus, op. cit., Lib. VIII, Cap. IX, n. 38.

[307]« . . . mediis ordinariis non admodum difficilibus . . . ».—Lessius, op. cit., Lib. II, Cap. IX, Dub. 14, n. 96.

[308]« . . . remediis ordinariis non valde difficilibus . . . ».—Bonacina, op. cit., Tom.. II, Disp. II, Quaest. ultim. Sect. I, punct. 6, n. 2.

[309]« . . . non tenemur per medium valde difficile . . . ».—Laymann, op. cit., Lib. III, Tract. III, P. 3, Cap. I, n. 4.

nary means because of the tremendous pain involved. But he also remarks that whenever «from the amputation, future pains of notable proportion will not arise but only moderate pains, then one is bound to suffer the abscission; for everyone is held to conserve his life by ordinary means and it is an ordinary means to suffer something to conserve this same life.»[310]

Roncaglia's phrasing is very clear. It is an ordinary means to suffer moderate pain for the conservation of one's life. Hence, we can say that for Roncaglia, if a means of conserving life involves only moderate difficulty, it is an ordinary means.

Even in the time of Tournely this fact was recognized. Tournely teaches that the proper care of one's life and health can involve difficulty which is only moderate and not excessive.[311] This author, therefore, holds that an individual has the duty of undergoing moderate pain in order to conserve his life. Furthermore, if the individual concerned refuses to suffer such pain, he can be forced to submit to it for the conservation of his life.[312]

The difficulty connected with employing a particular means of conserving life can arise not only from pain, but also from many other elements such as cost, danger to life, fear etc. The notion of difficulty is generic. Therefore, in a solution of a practical case, consideration should be taken of the possible factors which constitute a difficulty.

The theologians require that an individual exert definite effort in conserving his life, but they do not demand any endeavor which could not be expected of men in general. Certainly a means whose use, absolutely speaking, entails a difficulty which exceeds the strength of men in general is not an ordinary means. Furthermore, if a means involves great difficulty for a particular individual, even though men in general do not find any great difficulty in its use, it ceases to be ordinary for this individual. In other words, even if the great difficulty is only relative, not absolute, it is still sufficient to render a means extraordinary for a particular individual. We have mentioned earlier in this chapter that Vitoria applied the relative norm even to food, a very common means of conserving life. It will be profitable now, however, to note the words with which he describes this relative difficulty. Vitoria writes: « . . . if the depression of spirit is so low and there is present such consternation of spirit in the appetitive power that only with the greatest of effort and as

---

[310]«. . . ex abscissione non sint futuri dolores ingentes, sed moderati, tunc tenetur pati abscissione; nam unusquisque tenetur mediis ordinariis vitam conservare et medium ordinarium est aliquid pati pro eadem vita conservanda».—Roncaglia, op. cit., Vol. I, Tract. XI, Cap. I, Q. IV.

[311]Cf. Tournely, op. cit., Tom. III, Tract. de Decalogo, Cap. II, de Quinto Praec., Art. I, conc. 2.

[312]Loc. cit.

though by means of a certain torture can the sick man take food, right away that is reckoned a certain impossibility and therefore he is excused . . .».[313]

The dictate of the natural law that requires a man to conserve his own life is a serious one. It is based on the double importance of man's human life. His life is important as a divine gift over which God retains the ultimate dominion. Secondly, it is important as the means whereby man can merit his eternal salvation. Hence, self-conservation is no mere heroic act, which although laudable, is not obligatory. The conservation of one's own life is not just a desirable thing which entails no serious duty. In reality, the natural law imposes self-conservation as a very definite obligation from which the individual is excused only when such conservation is impossible for him either physically or morally.

The natural law therefore requires that definite effort be expended in the conservation of one's life even if this involves difficulty. The difficulty however must be proportionate. If self-conservation involves excessive difficulty or proportionately grave inconvenience, then certainly the individual is excused. The reason is that the obligation of conserving one's life is a positive precept and as such does not bind with such grave inconvenience and difficulty. We have explained this in Chapter One.

St. Thomas refers to law as an «ordinatio rationis»—an ordinance of reason.[314] A law, to be a true law, commands only what is within reason. Furthermore, the fulfillment of a law need be accomplished only in a reasonable way. Hence, while it is true that one is excused from fulfilling a positive precept when this fulfillment involves grave inconvenience or moral impossibility, he is not excused when he can fulfill it reasonably. Therefore, it is not beyond the bounds of moral obligation to suffer reasonable difficulty in the use of the means of conserving life.

In determining whether a means is reasonable or not, many factors must be considered. One must take into consideration the means contemplated, the objective difficulty involved and his own ability to make use of the means. But he must also weigh the importance of the dictate of the natural law which requires his self-conservation. Any decisions to be made in this matter should be products of a consideration of both the gravity of the law and the difficulty involved in the fulfillment of the law. To ignore the gravity of the law prepares the way for neglect of duty. To ignore the difficulty involved in fulfilling the law fosters scrupulosity.

---

[313]«. . . quod si animi dejectio tanta est et appetitivae virtutis tanta consternatio, ut non nisi per summum laborem et quasi cruciatum quendam, aegrotus possit sumere cibum, jam reputatur quaedam impossibilitas et ideo excusatur»—a Victoria, Relectio de Temp., n. 1.

[314]Summa Theologica, I: II, q. 90, art. 4.

In our discussions of the element of moral impossibility which we shall treat in the section concerning the nature of extraordinary means, we will refer to the element of difficulty again. The main point to emphasize here, however, is that the nature of ordinary means does not exclude the concept of reasonable difficulty. Hence, we say that an ordinary means is one that an individual can reasonably employ in the conservation of his own life.

e) Media facilia

The reader can notice from the outline of elements presented earlier in this chapter that it is not a common practice of the moralists to include the notion of *easiness* in their discussions of the ordinary means of conserving life. Patuzzi,[315] Waffelaert,[316] and Noldin-Schmitt[317] do mention it. However, in context, the writings of these authors indicate that they did not intend to require a complete lack of difficulty before terming a means ordinary. They seem to mean that ordinary means must be means that one can employ conveniently—in other words, reasonably.

To say that an ordinary means must be easy to use is an expression that can be open to misunderstanding. One might easily imagine that the concept of ordinary means must of necessity exclude any type of difficulty. In the light of the discussion given in the previous section, however, it would seem correct to say that the proper expression is *reasonable,* not, easy. Ordinary means are reasonable means. They are not necessarily easy means because they can entail moderate difficulty.

2) The nature of the extraordinary means of conserving life

In this section, we shall discuss the elements which are included in the concept of the extraordinary means of conserving life. As in the previous section, we have gathered these elements from the writings of the moral theologians concerning the means of conserving life. Very often these writers used more than one phrase in referring to a particular element of extraordinary means. In the outline presented earlier in this chapter, we have given the majority of those phrases. However, in our treatment of them here in this section, it would seem more precise to join the elements into five groups in order that we can accentuate the inconvenience involved in the elements, rather than the expression used to describe the inconvenience. Therefore, we

---

[315]Patuzzi, op. cit., Tom. III, Tract. V, Pars V, Cap. X, Consec. 7.
[316]Waffelaert, op. cit., Tract. II, Vol. II, n. 40.
[317]Noldin-Schmitt, op. cit., II, p. 308.

shall discuss the elements in the following order: 1.) Quaedam impossibilitas, 2.) Summus labor and Media nimis dura, 3.) Quidam cruciatus and Ingens dolor, 4.) Sumptus extraordinarius, Media pretiosa and Media exquisita, 5.) Vehemus horror.

a) Quaedam impossibilitas

The moral theologians are quite conscious of the distinction between avoiding evil and doing good. They understand clearly that a man is always bound to avoid evil but he is not always bound to do positive good. There is a limit to the duty of doing good. To the theologians this is a distinction of major importance. Hence, when the theologians discuss the problem of conserving life, they apply the distinction between avoiding evil and doing good to this problem. A man is always bound to avoid suicide because it is intrinsically evil. However, there is a limit to his obligation of conserving his life in a positive manner. The obligation of conserving one's life in a positive way certainly does not include using any possible means but rather, it would seem to extend itself to the use of reasonable or moderate means. Hence, the theologians apply the term «ordinary» to those means which are reasonable and the term «extraordinary» to those means which a man is not obliged to use in conserving his life. The reason that the extraordinary means are not obligatory is the fact that there is a *certain impossibility* connected with either obtaining or using them. Hence, the individual concerned is excused from employing such means.

We have seen clearly in Chapter Two, section seven of this dissertation that the excusing cause of impossibility can be licitly applied in regard to the precept of the natural law which binds a person to conserve his life. When an individual is unable to fulfill the law, he is not bound to fulfill it. This inability can be of a physical nature. If, for example, the means of conserving life are certainly unattainable or if the individual is physically unfit to make use of these means, he is excused from conserving his life, on the grounds of *physical impossibility.* On the other hand, the individual may be physically capable of fulfilling the law,. but unable to, here and now, because of some circumstance of fear, danger or grave inconvenience which renders the observance of the law extremely difficult for him. It is then said to be *morally impossible* for him to fulfill the law. Hence, if the means of conserving life are excessively difficult or gravely inconvenient to obtain or use, then the use of these means is morally impossible.

It is obvious that physical impossibility excuses from the precept which obliges a man to conserve his life. Everyone understands that no one is bound to use a thing which he can neither obtain nor use. *Nemo ad impossibile tenetur.*

However, in connection with the term moral impossibility, it is necessary to recall that theologians distinguish the negative and affirmative precepts of the natural law. Negative precepts, such as the prohibition of suicide, are always binding because they forbid something that is intrinsically evil. The application of the excusing cause of moral impossibility therefore, is illicit. It is only in regard to the affirmative precepts of the natural law that one can use the excusing cause of moral impossibility.

Self-conservation is an affirmative precept of the natural law and as such, binds *semper* but not *pro semper*. When, therefore, a means of self-conservation involves a proportionately grave inconvenience, it is not obligatory and the individual is excused from the present observance of the precept.

In their discussions of the means of conserving life, the moralists use the terms «certain type of impossibility,» «moral impossibility,» and «grave inconvenience.» For example, Vitoria[318] and Sayrus [319] employ the term «a certain type of impossibility.» Mazzotta uses the same expression.[320] On the other hand, Tournely[321] and more recently Marc-Gestermann,[322] Aertnys-Damen[323] and Kelly[324] make use of the term *moral impossibility*. Finally, the term *grave inconvenience* is used, for example, by Lehmkuhl,[325] Kelly[326] and Paquin.[327]

We know from the accepted axiom that an affirmative precept is not binding in the presence of a proportionately grave inconvenience. Whether or not the terms *proportionately grave inconvenience* and *moral impossibility* are synonymous is perhaps open to dispute. Most authors however, define moral impossibility as a proportionately grave inconvenience which excuses from the present observance of the law. For example, Rodrigo defines moral impossibility as a «proportionately grave inconvenience extrinsic to the observance of a law, but accompanying that observance.»[328] Prümmer says that moral impossibility is present when «the prescribed undertaking can not be accomplished

---

[318]a Victoria, Relectio de Temp., n. 1.

[319]Sayrus, op. cit., Lib. Vii, Cap. IX, n. 31.

[320]Mazzotta, op. cit., Tom. I, Tract. II, Disp. II, Quaest. I, Cap. I.

[321]Tournely, op. cit., Tom. III, Tract. de Decalogo, Cap. II, de Quinto Praec., Art. I, conc. 2.

[322]Marc-Gestermann, op. cit., I, p. 491.

[323]Aertnys-Damen, op. cit., I, n. 566.

[324]Kelly, «The Duty of Using Artificial Means of Preserving Life», p. 206.

[325]Lehmkuhl, op. cit., I, p. 344.

[326]Kelly, *Medico-Moral Problems*, V, pp. 8–9.

[327]Paquin, op. cit., p. 399.

[328]«. . . incommodum proportionate grave et legis observationi extrinsecum, eidem observationi adnexum».—L. Rodrigo, *Praelectiones Theologico-Morales Comillenses* (Santander, Sal Terrae, 1944), Series I, Theologia Moralis Fundamentalis, II, n. 430.

except through very extraordinary effort. »[329] Zalba refers to the «inconvenience . . . which implies great difficulty and lack of proportion in relation to the law concerning which there is question. »[330] Lehmkuhl writes that an affirmative law does not bind in the presence of inconvenience, but he notes that the gravity of the law will determine the required gravity of the inconvenience.[331]

The authors, when writing in regard to the extraordinary means of conserving life, seem to use interchangeably the terms *moral impossibility* and *proportionately grave inconvenience*. It is difficult to determine whether or not they consider them equivalent terms, or whether the expression *proportionately grave inconvenience* implies a difficulty of less magnitude than *moral impossibility*. Whatever be the term they use, the fact remains that these authors insist that the difficulty involved in using a means of conserving life must be of sufficient proportion to constitute an excusing cause before the means can be called extraordinary. It would seem allowable therefore, to use the terms interchangeably when referring to extraordinary means. Father Kelly writing in *Theological Studies,* says that «an extraordinary means is one which prudent men would consider at least morally impossible with reference to the duty of preserving one's life.[332] Then in *Medico-Moral Problems,* the same author writes: «If the inconvenience involved in preserving life was excessive . . . then this particular means of preserving life was called *extraordinary.* »[333] Therefore, it is in keeping with the tradition of theological writing in this matter to say that an extraordinary means is a means which is morally impossible because it involves a grave inconvenience not in proportion to the gravity of the precept demanding self-conservation.

We have referred to the words of St. Thomas in regard to law—«ordinatio rationis». Merkelbach commenting on these words, notes that the term *ordinatio* signifies a «dispositio ad finem per media proportionata . . . »[334] He further explains that *rationis* means that the «will of the superior, in order that there can be

---

[329]«. . . quando opus praescriptum fieri nequit, nisi adhibendo labores prorsus extraordinarios».—D. Prümmer, *Manuale Theologiae Moralis* (Friburgi Brisgoviae, Herder, 1933), I, n. 235.

[330]«. . . incommodum . . . quod magnam difficultatem et improportionem implicat relate ad legem de qua est questio».—Regatillo-Zalba, op. cit., I, n. 555.

[331]Lehmkuhl, op. cit., I, p. 108.

[332]Kelly, «The Duty of Using Artificial Means of Preserving Life», p. 204.

[333]Kelly, *Medico-Moral Problems,* V, p. 9.

[334]Merkelbach, op. cit., I, n. 222.

a law, must be regulated by reason or in conformity with reason, otherwise wickedness would result rather than law . . . ».[335]

A true law is in conformity with reason, and the means employed to fulfill the law must be in conformity with reason. Since the dictate of the natural law which commands a man to conserve his life is obviously a reasonable law, the means employed to fulfill it need only be within reason. Hence any inconvenience or difficulty that is unreasonable is not obligatory. We may ask how great must be the difficulty or inconvenience involved in self-conservation in order to be unreasonable. Merkelbach says: « How great a difficulty is required to be an excuse must be judged from the importance of the law, the quality of the persons and circumstances of places and times etc. »[336]

The inconvenience involved in using a particular means of conserving life is not just reasonable difficulty. It must be an inconvenience extrinsic to the observance of the law and of sufficient magnitude to be out of proportion to the gravity of the law. A means of conserving life that involves only moderate difficulty and inconvenience is certainly not an extraordinary means. When one has to decide whether or not a means is extraordinary by reason of proportionately grave inconvenience, he must consider both the gravity of the law and the factors involved in establishing the inconvenience. Noldin-Schmitt say that the question of which means are extraordinary must be decided from the common estimation of men.[337] Fr. Kelly phrases it best of all: « In concrete cases it is not always easy to determine when a given procedure is an *extraordinary* means. It is not computed according to a mathematical formula, but according to the reasonable judgment of prudent and conscientious men ».[338]

One further point in this matter of moral impossibility concerns the relative norm. Are means to be considered extraordinary only if they involve moral impossibility for men, absolutely speaking, or will relative moral impossibility suffice? A means of conserving life which involves relative moral impossibility must be considered extraordinary. This would be true even if the cause of moral impossibility were unfounded, e.g., irrational fear. Fr. Kelly writes: « My general impression is that there is common agreement that a relative estimate *suffices*. In other words, if any individual would experience

[335]« . . . voluntas superioris, ut lex esse possit, debet esse ratione regulata sue rationi conformis, secus esset magis iniquitas quam lex . . . ».—loc. cit.

[336]« Quanta autem difficultas requiratur ut excuset, moraliter aestimandum est ex legis momento, personarum qualitate, circumstantiis locorum, temporum, etc. »—ibid., n. 377.

[337]Noldin-Schmitt, op. cit., II, p. 308.

[338]Kelly, *Medico-Moral Problems*, V, p. 11.

the inconvenience sufficient to constitute a moral impossibility in the use of any means, that means would be extraordinary for him».[339]

We have seen in this discussion that an essential element of extraordinary means is moral impossibility. An extraordinary means of conserving life is one which is morally impossible due to some grave inconvenience out of proportion with the gravity of the law. The elements which we shall discuss in the following sections are actually the possible causes of moral impossibility in a particular means of conserving life. The elements will not always be present in a given means of conserving life. If they are present and render a means extraordinary, it is because they have been the cause of moral impossibility.

b) Summus labor and Media nimis dura

In our discussion of the moral teaching concerning the ordinary and extraordinary means of conserving life, we have noticed that the natural law requires a man to expend definite effort in order to conserve his life. Any effort which constitutes a moral impossibility however, is an extraordinary means. Hence, the moralists use such expressions as the *greatest of effort* or *too difficult* when they are describing an extraordinary means.

Tamburini notes that a man is not held to make use of extraordinary foods when this requires tremendous effort, because « . . . love of one's self does not demand such effort».[340]

Patuzzi recalls that Franzoja would oblige a man to employ means which are harsh and difficult and which would require great effort to use. Patuzzi says that this reply came from Franzoja because of Aristotle's teaching that a brave and strong man does not flee difficulty. However, Patuzzi is quick to note that Aristotle is speaking of those who commit suicide in order to flee difficulty and trouble, not about «those who refuse to avoid death at the cost of harsh and severe remedies . . . »[341] He adds then further on that « . . . an individual does not violate the natural law when for a good end and just cause he refuses to conserve his life by extraordinary, rather harsh and violent remedies».[342]

A means therefore which requires excessive effort involves a moral impossibility and thus, is an extraordinary means. There are many factors in con-

---

[339]Kelly, «The Duty of Using Artificial Means of Preserving Life», p. 206.

[340]« . . . quia cum tanto labore, nequaquam propria charitas obstringit».—Tamburini, op. cit., Lib. VI, Cap. II, Sect. II, n. 3.

[341]« . . . non vero de illis qui vitare mortem recusant mediis acerbis et aerumnosis . . . ».—Patuzzi, op. cit., Tom. III, Tract. V, Pars V, Cap. X, Consect. sept.

[342]«Non ergo legem naturae et caritatis violabit qui recto fine justaque de causa remediss extraordinariis, acerbioribus, et violentis vitam conservare recusarent».—loc. cit.

serving one's life which could cause this effort. In the writings of the earlier moralists, one of the examples of a non-obligatory effort is the example of a long journey to a more healthful land.[343] Many of the authors repeat this example. However, a modern example is given by Zalba. He notes that a man is not bound «to submit himself to a very dangerous operation or to a very burdensome convalescence».[344] Many modern medical and surgical remedies do not give any moral assurance of proportionate benefit. Thus they are extraordinary means. However, even where the technique involved in these procedures has been perfected so that they give definite hope of proportionate benefit, nonetheless, the very harsh or very troublesome convalescence which follows such procedures could render the remedy itself an extraordinary means. Any means of conserving life which involves the excessive expenditure of effort on the part of the individual concerned is an extraordinary means. Here again, the relative norm suffices. If the means involves effort which constitutes a grave inconvenience for the individual concerned, even though most men would find the means reasonable, the means is nevertheless, an extraordinary means for this individual.

c) Quidam cruciatus and Ingens dolor

One can readily understand that the element of pain can render a means of conserving life extraordinary. Very often, pain is involved in the remedies employed to cure sickness or disease. This is true with modern medical procedure but it was even more true before the days of anaesthesia. Hence, we note that pain is almost universally mentioned by the moralists as an element which can cause a means to be extraordinary. The pain involved in particular remedies can constitute a moral impossibility and therefore, the remedy is an extraordinary means of conserving life, even if the hope of benefit is certain.

The older moralists were very conscious of this fact. They all mention the element of pain. The common example which they give to emphasize this point is an amputation. Whenever they write concerning extraordinary means, invariably they mention pain and almost in the same line, cite the example of an amputation. This is not without reason. These authors were writing in the pre-anesthetic days when the pain involved in an amputation must have been excruciating. The abscission was painful enough but this was

---

[343]Cf. e. g., Sayrus, op. cit., Lib. VII, Cap. IX, n. 28. Paquin however, says: «. . . mais cet exemple, dans notre monde moderne, n's peut-??etre déjà plus une valeur absolue».—op. cit., p. 400.

[344]«neque operationi valde periculosae vel convalescentiae molestissimae se submittere . . .»— Regatillo-Zalba, op. cit., II, p. 269.

followed by cauterizing with hot irons in order to stop the bleeding. For example, the German surgeon Wilhelm of Fabry (1560–1624) is said to have used «a red hot knife for amputation in order to check bleeding!».[345]

Besides the fact that amputation without anaesthesia is so obvious as an example of intense pain, perhaps the older moralists cited this example so often because in those days amputation was the remedy for almost all compound fractures. The following lines from Guthrie's *History of Medicine* will help in understanding the conditions of surgical procedures at that time and also why the example of amputation is so constant in the writings of the moralists:

> These were the days in which hospital gangrene assumed epidemic proportions, and sepsis was an inevitable sequence of operations. Compound fractures were treated by amputation, with a mortality of at least twenty-five percent, while the surgeon wore an old blood-stained coat with a bunch of silk ligatures threaded through one of the buttonholes, ready for use . . . Small wonder, then, that a considerable degree of heroism was demanded from the unfortunate patient who, having endured the tortures of operation without anaesthesia, was still obliged to face the pains and dangers of a septic wound.[346]

Science has progressed since the days when there was no remedy for pain. In the Providence of God, the discovery of anaesthesia eventually came and brought with it an entirely new outlook in regard to surgical interventions. Contemporaneously, the great scientist Lister discovered «the principle involving the prevention and cure of sepsis in wounds».[347] In the course of years, as the antiseptic system was adopted in surgical procedure, the great danger of infection in operations was also eliminated, hence, surgical procedures in general today are not as painful or dangerous as they were in former times. Therefore many of the procedures which were extraordinary means, may possibly be ordinary means now. Consideration, however, must certainly be given to each individual case before determining a means as ordinary or extraordinary. It is true that pain is removed during operations by anaesthesia and it is somewhat lessened in convalescence by sedatives. However, pain and discomfort are still involved in many procedures and if these elements constitute a proportionately grave inconvenience, then the means is an extraordi-

---

[345]Guthrie, op. cit., p. 150.
[346]Ibid., p. 307.
[347]Ibid., p. 324.

nary means. Anaesthesia has lessened the influence of pain as a factor in causing a means to be an extraordinary means, but it has not eliminated the necessity of considering this element when judging whether or not a means is ordinary or extraordinary.

Furthermore, we must keep the relative norm in mind. The same pain that does not render a means extraordinary for one individual, could render it extraordinary for another individual. Hence, prudent judgment above all is necessary.

One must consider not only the pain involved in any surgical intervention—which these days can usually be eliminated—but also the post-operative pain, which usually can be lessened, if not eliminated. In this regard, however, the words of Capellmann are significant:

> Although the cure of wounds effected by an operation will bring post-operative pain, this pain is usually not more intense, and most often less intense, than the pain which the sickness which has caused the operation brings and which the patient would have to suffer even if he did not submit to the operation.[348]

It is well therefore, to remember that the element of pain must definitely be considered when determining whether a means is ordinary or extraordinary. The effect of anaesthesia should be considered. The operative and post-operative pain should be considered. The pain in relation to the individual concerned should be considered. If the pain involved would not exceed the strength of men in general, and does not constitute excessive inconvenience for this particular individual, the procedure is an ordinary means. Otherwise, it is an extraordinary means.

One further point in this regard refers to an opinion found in the Ballerini-Palmieri edition of Gury's *Compendium Theologiae Moralis*. The opinion suggests that one would not be bound to accept an artificial means of inducing sleep, «as long as such inducing of sleep is a dangerous thing . . . because . . . certainly it is an extraordinary means: really, the very loss for some time of the use of reason and of the mastery of his acts, such as occurs in this hypothesis seems an extraordinary thing».[349] One must readily

---

[348]«Quamvis deinde curatio vulnerum operatione effectorum postea dolores afferat, hi tamen generatim non atrociores, pleurumque minus sunt atroces, quam illi quod morbus ipse, quo operatio necessaria fiebat, excitavit, quosque aegrotus etiam sine operatione perferre debuit».— Capellmann, op. cit., p. 26.

[349]Gury-Ballerini-Palmieri, op. cit., n. 391. Cf. supra Chap. II, footnote 117 of this dissertation for the original text of this quotation.

admit that any excessive danger involved in the use of anaesthesia in a particular case would certainly render a procedure an extraordinary means. We have already treated this point when speaking of proportionate benefit. However, it does not seem that one could establish that the use of anaesthesia is always an extraordinary means on account of the loss of the use of reason and mastery of one's acts. We have stated that the inconvenience involved in a procedure must be out of proportion with the gravity of the law. Since we are discussing at this time, a means which is to be employed for the conservation of one's life, it does not seem that the inconvenience involved in the temporary loss of the use of reason would be out of proportion to the duty of self-conservation. Anaesthesia is hardly an extraordinary means on that account. A case is possible, though, in which a person would have an excessive fear of losing the use of reason. Then, the means might become extraordinary, not because of the loss of the use of reason however, but because of the excessive fear. We shall discuss this element of fear in another section of this chapter.

d) Sumptus extraordinarius, Media pretiosa and Media exquisita

The moral theologians have always taken into account the element of expense when discussing the ordinary and extraordinary means of conserving life. They have constantly taught that any means of conserving life which imposes an excessive hardship on an individual because of cost is an extraordinary means. In other words, unreasonable expense can constitute a moral impossibility and thus render a means extraordinary. To describe this excessive coast involved in conserving one's life, the moralists use such general terms as *sumptus extraordinarius, media pretiosa* and *media exquisita.*[350] We have noted earlier in this chapter that the authors speak very frequently of the relative norm in regard to expense. It is apparent from their writings that any expense which causes a grave inconvenience for a particular individual renders a means of conserving life an extraordinary means. We have noted also in this chapter that when the moralists speak of cost, they frequently use the expression *secundum proportionem status.* Hence, the relative norm in this matter suffices.

It is not the practice of these authors, even the recent ones, to establish a definite expense beyond which an individual is no longer obliged.[351] However, there is nothing in their writings which is opposed to establishing an absolute

---

[350]Banez, however, writes that 3,000 ducats is an extraordinary means, cf. op. cit., in II: II, q. 65, art. 1.

[351]Cf. supra, footnote 22 for reference to the suggestion of E. Healy, S. J. in this regard.

norm. In fact, if anything, their writings favor an absolute norm.[352] But one will not find the practice of stipulating a definite amount as an example of expense which is an extraordinary means, absolutely speaking. No doubt, the theologians are mindful that monetary values change and that the income of individuals changes. Furthermore, the amount of money that constitutes a moral impossibility, absolutely speaking, for people of one country might easily be reasonable for people of another country. Hence the authors leave the determination of absolute expense in this matter of extraordinary means to the contemporary and native moralists.

The history of the problem of the ordinary and extraordinary means of conserving life shows that expense has always been considered an essential factor in determining a means ordinary or extraordinary. This is no less true these days. The progress of science has brought about substantial improvements in medical procedures and technique. The cure of ills and the conservation of life has been greatly advanced. However, the question of expense is still a very real problem and in reality, is perhaps even a greater problem than before. Robert Cunningham, writing about an American private health insurance plan, says:

> The constantly growing complexity of medicine has made medical care increasingly expensive. Diagnosis today is far more exact than it was even twenty years ago, but it often requires many expensive laboratory tests. And many modern treatments also are costly . . . Other studies have shown that one fifth of the nation's families are in debt for hospital or medical bills, and that medical care commonly takes from 4 to 7 per cent of family income and, in a few cases, as much as 40 per cent.[353]**

The cost of medical and surgical treatments which require hospitalization vary. Some treatments are not too expensive. For example, one hospital estimates $133.00 as the cost of hospitalization for a case of acute appendicitis

---

[352]For example: «On the other hand, no one not even a very wealthy person is obliged, *per se*, to call in a very expensive physician . . . There is an absolute norm beyond which means are *per se* extraordinary».—J. Sullivan, *Catholic Teaching on the Morality of Euthanasia* (Washington, University of America Press, 1949), p. 64.

[353]R. Cunningham, *The Story of Blue Shield* (The Public Affairs Committee, 1954), p. 2.

**Cf. part II of this book (on *Feeding the Hopeless and the Helpless,* pp. 55, 56) for observations on the extent of medical and hospital insurance coverage in contemporary America.

with no complications.[354] The price includes the cost of the operating room, anaesthesia, medication and hospital ward accommodations for eight days. On the other hand, the cost of hospitalization for diabetes mellitus involving a gangrenous ulcer of the right foot and a low tibial amputation is estimated at $892.10.[355] The ward accommodations in this case are for sixty-one days. The price is broken down in the following way:

Operating Room	$ 17.50
Anaesthesia	30.00
Laboratory	257.50
Medication	154.10
Medical & Surgical Supplies	6.00
Board—61 days a $7.00 a day	427.00
	$892.10**

The reader will note that in both cases the cost is only for hospitalization and does not include the fees of either the doctor or surgeon.

We can see therefore that expense is involved even now in the conservation of one's life. However, there are additional factors in the question of cost that must be considered. Today, public hospitals exist and very often the cost of medical treatment, at least in full, does not have to be paid by the patient.[356] Secondly, some countries, such as England, have a Health Service plan whereby medical treatment is paid for from public funds. Thirdly, there are private insurance plans, as for instance in the United States. With such insurance, a patient is greatly aided in meeting a medical bill which would otherwise be impossible for him to pay. We can understand therefore, that medical expense must be considered in the light of the individual's financial condition.

---

[354]St. Joseph's Hospital, Reading Pennsylvania. The cost sheet was prepared by Sister M. Fridoline, O.S.F. and submitted to me for use in this dissertation.

[355]Loc. cit.

[356]Cf. Ubach, op. cit., I, n. 488 where he notes that extraordinary cost is often absent because a surgical operation is usually performed in a public hospital.

**Hospital charges today (1988) are based on Diagnostic Related Groups (or DRG's). Through the kindness of John W. Logue, President of Carney Hospital, Boston, MA, the following fitures have been made available for comparative purposes. According to the data base presently in effect at Carney Hospital, the average charge for an appendectomy without complications (DRG 167) would be $3,050.00 (3.7 days average length of stay). For any operation on the cranium for an individual under age 17—no trauma (DRG 001) the average charge would be $24,874.00 (36 days average length of stay).

The tradition of moral teaching in regard to the means of conserving life shows that consideration must be given to the question of expense. The cost involved will render the means an extraordinary means if it is excessive, at least for the individual concerned. Here again however, prudent judgment must be had in making the decision and consideration must be given not only to the expense but also to the gravity of the duty of self-conservation.

e) Vehemens horror

The final element which the moralists consider in their discussions of extraordinary means is *vehemens horror*. There are two main emotions to which the authors give attention. One is intense fear. The other is very strong repugnance.

The emotion of *fear* helps a man to protect his life. It is because of fear that a man withdraws from what is harmful or injurious. Fear causes a man to escape from danger. Yet, «fear is sometimes so intense that it paralyzes the subject and leaves him unable to move».[357] Fear, being a natural emotion, quite obviously is present when certain means of conserving life come into question. When an individual considers the pain or other inconveniences involved in a particular procedure, fear can cause him to shun this means of conserving life. In certain cases, the fear of a particular procedure can be so intense that it constitutes a moral impossibility. Thus, the procedure becomes an extraordinary means. There are medical procedures which can cause fear, even excessive fear, in most men. However, in any practical decision, one must consider the emotional or psychological condition of the individual concerned. If the fear is excessive and causes a grave inconvenience, the means in question is an extraordinary means.

Sometimes this excessive fear may be unfounded. It may be unwarranted by the objective danger or pain involved in a procedure. In this case, the individual concerned should rid himself of this unnecessary excessive fear. He should consider the matter objectively. Fear that is irrational should be eliminated, if possible, before determining whether or not a means is extraordinary. However, if the excessive fear remains, irrational and unwarranted though it be, it can constitute an extraordinary means. Thus, it provides a legitimate excuse from employing such a means of conserving life.[358]

Repugnance or distaste for a particular means is also mentioned by the moralists in their writings. Usually, in this connection, they give the example

---

[357] T. Gannon, Psychology—*The Unity of Human Behavior* (Boston, Ginn and Company, 1954), p. 254.

[358] Cf. Ubach, op. cit., I, 488.

of a maiden who is unwilling to submit to any medical treatment by a male doctor, when this is repugnant to her sense of modesty.[359] This resolve on the part of the maiden whereby she prefers the pains of illness, even death itself, to the inconvenience caused by repugnance to treatment by a male doctor is perhaps unwarranted. The fact remains, nonetheless, that this intense distaste can constitute a moral impossibility. Patuzzi does not agree. He calls this repugnance imprudent and inane. Furthermore, this author says that the maiden ought to subject her emotions to the law of charity and the law of nature.[360] However, it seems that most moralists would agree that if the maiden's repugnance causes a moral impossibility, then the treatment by a male doctor is for her an extraordinary means.

One final point in this section concerns another example in regard to the element of repugnance. We have mentioned before that the moralists cite an amputation as an example of an extraordinary means, due to the grave danger and intense pain involved. Science has improved the technique in operations and thus the amputation is no longer as dangerous as it was. Anaesthesia has removed the pain. Yet repugnance to living with a mutilated body could just as readily constitute a grave inconvenience. This point also should be remembered when determining such a procedure as an ordinary and extraordinary means for a particular individual.[361]

We can see therefore that the two factors, fear and repugnance, must be considered when judging whether a procedure is an ordinary or extraordinary means of conserving life. The relative norm is or particular importance in regard to this element. A procedure which causes no fear or repugnance at all for men in general, might easily be a source of grave fear or intense repugnance for another individual. If therefore, the fear or repugnance constitutes a moral impossibility, it renders the procedure an extraordinary means of conserving life.

C.
FORMULATION OF A DEFINITION OF THE TERMS ORDINARY AND EXTRAORDINARY MEANS OF CONSERVING LIFE

We have studied up till now the writings of the moral theologians in regard to the ordinary and extraordinary means of conserving life. We have

---

[359]For example, Busenbaum and St. Alphonsus. Cf. quotation supra, Chap. II, footnote 81.
[360]Cf. quotation supra, Chap. II, footnote 111.
[361]Cf. Ballerini-Palmieri, *Opus Theologicum*, II, p. 645, n. 868, footnote « b ». For the quotation of this reference cf. supra, Chap. II, footnote 118.

noticed that no set definition of these terms has been given, but that the authors simply described these means. From the descriptions and the examples given by these writers, we have been able to gather the essential elements involved in the terms ordinary and extraordinary means. We have collected the elements that are constantly used and have studied what is implied in these elements. Hence, we actually have the essential concepts which the tradition in moral writings requires for ordinary and extraordinary means.

Gerald Kelly, S. J. is one of the very few moralists to attempt a definition of these terms. He restricts it, however, to hospital procedures. This author writes: «As regards hospital procedures, *ordinary means* of preserving life are all medicines, treatments, and operations, which offer a reasonable hope of benefit for the patient and which can be obtained and used without excessive expense, pain or other inconvenience».[362] In reference to extraordinary means, he says: «By these we mean all medicines, treatments, and operations, which cannot be obtained or used without excessive expense, pain or other inconvenience, or which, if used would not offer a reasonable hope of benefit».[363]

Hospital procedures are not the only means of conserving life. Hence, a definition of ordinary and extraordinary means must be broad enough to include any means which is used for conserving life. Furthermore, an ordinary means is one which excludes the notion of moral impossibility, but it does not exclude the notion of reasonable difficulty.

The elements which we have noted to be included in the nature of ordinary means are: definite hope of proportionate benefit, the notion of being common, and reasonable effort. On the contrary, extraordinary means involve the notion of lack of proportionate benefit, and the notion of moral impossibility arising from unreasonable inconvenience in regard to pain, fear or expense etc.

Since all these elements have been shown to be constant in the moral teachings concerning the ordinary and extraordinary means of conserving life, we suggest the following definitions:

> *Ordinary means of conserving life* are those means commonly used in given circumstances, which this individual in his present physical, psychological and economic condition can reasonably employ with definite hope of proportionate benefit.
> *Extraordinary means of conserving life* are those means not commonly used in given circumstances, or those means in common

[362]Kelly, *Medico-Moral Problems*, V, p. 6.
[363]Loc. cit.

use which this individual in his present physical, psychological and economic condition can not reasonably employ, or if he can, will not give him definite hope of proportionate benefit.

The reader will note that these definitions are based on the relative norm. In this matter, the relative norm suffices in judging whether a means is ordinary or extraordinary. However, if there is a question of absolute grave inconvenience, then the same definition of extraordinary means is obviously valid. In regard to ordinary means, we have previously eliminated the use of an absolute norm.

3.2 THE OBLIGATION OF USING THE ORDINARY AND EXTRAORDINARY MEANS OF CONSERVING LIFE

Thus far in this chapter, we have been discussing the nature of the ordinary and extraordinary means of conserving life. We now intend to discuss the obligation of using these means. The usual manner of phrasing this obligations in: *per se* a man is obliged to use the ordinary means of conserving his life; *per se* he is not obliged to use extraordinary means, though the use of extraordinary means might be obligatory *per accidens*.[364]

A—The obligation of using the ordinary means of conserving life

Zalba expresses the obligation of using the ordinary means this way: «Cura vitae conservandae et administrandae imponit obligationem, ex genere suo gravem, positive procurandi et applicandi media congrua».[365] There is a grave obligation of employing the ordinary means of conserving one's life. Our life is a precious gift of God, and it provides an essential condition in this economy by which we can merit heaven. Hence, the care of our life is a serious obligation and imposes the duty of employing the ordinary means necessary for such care. Not to employ the ordinary means of conserving life is tantamount to suicide and thus a grave sin. One who refuses to employ the ordinary means of conserving his life, equivalently kills himself.[366]

---

[364]Cf. Kelly, «The Duty of Using Artificial Means of Preserving Life», p. 206.
[365]Regatillo-Zalba, op. cit., II, p. 268.
[366]Cf. Genicot-Salsmans, op. cit., I, p. 298.

We have included the notion of utility or proportionate hope of success and benefit as an essential part of our definition of ordinary means. Any means, therefore, that does not give definite hope of benefit is an extraordinary means. This element has been shown to be included constantly by the moralists in the concept of ordinary means. Sometimes, however, confusion on this point can occur. Some authors speak of ordinary means and hope of benefit as two separate entities. Then they join the two notions in order to determine the obligation of using the ordinary means. The implication is that one can determine a means as ordinary apart from the notion of proportionate benefit. For example, Fr. Kelly writes: «The patient is *per se* obliged to use only those means which are ordinary and which offer a reasonable hope of success».[367] The same author discussing a practical case, writes concerning a particular means of conserving life: «But even granted that it is ordinary, one may not immediately conclude that it is obligatory».[368] Fr. Kelly is actually carefully noting that all attendant circumstances must be weighed before a means of conserving life can be called ordinary and obligatory.

In order to avoid this confusion, we have based our definition on the relative norm. Thus, if a means of conserving life is ordinary in accordance with our definition, it is automatically obligatory. It is precisely because of this possible confusion that we have stated that an absolute norm for ordinary means cannot be admitted. Since the obligation of conserving life rests with the individual primarily, it would seem that the ordinary means should be determined in accordance with the conditions of the individual. Once the means are then determined as ordinary means for this individual, they are obligatory.

Again it is well to reacll that this method is in no way opposed to establishing a *general norm* whereby means are characterized as ordinary for most men. But, in the last analysis, the individual's own conditions will determine a means as ordinary or extraordinary. That is the reason we have based our definition on the relative norm; it is also the reason why we can say that ordinary means of conserving life are always obligatory.

B—The obligation of using the extraordinary means of conserving life

All authors admit that reasonable care of one's life does not include the use of extraordinary means. Hence *per se* extraordinary means are not obliga-

---

[367]Kelly, «The Duty of Using Artificial Means of Preserving Life», p. 216.

[368]Ibid., p. 218. In later writings, Father Kelly includes the notion of usefulness in his definitions of ordinary and extraordinary means; cf. supra the definitions cited from *Medico-Moral Problems* and also, «The Duty to Preserve Life», *Theological Studies*, XII (1951), p. 550.

tory. The moralists, however, do note that extrinsic circumstances can change a case. They admit that for some reason a person might be bound to take more than ordinary care of his life, particularly when there is question of prolonging one's life. For this reason, they say that an individual might be bound *per accidens* to employ even extraordinary means of conserving his life.[369]

The usual examples of the obligation per accidens of using extraordinary means are: 1) one who is especially necessary to his family or society,[370] and 2) one who should prolong his life for his spiritual welfare.[371]

For example, suppose that the father of a large family is dangerously ill. The doctors give him moral assurance that by means of a surgical intervention he can regain his health. However, the post-operative pain will be very intense and for him will constitute a moral impossibility. In this case the means of conserving life is considered extraordinary. Hence, the individual has *per se* no obligation to use this means to conserve his life. However, the extrinsic circumstance of a large family could change the case. The means of conserving life is still extraordinary; his duty ot his own life still does not demand the use of extraordinary means. But his duty to his family could oblige him to make use of a means which he would not otherwise be bound to employ. Hence, in such a situation, the individual is said to have the obligation per accidens of using an extraordinary means of conserving his life.

In regard to the second example, we may cite this case. A patient is dying in great pain. Death is certain and inevitable. He is a Catholic but has been away from the Sacraments for twenty years. He is willing to see a priest and receive the Sacraments. A certain drug may prolong his life for another hour or two. Must he take the drug in order to stay alive long enough to receive the Sacraments?[372] Our reply is as follows. The drug in question is an extraordinary means because the physical benefit to be derived from its use is negligible. Death is certain. There is no proportionate hope of benefit. Since the drug, therefore, is an extraordinary means, it is not obligatory per se. However, the patinet has the grave obligation of making his peace with God and receiving the Last Sacraments. Thus, the hour or so that will be given him by using the drug are necessary for him in order to see a priest. From the obligation, therefore, of caring for his soul, the obligation arises per accidens

---

[369]Cf. Regatillo-Zalba, op. cit., II, pp. 268-269.

[370]Loc. cit.

[371]Kelly, « The Duty of Using Artificial Means of Preserving Life », p. 206.

[372]This case is a modification of one presented for discussion by Fr. McFadden. Cf. C. McFadden, *Medical Ethics* (Philadelphia, Davis Company, 1955), p. 159, case 11.

of prolonging his life by using an extraordinary means. Hence, in this case, the patient is bound per accidens to use the drug in question.

The principle involved in this matter is very clear, namely: extraordinary means are obligatory only per accidens. Applications of this principle however, can be complicated because the circumstances of a case can be involved. Prudent judgment above all is necessary. It must be remembered that the common tendency of most men is to conserve their lives by any possible means. However, their moral obligation extends per se only to the use of the ordinary means, and only per accidens to the extraordinary means.

In this chapter, we have seen the nature of the ordinary and extraordinary means of conserving life. We have seen that the relative norm suffices in determining a means as ordinary or extraordinary. We have also mentioned that there can be an absolute norm in regard to extraordinary means according to which certain means are not obligatory for any man, per se. Furthermore, we stated that a *general norm* can be established whereby certain means are classed as ordinary means for most men, although we emphasized that in the last analysis only the relative norm will determine an ordinary means. Finally, we reviewed the principles involved in the obligation to use the means of conserving life. We noted that means which are ordinary according to our definition are obligatory means. Extraordinary means are not obligatory except per accidens.

CHAPTER IV

Practical Considerations in the Matter of the Ordinary and Extraordinary Means of Conserving Life

4.1 CONSIDERATIONS IN REGARD TO THE ELEMENT OF «RISK» IN MODERN OPERATING TECHNIQUE

In the previous chapter, we discussed the nature of the ordinary and extraordinary means of conserving life. In that discussion, we noted that one of the factors which must be considered in determining a means as ordinary or extraordinary is the notion of hope of success. This factor is very important, especially in the determination of modern surgical operations as ordinary or extraordinary means of conserving life. Certainly surgical interventions involve risk. This was true particularly in past ages, but it is also true today. Modern operating technique, with the advances and progress of medical science, has greatly reduced the risk of death, but it has not eliminated risk of death completely.

Traditionally, the moralists have listed amputations and incisions into the abdomen as constant examples of extraordinary means. Published rates of success in such operations today are not sufficiently broad in scope to enable the moralist to render a categoric opinion about the moral problem of «element of risk» in these operations. However, it is interesting to note by way of illustration that in sixty-three recorded cases of leg amputations, five deaths are reported; in 2,454 recorded cases of appendectomy operations, eight deaths are recorded, and finally in 1,382 reported cesarean sections, three deaths are reported.[373]

The indications of the reported causes of death are that complications extrinsic to the operating technique, as well as the physical condition and age of the patient have been generally the factors responsible for death in the cases cited here. In the report submitted by St. Joseph's Hospital, Reading, Pennsylvania, there is this important observation: «the individual patient must be considered with particular emphasis on old age. Mortality for example, listed under hip surgery more often is caused by age rather than the surgery, a. v., surgery is more the occasion than the efficient cause».[374]

Another observation from this same report mentions that:

> Operating techniques have not changed too radically. Lowering of mortality rates is due more to connected issues. Above all other such issues the one factor most responsible is the science of anaesthesia which has greatly advanced in the past 15 years. It is common practice now to have an M. D. specialist in anaesthesia rather than a nurse as formerly. With this set-up the operating surgeon has a freer mind and hand. Other connected issues are intravenous feedings, blood transfusions (plasma and direct); also antibiotics which greatly reduce danger of infection. Pre-operative

---

[373]These figures were contained in lists of operations obtained from the following hospitals: Lynn Hospital, Lynn, Massachusetts; St. Joseph's Hospital, Reading, Pennsylvania; St. John's Hospital, St. Louis, Missouri; St. Mary's Hospital, Decatur, Illinois; St. Elizabeth's Hospital, Belleville, Illinois; Sacred Heart Hospital, Eau Claire, Wisconsin. For their generous cooperation in preparing these figures and giving permission for the use of them, I am indebted to the authorities of these hospitals. I have made use also of the following article: C. Sullivan, M. D. and E. Campbell, M. D., «One Thousand Cesarean Sections in the Modern Era of Obstetrics», *Linacre Quarterly*, November 1955, pp. 117–126. In this article, the authors present a study of 1,000 consecutive cesarean sections performed by the staff of St. Elizabeth's Hospital, Brighton, Massachusetts. The authors report that: «In this series of 1,000 consecutive sections, 3 mothers died, a mortality of 0.3% . . . None of the 3 deaths was in any way associated with the technic of cesarean section, and all were emergency procedures». (ibid., p. 123).

[374]Report prepared by James Diamond, M. D. and R. Impink, M. D. of St. Joseph's Hospital, Reading, Pennsylvania and submitted to me for use in this dissertation.

checks especially for the aged also reduce mortality: electrocardiographs, chest x-rays, blood chemistry.[375]

The element of risk has been greatly reduced due to modern advances. However, every surgical operation contains a certain amount of risk and this should be considered in any classification of surgical procedures as ordinary or extraordinary means.

4.2 MODERN MEDICAL AND SURGICAL PROCEDURES AS ORDINARY OR EXTRAORDINARY MEANS**

The discussion of the element of risk in surgical operations leads directly to the consideration of modern medical and surgical treatments as ordinary or extraordinary means of conserving life. The reader will recall that we noted in Chapter Three that there is no *absolute norm* for designating a means of conserving life as an *ordinary means*. This is true because of the many relative factors involved in the medical treatment of each individual patient. However, we did admit that one could classify certain procedures as ordinary means, according to a *general norm*. In other words, there are some medical treatments which usually are ordinary means of conserving life for men in general, even though certain relative considerations may render them extraordinary means for particular individuals.

Many of the older moralists considered surgical operations extraordinary means because of the pain, expense and risk of death involved. We have mentioned in the previous chapters that anaesthesia has lessened the effect of the element of pain, and that expense also has been diminished because of public hospitals and insurance plans. However, these factors must be considered because there is still an element of danger in the use of anaesthesia and

---

[375]Ibid.

**As a postscript to the publication of his dissertation in 1958, Bishop Cronin mentioned the "Statement on Reanimation" of Pope Pius XII (Nov. 24, 1957) as an "important discussion" which appeared since the writing of his dissertation. That address of Pope Pius XII is presented in Appendix IV of this book. and would validate, in general, the discussion in this section 4.2 with regard to the obligation to "use only ordinary means." Cf. also the *Declaration on Euthanasia,* Appendix I of this book, with particular attention to the statement on p. of this book: "It is also permissible to make do with the normal means that medicine can offer. Therefore one cannot impose on anyone the obligation to have recourse to a technique which is already in use but which carries a risk or is burdensome . . . ."

post-operative pain and inconveinence can constitute even now a moral impossibility. Furthermore, the inconveinence of expense has by no means been removed completely; expense can still constitute a moral impossibility.

The element of risk has been lessened also, but it is still present, particularly in operations performed on elderly patients or on those patients who have a relatively weak constitution. It would seem however, that *as regards the operating technique,* most common operations offer sufficient hope of success *in the case of young patients* to be termed ordinary means of conserving life. For example, a leg amputation, from the aspect of *operating technique,* does not involve excessive danger for a young patient in the normal case, and hence from that viewpoint, the procedure would be an ordinary means. On the other hand, the danger involved in this operation in the case of an elderly patient is much greater, and in most circumstances, such a procedure would be an extraordinary means of conserving life.

Furthermore, the circumstances of the operation affect the situation. The risk ordinarily involved in a cesarean section or an appendectomy performed in a modern hospital with all the advantages of skilled surgeons, anaesthesia-specialists, and antiseptic facilities would not be sufficient to render these procedures extraordinary means on that account. However, the same procedures performed in one's home, in a less modern or rural clinic, or by a less capable doctor could easily be an extraordinary means due to the risk involved.

Major surgery of the more radical type still remains today an extraordinary means of conserving life and health because of the danger involved. For example, the various types of neurosurgery are not morally obligatory for the patient.

A practical summary of the classification of modern surgical interventions as *moral* ordinary or extraordinary means, *from the aspect of the operating technique alone,* would be: 1) Common surgery, even though major surgery, performed on patients of relatively young age and relatively strong constitution, and in surroundings which offer the advantages of modern hospital skill, precautions and equipment is *generally* an ordinary means of conserving life. 2) Major surgery, even though common surgery, performed on patients of advanced age or of relatively weak constitution, cannot be classed *generally* as an ordinary means of conserving life. 3) Major surgery, even though common surgery, performed on the young or the old, in surroundings which do not offer the advantages of modern hospital skill, precautions and equipment cannot be classed *generally* as an ordinary means of conserving life. 4) Radical surgery which involves great risk and danger, or which is still insufficiently tested is an extraordinary means of conserving life both for the young and the old.

The above summary is only in regard to the *operating technique,* so that expense, pain and repugnance can still determine a means as ordinary or extraordinary. It is on the basis of repugnance that leg amputations probably still remain extraordinary means of conserving life for most people even in these days. This certainly is true in the case of the amputation of both legs.

From the viewpoint of medical treatment, we may say that the initial visit to or calling of a doctor and the examination by him[376] are ordinary means in the case of a person who is seriously ill, as is also ordinary nursing care. However, repeated expense in this matter can render the means extraordinary. The basic medicines, intravenous feedings, insulin, the many types of antibiotics, oxygen masks and tents, preventative medicines and vaccines are ordinary means of conserving life. However, even in these treatments, the relative physical, psychological, and economic condition of an individual can change the case. For example, an extreme horror of needles could easily render repeated injections as extraordinary means for a particular individual. Furthermore, the relative benefit to be derived from an intravenous feeding can be slight in an individual case, and thus the intravenous feeding will be an extraordinary means, as we shall see further on in this chapter.

Blood transfusions *in general* are ordinary means of conserving life unless the expense involved renders them extraordinary means, or unless the condition of the patient provides little hope of benefit in making use of the transfusions. An interesting aspect of blood transfusions is discussed by Father John Ford, S. J. in *Linacre Quarterly.*[377] The author studies the refusal of blood transfusions by Jehovah's Witnesses. Jehovah's Witnesses believe that such transfusions involve eating blood, which is contrary to the biblical prohibition found in the Old and New Testaments (Leviticus. 3:17; Acts, 15:29). Hence, they will refuse such treatment. The question arises then as to whether a blood transfusion should be considered an ordinary means of conserving life for the Jehovah's Witness. Father Ford maintains that the mistaken frame of mind which the Jehovah's Witness possesses in this matter makes the blood transfusion for him an extraordinary means of conserving life. Father Ford writes:

> With a sincere Jehovah's Witness who is firmly convinced that a transfusion offends God, we are dealing with a case where his conscience absolutely forbids him to allow the procedure. In

---

[376]Note, however, the exception made in the case of the maiden whose sense of modesty would render an examination by a male doctor extremely repugnant and hence, for her such an examination could be an extraordinary means.

[377]J. Ford, S. J., « The Refusal of Blood Transfusions by Jehovah's Witnesses », *Linacre Quarterly,* February, 1955, pp. 3–10.

this mistaken frame of mind, he would actually commit sin if he went against his conscience and took the transfusion. I see no inconsistency in admitting that this frame of mind is a circumstance which makes the transfusion for him an *extraordinary* means of preserving life.[378]

In general, however, blood transfusions are to be considered ordinary means of conserving life, in the theological sense, just as they are certainly an ordinary medical procedure.

4.3 PRACTICAL APPLICATIONS IN REGARD TO THE DOCTOR

Up till now, our study of the ordinary and extraordinary means of conserving life has been limited to a consideration of the duty of *each individual* to conserve his own life. In other words, we have prescinded, thus far, from any discussion of the extension of this duty to those persons who may be charged with the conservation of another's life, e.g., relatives, physicians and surgeons etc. In this present section, therefore, we shall consider the duty of employing the means of conserving life, as it applies to the *doctor*—(we are including physicians and surgeons under the term «doctor»).

The Obligation of the doctor to Take Care of the Sick

There are many obligations which are binding on the doctor by reason of his professional calling. These obligations begin even in medical school where he has the duty of learning the science of medicine.[379] What concerns us here, however, is the doctor's particular duty to heal and cure. We are interested in the *source* of this obligation and the *content* of the obligation.

A—The source of the obligation

The doctor is bound, in general, by the law of God and his professional oath to take care of the sick, although *per se*, he is free to accept or not accept a

---

[378]Ibid., p. 6. J. Connery, S. J. prefers to consider the blood transfusion as an ordinary means for the Jehovah's Witness and excuse such a patient from using it on the basis of invincible ignorance—cf. «Notes on Moral Theology» *Theological Studies*, XVI (1955), p. 571.

[379]Cf. A. Bonnar, *The Catholic Doctor* (London, Burns Oates and Washbourne Ltd., 1952), pp. 157–162 for a discussion of «The Doctor in His Practice».

particular person as a patient. This obligation to take care of the sick can stem immediately from the *virtue of charity* and the *virtue of justice*.

1) The virtue of charity

The virtue of charity obliges all men to aid their neighbors who are in need. This need may be spiritual or temporal, and both may be extreme, grave or ordinary. Jone-Adelman describe the obligation this way:

> *In extreme spiritual necessity* we must assist our neighbor even at the risk of our life . . . In *extreme temporal necessity* our neighbor must be helped even at our great personal inconvenience, but not at the risk of our life, unless our position or the common welfare demand the safety of the threatened party . . . In *grave spiritual or temporal need* our neighbor must be helped in as far as this is possible without a serious inconvenience to ourselves . . . In *ordinary spiritual or temporal necessity* one is not obliged to help his neighbor in each and every case.[380]

The virtue of charity, therefore, obliges all men to aid their neighbors who are in need. The doctor's obligation from charity to assist the sick is but a simple application of the general demands of the virtue of charity. Hence, a doctor is bound to take care of a sick man who is ill and needs medical attention, if no other doctor is nearby who can and will aid this sick individual.[381] The gravity of the obligation depends, naturally enough, on the degree of necessity in which the sick man finds himself. The doctor's obligation, therefore, can be very grave, serious or slight according as the urgency of the sick man's illness is extreme, grave or ordinary.

Since the duty of charity is a positive obligation, it is not binding in the presence of a proportionately grave inconvenience. « The proportion can be less rigorous when the demands of charity are less strict. » Hence, only a very grave inconvenience will excuse a doctor from taking care of a sick man in extreme need; only a grave inconvenience will excuse him if the person is in grave need, and any real inconvenience will be sufficient to excuse him from caring for a person in ordinary need.

---

[380]Jone-Adelman, op. cit., pp. 85–86, nn. 138–139.

[381]Cf. F. Hürth, S. J., *De Statibus* (Romae, Pont. Universitas Gregoriana, 1946), p. 106.

[382]« La proportion peut même être ici moins rigoureuse, puisque les exigences de la charité sont moins strictes ».— Paquin, op. cit., pp. 102–103.

Furthermore, besides this obligation of charity to our neighbor in general, we are bound in a special way to help the poor. Jone-Adelman describe this obligation in the following way:

> In a case of *extreme necessity* one is obliged under grave sin to help the poor even by sacrificing things necessary for our state of life . . . In a case of *grave necessity* one must help the poor if it can be done without sacrificing things necessary for one's state in life . . . In their *ordinary need* one must help the poor in general from one's superfluous possessions . . . .[383]

This obligation obviously enough applies to the doctor too. Hence, the doctor has the very grave duty to assist gratuitously a poor person in extreme need. He also has the grave obligation to assist gratuitously a poor person in grave need; a slight obligation to help a poor man in ordinary need. In these cases also, we suppose that the man in question is the only doctor available who is willing and able to take care of the sick man, and that the doctor can render his services without a proportionately grave inconvenience.

2) The virtue of justice

Besides the obligation which the virtue of charity imposes on the doctor, a duty can also arise from the virtue of justice. The doctor is bound in justice to visit and take care of the sick with whom he has a contract or a quasi-contract.

A contract exists when the services of the doctor are engaged, orally or by writing, for the purpose of caring for a particular person or group of persons.[384] A quasi-contract exists when the doctor responds to the «call» of a sick person and implicitly agrees, on the promise (at least implicit) of payment, to continue his services as long as the condition of the patient requires them.[385] In these instances, the patient has a strict right to the services of the doctor and the doctor is bound in justice to render the services. A proportionately grave inconvenience, however, can excuse a doctor from his obligation, as long as the inconvenience is one which is not inherent in the professional work itself.[386] For example, a doctor's own illness will excuse him, even though his obligation in the matter is one of justice. However, the danger of a conta-

---

[383]Jone-Adelman, op. cit., pp. 86–87, n. 141.
[384]Cf. J. Paquin, op. cit., p. 101.
[385]Loc. cit.
[386]Ibid., p. 102.

gious disease will not excuse him from caring for a person whom he is obliged in justice to assist.

B—The content of the obligation

Since the doctor is bound to take care of the life and health of the sick, he is obliged to employ the means of conserving life. Hence, the next point is in regard to the doctor's obligation to use the *ordinary and extraordinary means of conserving life.*

1) The doctor's obligation of employing the ordinary means of conserving life

Certainly, the doctor has the obligation *per se* of using the ordinary means of conserving life when he treats a patient. Otherwise, he would have no obligation at all. If the doctor were not bound to employ the ordinary means, *a fortiori,* neither would he be bound to employ the extraordinary means. Thus, the question would be closed, and no further discussion would be warranted here. The doctor's basic duty is described very well by Father Connell: « The doctor is bound by the law of God, as well as by his Hippocratic oath, to preserve the life of a patient as long as is reasonably possible. This means that ordinary measures must be employed even in the case of one who will continue to be, naturally speaking, merely an unprofitable burden on society. »[387]

The moralists recognize this obligation of the doctor, although some phrase it in a manner different from Father Connell's description. For example, Genicot-Salsmans write: « The doctor is bound in justice to furnish the safer or better remedy to a sick person. »[388] Implicitly contained in this statement is the obligation of using ordinary means. If the doctor is bound to use the safer or better remedies, *a fortiori,* he is bound to supply the ordinary remedies. There are other moralists, however, who write in a manner similar to Father Connell. For example, Father McFadden says: « It is never permissible to hasten the death of any product of human conception. The degree of deformity does not change the situation . . . the *ordinary* steps to conserve life/

---

[387]F. Connell, *Morals in Politics and Professions,* (Westminster, The Newman Press, 1951), p. 121.

[388]« Medicus ex *justitia* tenetur ad *remedium tutius* seu melius aegroto praebendum ».—Genicot-Salsmans, op. cit., I, n. 701. Similarly, Vermeersch, *Theol. Moralis,* II, n. 492; Aertnys-Damen, op. cit., I, n. 1250; Noldin-Schmitt, op. cit., II, nn. 743–744; Capellmann, op. cit., p. 35; G. Payen, *Déontologie Médicale D'Après Le Droit Natural, Résumé,* (Zi-ka-wei, Imprimerie de la Mission Catholique, 1928), p. 40.

must be taken.»[389] Father Davis writes that doctors sin seriously if they «. . . do not use reasonable and ordinary precautions, for their duty is to keep patients alive, and they have no privilege of killing them.»[390] Father Hürth notes that «even if a doctor has assumed the care of a sick person from charity alone, he is bound in strict justice to ordinary diligence.»[391]

In other words, just as the patient himself is bound to accept the ordinary means of conserving life, so also the doctor is bound to employ the ordinary means of conserving life when he is treating his patient. The patient's refusal to furnish the ordinary measures is equivalent to suicide. The doctor's refusal to furnish the ordinary measures is equivalent to murder. That is why in the *Code of Ethical and Religious Directives for Catholic* Hospitals, one reads: «The failure to supply the *ordinary means* of preserving life is equivalent to euthanasia.»[392]

We have stated that a proportionately grave reason will excuse the doctor from administering to a patient. This teaching applies to the use of ordinary means. A proportionately grave inconvenience which is not inherent in the doctor's professional work will excuse him from his obligation in justice to supply the ordinary means of conserving life. (Recall that this applies also to the care of a patient whom the doctor accepts *ex caritate sola,* since the doctor even in this case is bound *in justice* to employ the ordinary means of conserving life.)

The determination of the doctor's obligation to heal and cure is sufficiently clear in the common case in which ordinary means is all that is necessary for the patient's recovery. Obviously, the doctor is obliged to employ the ordinary means in such a case. However, the difficulty arises in the case in which a patient's illness requires treatment by extraordinary means, or in cases of incurable illness or old-age. In cases of this type, one may ask whether the doctor is obliged to go beyond the use of ordinary means and employ also the extraordinary means in order to conserve his patient's life and health. Thus, we come to the doctor's obligation of using the extraordinary means of conserving life when he is treating a patient.

---

[389]McFadden, op. cit., p. 151.

[390]Davis, op. cit., II, p. 127.

[391]«Etsi vero medicus curam aegroti ex sola caritate assumpsit, tamen ad diligentiam ordinariam tenetur ex justitia stricta».—Hürth, *De Statibus,* p. 107.

[392]*Code of Ethical and Religious Directives for Catholic Hospitals* (St. Louis, The Catholic Hospital Association of the United States and Canada, 1949), p. 5. In the current Catholic directives, entitled *Ethical and Religious Directives for Catholic Health Facilities,* as approved by the National Conference of Catholic Bishops as the national code "subject to the approval of the bishop for use in the diocese," November, 1971, the phrase above is found in Directive No. 28.

2) The doctor's obligation of employing the extraordinary means of conserving life

It might appear at first glance that the doctor's obligation of employing the means of conserving life is coextensive with the patient's obligation of using these means. A deeper investigation of this problem, however, reveals that this opinion is not complete. Father Kelly writes in this regard:

> It is easy to show that this statement is inaccurate. The patient is *per se* obliged to use only those means which are ordinary and which offer a reasonable hope of success. But he may use other means and if he reasonably wishes to use them the relatives and physicians are strictly obliged to carry out his wish.[393]

The patient and the doctor are bound to use ordinary means. The patient can refuse to use extraordinary means. If, however, the patient chooses to employ the extraordinary means of conserving his life, the doctor has no choice but to follow the patient's wishes. Hence, we can see that in determining the doctor's obligation to employ the extraordinary means, the first step is to ascertain the patient's own desires in this regard. In the last analysis, it is the patient who has the right to say whether or not he intends to use the extraordinary means of conserving life. Therefore, the patient's refusal to accept the extraordinary means immediately releases the doctor from any obligation of employing these means. However, when the patient desires the use of extraordinary means, the situation is different.

Before we attempt to determine the doctor's obligation when the patient desires the use of extraordinary means, it will be helpful to have the following distinctions in mind. 1) *The patient accepted ex caritate and the patient to whom the doctor is bound ex justitia to assist.* This distinction has been sufficiently explained earlier in this chapter. 2) *The expressed request of the patient (explicit or implicit) and his unknown desire.* The patient can expressly request the use of extraordinary means, either explicitly himself or through others, or implicitly by his general attitude in regard to caring for his health. Perhaps, however, his desire of using or not using extraordinary means is entirely unknown. For example, he may be unconscious or delirious. 3) *Absolute extraordinary means and relative extraordinary means.* The absolute extraordinary means are considered morally impossible for all men. The relative extraordinary means are those means

---

[393]Kelly, «The Duty of Using Artificial Means of Preserving Life», p. 216.

which are extraordinary either for the patient alone, or for the patient and doctor both. 4) *Useful extraordinary means and useless extraordinary means.* The former give definite hope of proportionate success and benefit, whereas the latter do not.

Case I

The first possibility is the case which involves a patient ex caritate, who needs extraordinary means to conserve his life. He requests the doctor to employ these means. In this case, if the extraordinary means are absolute extraordinary means, the doctor is not bound to employ them in order to conserve the life of the patient. There is no obligation in charity to do for others what one is not obliged to do to save his own life.[394] If the extraordinary means is extraordinary relative only to the patient (for example, an operation that is extraordinary by reason of the extreme pain that it causes to the patient), and will be of benefit to the patient, then the doctor is bound to employ such a means. The reason is that charity demands that one assist his neighbor in extreme need even at the cost of serious inconvenience to one's self. However, if this means of conserving life is useless, or if it will be of benefit to the patient but will cause a proportionately grave inconvenience to the doctor, then the doctor is not obliged to supply the means. The doctor need not supply a useless means because no one is bound to use what is useless. The doctor is excused in the second case because we are not bound in charity to employ extraordinary measures to help our neighbor when this is a source of proportionately grave inconvenience to us. This is true, even if the means will be of benefit to our neighbor.

The particular obligation of charity to the poor can present even a more specialized problem for the doctor. Imagine the case of a poor man for whom a necessary medical treatment is an extraordinary means by reason of the expense involved. The poor man requests the treatment. In this case, if the doctor can supply the treatment without a proportionately grave inconvenience to himself, he is obliged to supply it. However, a proportionately grave personal inconvenience would excuse him from his obligation. Hence, «a surgeon need not perform an extraordinary operation gratis.»[395]

---

[394]Jone-Adelman, op. cit., p. 87, n. 141.
[395]Loc. cit.

Case II

The second possibility involves the patient ex caritate who needs an extraordinary means to conserve his life. His desires, even implicit, however, in regard to the use of the extraordinary means are unknown. Is the doctor bound to use these extraordinary means?

If the means will not be of benefit to the patient, the doctor's obligation extends only to the use of ordinary means and he need not employ the extraordinary means. However, if the means would be of proportionate benefit to the patient, the doctor should make a reasonable attempt to determine whether or not the patient would desire the use of extraordinary means. After this investigation, if the doctor believes that the patient would want the extraordinary means, then the doctor should follow the norms given in *Case I*. If however, it is entirely unknown what the patient himself would want, and this cannot be determined, then the doctor's duty of charity does not bind him to employ the extraordinary means, even though such means would be of benefit to the patient. We are not bound in charity to force a neighbor to save his life by means which he personally is not bound to use to save his own life. A doctor who would use extraordinary means to save a person's life when the doctor has not ascertained the patient's own wishes, would be in effect forcing the patient to use means which the patient himself is not morally obligated to use.

Case III

The third possibility involves the patient *ex justitia* who reasonably wishes the use of an extraordinary means to conserve his life. In this case, the doctor is strictly obliged to carry out the patient's wish. We may phrase the obligation of the doctor in the case of a patient *ex justitia* this way. The doctor is obliged to supply those means which the patient is bound to use and reasonably wants to use.[396]

Case IV

The fourth possibility involves the patient *ex justitia* who needs an extraor-

---

[396]Cf. Paquin, op. cit., p. 402.

dinary means to conserve his life. It is unknown, however, whether or not he wishes to use this extraordinary means.

Since the doctor is unable to ascertain the patient's own wishes in the matter, he should make a reasonable effort to determine what the patient's wish would be if the patient personally could respond. In the event that relatives are present, they should try to make the decision in the name of the patient, and the doctor is obliged to follow their wishes. If there are present no relatives nor persons entrusted with the care of the patient's welfare, then it is up to the doctor to make the decision. His obligation in justice to the patient binds him to take reasonable care of the patient. He must consider the spiritual, physical, financial and social condition of the patient. Perhaps, the doctor will require the aid of others in making this consideration, but in the last analysis, it is the doctor's duty to do what he thinks will bring about the greater good of the patient. If the doctor judges that the use of extraordinary means is not the better course to take, then he should feel free in conscience to follow out his judgment.

Quite often, it is the doctor alone who really can judge the benefit of using an extraordinary means anyway. Even when the patient is able to make the decision, he is not always capable of it either because of lack of knowledge or emotional upset. The relatives and friends may be disturbed; they may lack good judgment; they may shun the responsibility of making the decision. The doctor can be level-headed in a situation where the patient or relatives of the patient may not be. If the patient and relatives rely on the doctor's judgment when they *themselves* are responsible for the decision, then the doctor should make a reasonable judgment and feel free to follow it, when *he alone* is responsible. The failure to use extraordinary means when the doctor judges this the better course of action is not euthanasia. The doctor, having considered the aspects of the problem reasonably and conscientiously, should feel that he has satisfied his duty in charity and justice to his patient. He has satisfied also his oath to « . . . use treatment to help the sick according to my ability and judgment . . . »[397]

There are cases in which the doctor does not experience too much difficulty in deciding what he should do. The moral issues are clear. For example, Father Connell mentions the following case and gives a solution with which moralists and doctors would agree:

If the child whose physical constitution is so defective that he will grow up to be a drivelling idiot is seriously ill with pneumonia, the physician must employ the most effective remedies he

---

[397]Cf. the Hippocratic Oath in McFadden, op. cit., p. 456.

knows in order to cure him, provided they can be reckoned as ordinary means. There is no obligation to use extraordinary remedies to preserve a life so hampered. Thus, if this child needed a very difficult and delicate operation, which only a specialist could perform, in order to prolong its life, there would be no obligation on the parents or on the doctor to provide such an operation.[398]

However, the doctor, forced to make a decision personally, can find himself involved in a situation more complicated than the one which Father Connell describes. In his doctoral dissertation, *Catholic Teaching on the Morality of Euthanasia*, Father Sullivan gives the following case.[399] A patient is dying of cancer. He is in extreme pain and drugs no longer offer him any extended relief from the pain because he has developed a «toleration» of any drug given him. Since the disease is incurable, and the patient is slowly dying, the doctor wants to stop the intravenous feeding in order to end the suffering. The doctor believes that otherwise, since the patient has a good heart, he will linger on for several weeks in agony. He therefore stops the intravenous feeding and the patient dies. A similar case is presented by Father Donovan in the *Homiletic and Pastoral Review.*[400] Neither author specifically mentions whether or not the patient is conscious, or whether or not there are relatives who can make the choice. In his reply, Father Sullivan says:

Since the cancer patient is beyond all hope of recovery and suffering extreme pain, intravenous feeding should be considered an extraordinary means of prolonging life. The physician was justified in stopping the intravenous feeding. He should make sure first, however, that the patient is spiritually prepared.[401]

Contrary to this opinion, Father Donovan writes:

I fear that to neglect intravenous feedings is a form of mercy killing rather than a means of sustaining life that is morally impossible to use. Here is a cancerous person given three months to live, and he cannot be nourished except by intravenous means, is he therefore to be let starve to death, even if he is willing?[402]

---

[398]Connell, op. cit., p. 121.

[399]Sullivan, op. cit., p. 72.

[400]J. Donovan, «Question Box», *Homiletic and Pastoral Review*, XLIX (August, 1949), p. 904.

[401]Sullivan, loc. cit.

[402]Donovan, loc. cit.

Father Sullivan has carefully mentioned many conditions in his presentation of the case. It would seem, therefore, that the intravenous feeding is an extraordinary means for the cancerous patient concerned. Even in the situation related by Father Donovan, it would be licit to consider the intravenous feeding an extraordinary means of conserving life. However, recall that we based our definition of ordinary and extraordinary means on the relative norm. In the presumption, therefore, that a doctor alone has the responsibility to make a decision in a particular case, he should consider all the conditions of the patient, because intravenous feeding cannot be called an ordinary means of conserving life, *absolutely speaking,* even though according to a *general norm,* it may be an ordinary means for most men.

If, after due consideration of the particular case before him, the doctor decides that the intravenous feeding is an extraordinary means for the patient concerned, he should then follow out the norms we have given above for the doctor's use of extraordinary means in the treatment of patients. Cases of this nature must be solved in individual instances after prudent consideration of the condition of the patient concerned. General norms are guides and helps, not the definitive solutions of each similar case. The doctor must use great prudence, but he must also feel free to follow out his considered judgment. Euthanasia is illicit and intrinsically evil. However, prolonging a patient's life by an extraordinary means, when all that the doctor can do to cure the person has been done, is not the only morally justifiable alternative. It is licit *per se* to refrain from using an extraordinary means of conserving life.

Even more intricate than the cases just mentioned is the problem presented by Father Ford, S. J. in his article on the refusal of blood transfusions by Jehovah's Witnesses. We have seen that Father Ford rightly judges blood transfusions as extraordinary means for Jehovah's Witnesses. Since blood transfusions are extraordinary means in such cases, they are not obligatory. Father Ford then makes this application to the doctor's obligation in the matter:

> The consequence of this opinion for the physician is obvious. Where the patient is not morally obliged, objectively to make use of a procedure, and actually refuses it, the physician is not morally obliged to give it to him; nor do the hospital administrators have a moral obligation to see that he gets it.[403]

Father Ford next discusses the doctor's position when faced with the care of child who needs a transfusion, but whose parents are Jehovah's Witnesses.

---

[403]Ford, « The Refusal of Blood Transfusions by Jehovah's Witnesses », p. 7.

Must the doctor regard the blood transfusion as an extraordinary means for this child, even as he would consider it such for the child's parents? Is it licit for the doctor to refrain from giving the transfusion in such a case? Or, must the the doctor consider the transfusion as ordinary means, as it is for most men, according to the general norm? Is the doctor, therefore, bound to give the blood transfusion to the child of Jehovah's Witnesses? Father Ford replies:

> In this case of a young child, therefore, it would be morally wrong to make an agreement not to administer a transfusion in cases of serious need; and if such an agreement were made, one would have no obligation to honor it. The obligation of physicians and others who have actually undertaken to care for the child would ordinarily be an obligation of justice as well as charity. Others who have not actually undertaken the care of the child might have an obligation of charity to intervene in order to see to it that a neglected child is properly cared for.[404]

Father Ford adds, however, that many factors must be considered which could render quite difficult the possibility of the doctor's carrying out his obligation in this regard. Hence, this author notes further: «after all his (the doctor's) legal position is far from clear; and it is no small matter to undertake a surgical procedure on a young child contrary to the express refusal of the parents to allow it».[405]

3) Additional Factors to be Considered in Determining the Doctor's Obligation of Employing the Extraordinary Means

Father Ford's consideration of the doctor's legal position leads directly to our next point. Up till now, we have been treating of the doctor's obligation merely from the aspect of his duty in charity or or justice or both to his patient. We have seen his obligation of charity to his neighbor in general, and to the poor in particular. We have also seen his obligation in virtue of the patient-physician contract, namely a duty in justice. However, a question arises as to whether or not the doctor's complete duty in the matter of using the extraordinary means of conserving life is sufficiently explained merely from his moral obligations of charity and justice in regard to his patient. Are the moral obligations of charity and justice to the patient the only obligations that bind a doctor in this matter?

---

[404]Ibid., p. 8.
[405]Ibid., p. 9, parentheses mine.

Father Kelly, S. J. in his writings on medical ethics, has emphasized, on more than one occasion, the need of considering the doctor's professional ideal whenever we discuss the doctor's obligation of using the extraordinary means of conserving life when he is treating a patient. Father Kelly first makes reference to this point in his article, «The Duty of Using Artificial Means of Preserving Life», when he writes:

> As for the physicians, there may be another, and perhaps more important difference. I have spoken of this matter occasionally with very conscientious physicians, and I have found that they consistently express a professional ideal to the effect that they must use all means in their power to sustain life, and that they must use any remedy which offers any hope, even a slight hope, of cure or relief . . . I do not know how common this professional ideal is. But from my own experience with physicians and from many recent statements of the medical profession against euthanasia I would conclude that it is very common among conscientious physicians.[406]

In a later article in *Theological Studies*, «The Duty to Preserve Life», Father Kelly writes more at length on the same subject—namely, the suggestion that the physician's professional ideal may create obligations that extend beyond the duties and wishes of the patient.[407] This last article is reprinted substantially in another article written by the same author in *Medico-Moral Problems*, «The Extraordinary Means of Prolonging Life».[408] The influence of Father Kelly's writing on theological discussions of this subject cannot be denied. He has emphasized the need of investigating the duty that arises for the doctor from his obligations to the common good and his professional ideal and standard.

The subject of the doctor's duty to conserve life by extraordinary means was brought up and discussed at the 1952 meeting of the Catholic Theological Society of America in Notre Dame, Indiana. Father John Goodwine, writing in *Proceedings*, reports on the seminar discussion had at that time.[409] He notes that it was generally felt by those present that «the physician-patient contract

---

[406]Kelly, «The Duty of Using Artificial Means of Preserving Life», pp. 216–217.

[407]Kelly, «The Duty to Preserve Life», pp. 550–556. Fr. Kelly does not state whether he considers this an obligation in the *strict sense* or merely a professional preference.

[408]Kelly, *Medico-Moral Problems*, V, pp. 11–15.

[409]J. Goodwine, «The Physician's Duty to Preserve Life by Extraordinary Means», *Proceedings of the Seventh Annual Convention* (The Catholic Theological Society of America, 1952), pp. 125–138.

alone is not sufficient to explain the obligation which physicians feel is theirs, viz., to do more than use ordinary life-saving means».[410] This author then notes that «it is extremely difficult to find a definite and clear statement of the duties physicians owe to their profession».[411]

In order to obtain some idea of what possible obligations may be binding on the doctor in virtue of his duty to the common good and his profession, Father Kelly has recourse to the medical profession itself. He has examined the ideals which conscientious doctors themselves enunciate. From his findings, Father Kelly has been able to group these ideals under two standards. One he calls the «strict professional standard» and the other, the «moderate standard».[412] The first group believes that «the doctor's duty is to preserve life as long as he can, by any means at his disposal, and no matter how hopeless the case seems to be.»[413] These doctors think that «. . . insofar as the judgment is left to the doctor himself he must simply keep trying to prolong life right to the very end».[414] The moderate standard is embraced by those doctors who:

> . . . try to effect a cure as long as there is any reasonable hope of doing so; they try to preserve life as long as the patient himself can reap any tangible benefits from the prolongation. But they also think there is a point when such efforts become futile gestures; and they believe that at this point the sole duty of the doctor is to see that the patient gets good nursing care and that his pain is alleviated.[415]

The strict standard certainly avoids any type of «euthanasia mentality.» However, Father Kelly notes that the moderate standard has many good features: 1) it is consistent with the policy of the theologians by which they place a reasonable limit on obligations; 2) it is in harmony with the «good Christian attitude» toward life and death; 3) it is less likely to burden the relatives of the patient with excessive strain and expense.[416]

Since the publication of the above-mentioned articles, a very significant statement has appeared in print. Dr. A. E. Clark-Kennedy delivered the in-

---

[410]Ibid., p. 133.
[411]Ibid., p. 134.
[412]Kelly, *Medico-Moral Problems*, V, pp. 12–13.
[413]Loc. cit.
[414]Ibid., p. 13.
[415]Loc. cit.
[416]Ibid., pp. 13–14.

augural address at the opening meeting of the 218th Session of the Royal Medical Society of Edinburgh and this address is reprinted under the title, «Medicine in Relation to Society», in the British *Medical Journal*. In this address, Dr. Clark-Kennedy says:

> Now, it is always easier to perform a palliative operation or put the patient on deep x-ray treatment or chemotherapy; easier, in fact, to do something than to do nothing. Some course of action will probably relieve his immediate symptoms, and often it prolongs his life. It will raise hopes and sometimes clear the bed for the admission of another case for whom more might be done. But what happens to the patient in the end? . . . The Roman Catholic doctor in dealing with his Roman Catholic patient has firm guidance from his Church in these matters, and some may hold the view that it is always our duty to prolong life so far as is possible, but my experience teaches me that most of the non-Catholic laity would, if they knew the truth, wish doctors to exercise more moral courage than in point of fact is, I think, their practice in these situations. If the patient or his relatives really could be told the facts, they would have their doctor withhold treatment when «the game is up», and let nature take its course . . . It is written «Thou shalt not kill». But letting nature take its course when nature cannot be stopped is not killing. Nor in my judgment is a patient committing suicide when he refuses palliative or problematical, as opposed to a reasonably certainly curative, medical or surgical treatment. Never before in the history of medicine has it been so important to remember Clough's oft-quoted rider . . . . « But needst not strive officiously to keep alive» . . . If I really thought that I was either under a moral obligation to keep all my patients alive as long as possible, or under a legal obligation always to apply the textbook treatment for the textbook disease, I would give up medicine to-morrow![417]

The statement indicates the vexation that besets the doctor when he faces the problem of prolonging a patient's life. Dr. Clark-Kennedy betrays a lack of complete understanding of the Catholic teaching in this matter; the Catholic Church does not demand that the doctor preserve life as long as possible.

---

[417]A. E. Clark-Kennedy, «Medicine in relation to Society», *British Medical Journal*, March 12, 155, pp. 620– 621.

However, the Doctor has very skillfully presented a legitimate problem; a problem which at times can be very disturbing to the physician. Science has progressed in the treatment of some diseases—only far enough, however, to prolong the patient's life, not cure the disease. Dr. Clark-Kennedy's statement also reveals that evidently there is no agreement among doctors themselves as to a course of action which might be called a general rule in this matter.

A similar statement has been made by an American general practitioner. Dr. Francis T. Hodges of San Francisco, California writes:

> The hopelessly ill patient need not, through a distorted sense of professional duty, be subjected to heroic and extraordinary measures, whose only purpose can be prolongation of an existence that has become intolerable. But it must be the patient himself who declines the measures . . . Let us sense those times when we must not reach into the bottom of our medicine bags for agents to whip into a body tired unto death a final, additionally exhausting further fight against death, a death for which the patient is already prepared . . . There are times when the patient has legal, ethical, moral and religious justification of his request to be allowed to die in peace.[418]

The medical profession itself realizes the problem, but «as yet there is no clear-cut professional standard regarding . . . the 'fine points' of care of the dying».[419] The medical profession may very well look to the moralists for the answer, just as Father Kelly has consulted doctors in order to attempt an appreciation of their ideals. However, when this problem of the doctor's obligation (arising from his duty to his profession and the common good) of using extraordinary means was discussed at the seventh meeting of the Catholic Theological Society of America, «it was generally felt that until more is known about the doctor's obligation to society no satisfactory and clear-cut statement of their duty to use extraordinary means can be drawn up».[420] Father Kelly notes that «among moral theologians a somewhat similar condition prevails; up to a certain point duties are clear and there is agreement on what must be done; beyond that point the rules of obligation become obscure and there is room for differences of opinion».[421]

---

[418]Dr. Francis T. Hodges, quoted in *Time*, (Atlantic ed.), January 9, 1956, p. 31.
[419]Kelly, *Medico-Moral Problems*, V, p. 14.
[420]J. Goodwine, op. cit., p. 138.
[421]Kelly, *Medico-Moral Problems*, V, p. 14.

Conceivably, the doctor may believe that the advancement of medical science requires him to do all in his power to prolong life and to attempt a cure even though at the time, all seems hopeless. Confronted with an apparently hopeless case, the doctor realizes that even the present advances of science do not enable him to cure his patient. Certainly, ordinary means will not cure the patient; perhaps even extraordinary means will not effect a cure. Yet, the doctor senses the ignominy of giving into death and he finds himself constrained to fight the disease to the best of his ability, perhaps even by employing insufficiently tested methods and procedures. He realizes that medical knowledge has grown over the years and in great measure this has been due to experience with patients. Hence, the doctor is not content to let his patient refuse the extraordinary means of conserving life. To do so, he considers a betrayal of his duty to the furthering of medical science.

Furthermore, the doctor may be confronted with a patient whose life he could almost surely save if the patient would accede to the use of extraordinary means. The doctor believes though that agreement with the patient's wishes is euthanasia and therefore, contrary to his professional oath and ideal.

Yet the doctor must realize that although the advancement of medical knowledge is good in itself, there are other factors that must be considered. The conquest of medical problems is not the only duty of the doctor. He has the primary duty of *treating the patient* lying before him—that human being weak with illness who wants his help and his services, but who perhaps does not want health at the price of using clearly extraordinary measures. The advancement of medicine is a worthy motive, but it is a motive clearly limited, and it can never justify the doctor's forcing a patient to the use of extraordinary means of conserving his life.

The doctor must use the ordinary means of conserving life. He must also use those extraordinary means which the patient wants to use. He must continually study and attempt to find a remedy to the disease which afflicts his patient, but he must also remember that his prime duty is to his patient, not to his profession. Hence, any extraordinary procedure which the patient refuses, or which the doctor believes the patient would refuse if he were able to understand the problem more competently, is not obligatory for the doctor because it is not obligatory for the patient, and the advancement of science or the doctor's professional ideal does not change that fact.

The duty of conservation of a patient's life rests primarily with the patient himself. Since the patient is not morally obligated to use an extraordinary means, it seems highly unlikely that a doctor's profession can make him force the use of an extraordinary means on a patient. Clearly too, the non-use of extraordinary means, when the patient refuses them, is not euthanasia.

This same manner of thinking must guide the doctor in treating a patient who cannot make a decision in regard to the use of extraordinary means, and who has no one to make the choice for him. The doctor should judge the case reasonably and decide what will effect the greater good for the patient and then act accordingly. But he should never judge that an unconscious patient, or a charity patient, or a mentally ill patient, whose lives are in extreme danger, should be given treatment by extraordinary measures merely for the advancement of scientific and medical knowledge, or because he believes his professional ideal requires him to fight death right to the end. The doctor should treat the patient, not just the disease. Euthanasia is illicit, but so also is surreptitious experimentation carried on by using extraordinary means of conserving life without the consent of the patient.

The doctor may also believe that the common good requires him to employ the extraordinary means of conserving his patient's life. However, the doctor must remember that while it is incumbent on all to work for the common good, in this problem we are dealing with the question of a man's life. The prime responsibility for the conservation of one's life rests with the individual. The individual, per accidens, may be peculiarly necessary for the common good, and thus, be bound to conserve his life even by using extraordinary means. In this case, the doctor would be bound to employ these extraordinary means. However, when the common good does not demand that the patient himself use the extraordinary means of conserving life, it is difficult to see how the doctor can be bound, on account of the common good, to employ extraordinary means when he is treating this same individual.

Father Paquin writes:

> It is evident that the doctor must avoid the appearance of negative euthanasia, that he ought to avoid giving the impression of letting his patients die. But it is not opposed to the common good that a doctor, in certainly incurable cases, cease costly treatments which have no other effect than to prolong for a while a life, at times, already unconscious.[422]

In practice, therefore, a doctor should take his norm from the obligations of the patient himself. The doctor must employ the ordinary means of con-

---

[422] « Il est évident que le médecin doit éviter l'apparence de l'euthanasie négative, qu'il doit éviter de donner l'impression de laisser mourir ses malades. Mais le bien commun ne s'oppose pas à ce qu'un médecin, dans des cas certainement incurables, cesse des traitements couteux qu n'auraient pas d'autre effet que de prolonger très peu une vie parfois déjà inconsciente ».— Paquin, op. cit., p. 402.

serving life and then those extraordinary means which, *per accidens,* are obligatory for the patient or which the patient wants to use. He must never practice euthanasia and he must conscientiously strive never to give the impression of using euthanasia. Furthermore, he must strive to find a remedy for the disease. However, when the time comes that he can conserve his patient's life only by extraordinary means, he must consider the patient's wishes, expressed or reasonably interpreted and abide by them. If the patient is incurable and even ordinary means, according to the *general norm,* have become extraordinary for this patient, again the wishes of the patient expressed or reasonably interpreted must be considered and obeyed. Father Kelly gives this practical norm:

> When a doctor and his consultants have sincerely judged that a patient is incurable, the decision concerning further treatment should be in terms of the patient's own interest and reasonable wishes, expressed or implied. Proper treatment certainly includes the use of all natural means of preserving life (food, drink, etc.), good nursing care, appropriate measures to relieve physical and mental pain, and the opportunity of preparing for death. Since the professional standards of conscientious physicians vary somewhat regarding the use of further means, such as artificial life-sustainers, the doctor should feel free in conscience to use or not use these things, according to the circumstances of each case. In general, it may be said that he has no moral obligation to use them unless they offer the hope of some real benefit to his patient without imposing a disproportionate inconvenience on others, or unless, by reason of special conditions, failure to use such means would reflect unfavorably on his profession.[423]

The common good and a doctor's professional ideal do oblige him to keep trying to find a remedy for disease. What we have said about the doctor's obligation to follow the wishes of the patient is, therefore, not to be interpreted as a hindrance to further medical knowledge. Hence, a doctor should not interpret this teaching as being opposed to the trial of new medical procedures or cures. Within certain limits, it is licit to attempt a cure with extraordinary means—even though they be entirely new. As a matter of fact, such a method of action oftentimes redounds to the good of the patient himself. Pope Pius XII, speaking on September 13, 1952, to the First International Con-

---

[423]Kelly, *Medico-Moral Problems,* V, pp. 14–15.

gress on the Histopathology of the Nervous System, said in regard to this point:

Without doubt, before the employment of new methods can be morally permitted, one cannot demand that every danger and every risk be excluded. This goes beyond human possibilities; it would paralyze all serious scientific research and would return, very often, to the detriment of the patient. The estimate of the danger ought to be left in these cases to the judgment of the experienced and competent doctor. There exists, nonetheless, and Our explanations have demonstrated it, a series of dangers which morality cannot allow to be caused. It can happen in some dubious cases, all known means having failed, that a new method, still insufficiently tested, will offer, besides the very dangerous elements, good probability of success. If the sick person gives his assent, the application of the procedure in question is licit. But this manner of procedure cannot be established as the norm of conduct for normal cases.[424]

Here again, we note that an essential factor in this problem is the necessity of obtaining the patient's consent. A doctor may use a new method when all known and sure methods have failed, provided that the new method offers some good probability of success and provided that the patient freely consents to the use of the new method. Furthermore, it is necessary to emphasize that the doctor must make the patient fully apprised of the risk and dangers involved in the new procedure before he obtains the patient's consent. If the patient refuses to submit to the new cure or the new medical procedure, then neither the doctor's professional ideal nor the common good requires him to employ such a new cure or procedure.

---

[424]« Sans doute, avant d'autoriser en morale l'emploi de nouvelles méthodes, on ne peut exiger que tout danger, tout risque soient exclus. Cela dépasse les possibilités humaines, paralyserait toute recherche scientifique serieuse, et tournerait tr'es souvent au détriment du patient. L'appréciation du danger doit être laissée dans ces cas au judement du médecin expérimenté et compétent. Il y a cependant, Nos explications l'ont montré, un degré de danger que la morale ne peut permettre. Il peut arriver, dans des cas douteux, quand échouent les moyens déjà connus, qu'une méthode nouvelle, encore insuffisamment éprouvée, offre, à côté d'éléments très dangereu, des chances appréciables de succès. Si le patient donne son accord, l'application du procédé en question est licite. Mais cette manière de faire ne peut être érigée en ligne de conduite pour les cas normaux ».—Pius XII, « Address to the First International Congress on the Histopathology of the Nervous System ». The original text is taken from *Discorsi e Radiomessaggi di Sua Santità Pio XII* (Typographia Polyglotta Vaticana, 1953), XIV, pp. 329-330.

The doctor, therefore, stands between his patient and his profession. In the last analysis, however, it is his patient that should be his prime concern. The doctor should treat the human being. He should reasonably judge what will bring about the greater good for his patient in accordance with his professional ideal and the patient's wishes and then the doctor should feel free to follow out his judgment.

CONCLUSIONS AND RESUMÉ

1) God retains the radical possession of the rights over man's life. Man has full rights to the *use* of his life but to this only. Hence, any form of non-conservation of self, directly intended by an individual on his own authority, is illicit.

2) Likewise, man has the serious positive obligation of caring for his bodily life and health.

3) It is possible that an individual could be invincibly ignorant, for a time, of this obligation but certainly not for any extended length of time. However, it is possible that one might realize his obligation to conserve his life, but err in the practical application of the obligation to his status here and now.

4) There is no licit application of epikeia in this matter. Neither is a dispensation possible. However, an individual could receive the command from God to take his own life by some form of non-conservation of self. In such a case, the individual would then have permission to exercise a faculty ordinarily reserved as a divine prerogative.

5) The obligation to conserve one's life, being an affirmative precept of the natural law, does not require fulfillment under all circumstances. Hence, a moral impossibility would excuse.

6) The means to fulfil this precept of self-conservation are obligatory. Those means binding everyone in common circumstances are ordinary means. Those means involving a moral impossibility are extraordinary means.

7) There is a clear distinction between *natural* means of conserving life and *artificial* means of conserving life, Natural means of conserving life are *per se* intended by nature as the basic means whereby man is to conserve his life, whereas artificial means of conserving life are *per se* intended by nature as a means whereby man can *supplement* the natural means of conserving life. Both the natural means and the artificial means of conserving life are obligatory if they are *ordinary* means of conserving life.

8) There is a clear distinction between the terms, «ordinary means of conserving life» and «ordinary medical procedures» what is clearly an ordinary medical procedure is not necessarily an ordinary means of conserving life, in the theological sense.

9) The elements used by the moralists in their descriptions of the term, «ordinary means» are: spes salutis, media communia, secundum proportionem status, media non difficilia, and media facilia.

10) The elements used by the moralists in their descriptions of the term, «extraordinary means» are: quaedam impossibilitas, summus labor, media nimis dura, quidam cruciatus, sumptus extraordinarius, media pretiosa, ingens dolor, vehemens horror, and media exquisita.

11) A *relative norm* suffices in determining a means as an ordinary or an extraordinary means of conserving life.

12) There is no *absolute norm* according to which certain means of conserving life are clearly *ordinary* for all men. A relative norm must be applied.

13) It does seem that an *absolute norm* can be established according to which certain means of conserving life are clearly *extraordinary* means of conserving life.

14) It would be allowable to establish a *general norm* in regard to *ordinary* means, by which certain means of conserving life are characterized as ordinary means of conserving life for most men.

15) *Ordinary means of conserving life* may be defined as those means commonly used in given circumstances, which this individual in his present physical, psychological, and economic condition can reasonably employ with definite hope of proportionate benefit.

16) *Extraordinary means of conserving life* may be defined as those means not commonly used in given circumstances, or those means in common use which this individual in his present physical, psychological and economic condition cannot reasonably employ, or if he can, will not give him definite hope of proportionate benefit.

17) Ordinary means of conserving life, understood according to the above definition, are always morally obligatory.

18) Extraordinary means of conserving life, *per se* are not morally obligatory, however, *per accidens,* a particular individual may be bound to employ such means.

19) Even though advances in the field of medical science have reduced greatly the risk involved in surgical interventions, nonetheless, the element of risk must still be considered today in determining surgical procedures as ordinary and extraordinary means, particularly in cases involving patients of advanced age and weakened physical condition.

20) From the aspect of operating technique alone: *a*) common surgical interventions, even though major surgical interventions, performed on patients of young age and relatively strong physical constitution, and in surroundings which offer the advantages of modern hospital skill, precautions and equipment are *generally* ordinary means of conserving life. *b*) Major surgical interventions, even though common surgical interventions, performed on patients of advanced age or of relatively weak constitution, cannot be classed *generally* as ordinary means of conserving life. *c*) Major surgical interventions, even though common surgical interventions, performed on the young or the old in surroundings which do not offer the advantages of modern hospital skill, precautions and equipment cannot be classed *generally* as ordinary means of conserving life. *d*) Radical surgery which involves great risk and danger, or which is still insufficiently known is an extraordinary means of conserving life both for the young and the old.

21) The amputation of a leg probably remains an extraordinary means of conserving life, due to subjective abhorrence. This is certainly true in the case of the amputation of both legs.

22) The basic medicines, intravenous feedings, insulin, the many types of antibiotics, oxygen masks and tents, preventative medicines and vaccines, and blood transfusions are *generally* ordinary means of conserving life.

23) *Per se*, the doctor has the obligation of using the ordinary means of conserving life when he treats a patient *ex caritate* or *ex justitia*. A proportionately grave inconvenience excuses from this obligation.

24) The doctor must employ the extraordinary means of conserving life which the patient, accepted *ex justitia*, is bound to employ or reasonably wishes the doctor to use.

25) Extraordinary means must be used by the doctor in the case of the patient *ex caritate* who needs and wishes such measures, provided the doctor can furnish them without a proportionately grave inconvenience to himself.

26) If the wishes of a patient *ex caritate* in regard to the use of extraordinary means are entirely unknown and a reasonable investigation will not reveal these wishes, the doctor need not employ the extraordinary means of conserving life.

27) If the wishes of a patient *ex justitia* in regard to the use of extraordinary means are entirely unknown and cannot be determined after a reasonable investigation, the doctor, in virtue of his contract with the patient, should make a prudent decision in this regard in the name of the patient which will effect the greater good for the patient.

28) The doctor should feel free in conscience to use or neglect, according to the circumstances of each case, relatively useless artificial life-sustainers.

29) The doctor does not have the obligation of using all means in his

power to sustain life, nor does he have the obligation in all circumstances of prolonging life until such prolongation is no longer possible.

30) The doctor must try to effect a cure as long as there is any reasonable hope of doing so.

31) The doctor must try to find a remedy for disease. Hence, he may employ extraordinary means of conserving life, even hitherto insufficiently tested procedures, provided that all known and secure measures have failed, and the new procedure gives good probability of success and the doctor obtains the patient's consent.

Conserving Human Life

Part II

AN APPLICATION OF THE PRINCIPLES
AS PRESENTED AND DISCUSSED IN
PART I OF THIS BOOK

TO THE SUBJECT
OF

FEEDING THE HOPELESS AND THE HELPLESS

By MONSIGNOR ORVILLE N. GRIESE, STD, JCD
Director of Research, Pope John Center**

Feeding the Hopeless
and the Helpless

Introduction

Bishop Daniel Cronin begins this book with a chapter entitled "The Duty to Conserve Life," and emphasizes God's dominion over all mankind by quoting the following text from St. Paul's Epistle to the Romans (14:7 and 8):

> None of us lives as his own master and none of us dies as his own master. While we live we are responsible to the Lord, and when we die we die as his servants. Both in life and in death we are the Lord's.

The words of God's loyal servant Job (1:21), "The Lord gave and the Lord has taken away," refer also to physical life and death. No human individual has the right to challenge God's dominion by saying, "Let me starve to death!" (cf. also Wisdom, 16:13).

It is still against the law in the United States of America to commit suicide, or to help another in taking his or her own life. Within the past twenty years, however, U.S. courts have invoked the nebulous constitutional "right to privacy" to establish the right to use contraceptive devices (Griswold v. Connecticut, 1966), the right to have an abortion (Roe v. Wade, 1976), and the right to suicide (Bouvia, 1986). In the latter case, the concurring opinion of Judge Compton was worded as follows:

> The right to die is an integral part of our right to control our own destinies so long as the rights of others are not affected. That right should, in my opinion, include the ability to enlist assistance from others, including the medical profession, in making death as painless and quick as possible.[1]

Such an opinion would clash with the living will legislation in states throughout the nation. All thirteen of the living will laws passed in 1985, for example, do not allow the omission of nutrition and hydration.[2] It must be admitted, however, that there is evidence of a clear trend in the courts to accept starvation as a means of euthanasia. The "right to privacy" tactic has established a solid beachhead on the judicial front.

The most fundamental fallacy in the current campaign to justify the option of death by starvation is the claim that the patient who is in imminent danger of death has a right to make such a choice, or to empower others to make such a choice for him (her) when deprived of competency. It is axiomatic in hospital practice (as it should be) that the expressed wishes of the patient must prevail. This imperative is limited, however, by the phrase "within his rights." The basic truth is that no human individual has the right to terminate his own life or have others terminate his life at his request. This basic truth has been researched, discussed, established and corroborated so completely and effectively in Bishop Cronin's dissertation (now republished in this volume), that any effort to tamper with his scholarship would be an exercise in folly and in futility. Throughout this present study, Bishop Cronin's dissertation will be referred to as *Conserving Human Life*.

In order to avoid confusion and misunderstanding, it must be emphasized at the outset that the primary focus throughout this discussion is not on the *prolongation of life* (in the sense of the desire to add some years to an individual's allotted span of life beyond the ordinary course of life), but on the preservation or *conservation* of life from birth until natural death in the ordinary course of events. Bishop Cronin refers to an 18th century theologian, C. La Croix, who explains the difference between the two concepts by saying

---

[1]Cf. article by Edward R. Grant, J D, and Clarke D. Forsythe, J D, in the January, 1987 issue of *Issues In Law and Medicine*, p. 290.

[2]*Handbook of 1985 Living Will Laws* (New York, N.Y. :Society for the Right to Die, 1986), pp. 48–119. Note specific comments, pp. 6 and 16.

that the former (prolongation) implies efforts beyond the ordinary "to which we are not held," whereas the latter (conservation) implies a common or ordinary diligence "to which we are held." This author also portrays the concept of conservation of life as the "non-abbreviation" of life (*Conserving Human Life*, p. 62). Any needless shortening of life would be a violation of the fifth commandment: "Thou shall not kill."

In other words, all human individuals are obligated to use available common or ordinary means so as conserve or live out what might be called the "allotted span of years", without needlessly shortening that span in any way. No one is obligated, however, to strive anxiously to exceed that span. There would be no obligation, for example, to take up residence in a more favorable climate, or to shop around for the most unusual and nourishing foods and food supplements, or to take out an active membership in an athletic health club, or to travel far to obtain the services of the most outstanding physicians and surgeons, etc. This general guideline would apply even if the individual who is seeking these obvious health advantages is extremely wealthy, and well able to pay whatever price without neglecting financial obligations to his own family.

The first chapter of Bishop Cronin's dissertation entitled "The Duty to Conserve One's Life," constitutes a clear vindication of God's "radical possession of the rights over man's life," and also a most emphatic denial of any human individual's right to "any form of non-conservation of self, directly intended by an individual on his own authority" (*Ibid.*, p. 32). These conclusions are corroborated in chapter two (pp. 33–76) in a survey and analysis of opinions of theologians from the 13th century up to contemporary times. Chapter three (pp. 77–116) presents an enlightening discussion of "The nature of the ordinary and extraordinary means of conserving life, and the moral obligation of using these means . . . "(*Ibid.*, p. 77). Chapter four (pp. 117–152) explores further on the teaching of theologians on ordinary and extraordinary means, particularly with regard to modern medical and surgical procedures. it provides valuable guidance to physicians in arriving at decisions on ordinary and extraordinary means from an ethical viewpoint.

This fundamental point, therefore, on the lack of an individual's right to say "let me starve to death," or "help me starve to death," will not be pursued further in this study. As a matter of fact, the decision to append this discussion on the nutrition/hydration question to the publication of Bishop Cronin's dissertation was made in consideration of the *excellent foundation* for such a discussion as provided by Bishop Cronin's outstanding dissertation on the obligation of every individual to conserve his or her life. This fundamental truth, therefore, is accepted as already established and confirmed.

The following questions remain to be investigated in the survey of Church documents on the issue of providing nutrition and hydration to the needy and the helpless:

(1) Is it necessary to make a distinction between *medical treatments* and *ordinary nursing care*?
(2) Is the provision of nutrition and hydration included essentially in the concept of ordinary nursing care?
(3) Must nutrition and hydration be provided if the only alternative is to have recourse to some *artificial* means of feeding the patient.

If the answer to all of the questions stated above is in the affirmative (with proper modifying distinctions), it is logical to establish a general rule that nutrition and hydration must be provided to all sick individuals, including those who are in imminent danger of death due to a terminal condition or an irreversible condition. In other words, the obligation to continue to provide nutrition and hydration applies not only to those who are in a *hopeless* condition due to a terminal or irreversible condition and an imminent danger of death, but also to those who are in a *helpless* condition (but neither terminal nor in danger of death) due to advanced mental retardation, insanity, senility, etc. The three questions stated above will be pursued in an analysis of Church pronouncements on the subject. This will be followed by a discussion of possible exceptions to the general rule (Chapter II), and a discussion of the unique situation of patients who are permanently unconscious, but are neither terminal (in the strict sense of the word) nor in imminent danger of death (Chapter III).

CHAPTER I

Church Pronouncements on Feeding the Hopeless and the Helpless

The documents to be listed below represent various degrees of teaching authority. This factor will be resolved preliminary to the discussion of each pronouncement.

1.1 THE DECLARATION ON EUTHANASIA, CONGREGATION FOR THE DOCTRINE OF THE FAITH (Entire text presented in Appendix I of this book)

This document, which was approved personally by Pope John Paul II, constitutes the official position of the living magisterium of the Church on the subject of euthanasia and voluntary suicide. As such, it merits the "religious submission of will and mind" of every loyal Catholic as mentioned in Vatican II's *Dogmatic Constitution on the Church*) n. 25. Cf. also Canon 752, Code of Canon Law). Since the Declaration on Euthanasia originated from the Congregation for the Doctrine of the Faith, it shares the prestige of pronouncements such as papal encyclicals and responses of the Biblical Commission, as expressions of official Church doctrine.[3]

This important document is very clear with regard to the lack of any moral obligation to initiate or continue *medical treatments* which (when death is imminent and cannot be prevented by such measures) can yield only a precarious and painful prolongation of life." Unfortunately, one of the popular translations into English of that document failed to note the basic distinction in that document between *medical treatments* and *ordinary nursing care*. This translation rendered both phrases simply as "treatment".[4] The original Latin of the document compares with the proper English translation as follows:

LATIN (Italian in parentheses)

Imminente morte, quae remediis adhibitis nullo modo impediri potest, licet ex conscientia concilium inire *curationibus* (trattamenti) renuntiandi, quae nonnisi precariam et doloris plenam vitae dilationem afferre valent, haud intermissis tamen *ordinariis curis* (le cure normali) quae in similibus casibus aegroto debentur.[5]

ENGLISH Translation

When death is imminent and cannot be prevented by the remedies used, it is licit in conscience to decide to renounce *treatments* that can yield only a precarious and painful prolongation of life, but without interrupting in any way the *ordinary cares* which are due to the sick person in such cases.

Although the painful and precarious *prolongation* of life with regard to medical *treatments* in the circumstances mentioned above is not a moral imperative, the document is affirming, as a general rule, that *conserving* the life of the sick and the helpless is a binding moral obligation. The word "treatment" (*curatio, trattamenti*) implies that some relief from suffering, or some improvement in health, or even a cure of some significance is within the realm of possibility. When there is no longer any reasonable basis for such a hopeful prognosis, there is no longer any binding moral obligation for an individual who is in imminent danger of death to treasure the prolongation of life. At

---

[3]Cf. an article by Jesuit theologians John C.Ford and Gerald Kelly "Doctrinal Value and Interpretation of Papal Teachings," in *Moral Theology N.3*, Charles E. Curran and Richard A McCormick, S.J., eds. (New York, N.Y.: Paulist Press, 1982), pp. 4–5.

[4]This particular translation appeared in *The Pope Speaks*, 1980, p. 295.

[5]Cf. *Enchiridion Vaticanum*, VII (Bologna, Italy: Edizioni Dehoniane Bologna, 1982), n. 371, p.348. The date of issue was May 5, 1980. Cf.also a passage of Vatican II's document, *The Church Today*, n.69, which refers to the obligation of individuals and of groups to "feed the man dying of hunger, because if you have not fed him, you have killed him." This is mentioned as a "saying of the Fathers." A footnote traces the "saying" to the *Decree of Gratian*, and indicates that it was found even before the time of Gratian.

this critical juncture in life, faithful Christians are justified in saying with St. Paul: "We . . . would much rather be away from the body and at home with the Lord" (II Corinthians, 5:8). On the other hand, the phrase "ordinary care" (*ordinariae curae, le cure normali*) refers to the obligation, common to all members of the human race, to *conserve and sustain* their lives. There are circumstances when long-suffering individuals are justified in praying, in the spirit of the Book of Revelations, 22:20, "Come, Lord Jesus, take me now;" but no human mortal has the right to say: "Let me starve to death," or to expect others to take effective measures to that end.

Ordinary nursing care would include hygiene and cleanliness, comfort medications, warmth and proper temperature, TLC (tender, loving care) and, of course, the staff of life, nutrition and hydration. There is no logical basis for saying that the Declaration on Euthanasia does not include nutrition and hydration merely because those two items are not mentioned expressly. Surely "allowing nature to take its course" by denying food and drink to the sick and needy with death by starvation as the end result, is even more criminal than the reputed practice of some Eskimo tribes who deny warmth and TLC to ailing and aged members of the family by urging them to sit outside in the sub-zero cold to "allow nature to take its course" with the end result of death by freezing.

It is clear from the extensive survey and analysis of opinions of theologians from the thirteenth through the nineteenth centuries in Bishop Cronin's dissertation that those distinguished moralists rarely project the need of a distinction between *medical treatments* and *ordinary nursing care* (cf. pages 33–116). Hence it would appear that a terminal patient would have no obligation to take food and drink (and that others would have no obligation to provide it for the terminally ill) if eating and drinking afforded no positive hope of *conserving* life, or involved the procurement of unusual and uncommon foods, or if common foods could be procured only with excessive difficulty, etc. (cf. pages 85–111). In other words, eating and drinking in such circumstances would constitute an extraordinary means of conserving life (hence, non-obligatory) Typical of such a view is the following quotation from Dominican theologian, Francis de Vitoria (died 1546):

I would say . . . that if a sick man can take food or nourishment with a certain hope of conserving life (" . . . cum aliqua spe vitae . . ."), he is held to take the food, as he would be held to give it to one who is sick . . . One is not held to protect his life as much as he can by means of foods. This is clear because one is not held to use foods which are the best, the most delicate and most expensive, even though these foods are the most healthful, . . .

Likewise, one is not held to live in the most healthful place, therefore neither must he use the most healthful food . . . (cf. pp. 35–36)

It is not surprising to note that these theologians did not see the need of a distinction between treatments and ordinary nursing care. Throughout most of those centuries, hospital ministrations consisted mostly of providing food and drink, comfort medications and simple analgesics to the patients. Hospitals were designed as large enclosures with row upon row of beds for the poor, the sick and the needy. In 1198, for example, Pope Innocent III ordered the construction of a 200-bed hospital for "feeding daily a thousand poor." It was not until the 18th century that the trend in hospital design went from large wards to smaller rooms with just a few beds.[6] Except for repeated discussions of the obligation to submit to the painful removal of an arm or a leg, surgical treatments did not come into prominence until late in the 19th century when anesthetics (first used in Boston in 1849) gained acceptance as a standard means of providing painless surgery.

Another reason for not making a distinction between treatments and ordinary nursing care could be based on the tendency among theological scholars to simply repeat the opinion of a previous distinguished scholar; quoting, for example, St. Thomas Aquinas, or Francis de Vitoria, O.P., or Cardinal de Lugo, and later quoting the influential Busenbaum or the master moralist, St. Alphonse de Liguori. This tendency is noted well into the beginning of the 20th century. When invasive medical procedures such as kidney dialysis, brain surgery, resuscitation after cardiac or respiratory arrest, heart bypass, human organ transplants, etc. became standard in major health facilities throughout the land, however, theologians were equal to the challenge of providing a moral assessment of such wonders of medical technology. This was indicated by the many excellent addresses on matters medical as delivered by Pope Pius XII to various groups in the 1940's and 1950's, and by the publication of the application of traditional principles to new problems as presented in books such as the two volume *Contemporary Moral Theology* by Jesuit Fathers John C. Ford and Gerald Kelly (1958).

In view of the astounding advances in medical and surgical technology, a clear distinction between medical treatments and ordinary nursing care became not only defensible, but a practical necessity. For patients who are in imminent danger of death, the same latitude in refusing medical treatments "that can yield only a precarious and painful *prolongation* of life" cannot be

---

[6]*Dictionary of Moral Theology*, Francesco Cardinal Roberti and Monsignor Pietro Palazzini, eds. (Westminster, Md.: The Newman Press, 1962), pp. 577–580.

extended to the very *conservation* of life as dependent upon the provision of the very staff of life, nutrition and hydration, and the other comfort and hygienic aspects of ordinary nursing care. That testimonial of basic respect for human dignity (food and drink) cannot be omitted unless the effort to provide such basic care either is useless in terms of conserving the life of the patient, or adds excessive pain or burden for the patient, or if the administration of food and drink in a particular situation amounts to a virtual impossibility. These exceptional situations will be discussed at length in the second chapter of this study. The general rule, therefore, as stated in the *Declaration on Euthanasia,* is that when death is imminent, the "ordinary cares which are due to the sick person" are not to be interrupted.

A—Misinterpretation of the Address of Pope Pius XII (1957) (Cf.Appendix IV of this book)

In his address to the anesthesiologists on November 24, 1957, Pope Pius XII spoke of the individual's "right and duty in case of serious illness to take the necessary treatment for the preservation of life and health," and added (with obvious reference to *treatment*):

> But normally one is held to use only ordinary means—according to circumstances of persons, places, times and culture—that is to say, means that do not involve any grave burden for oneself or another. A more strict obligation would be too burdensome for most men and would render the attainment of the higher, more important good too difficult. Life, health, all temporal activities are in fact subordinated to spiritual ends . . . [7]

Some authors interpret these words of Pius XII as justification for withdrawing tube feeding from a terminal patient as a step in the pursuit of the "purpose of life."[8] First of all, such an interpretation clearly is out of context. Even

---

[7]The Pope Speaks, spring, 1958, pp.395, 396.

[8]Cf. "The Brophy Case: The Use of Artificial Hydration and Nutrition," by Philip Boyle, O.P., in the *Linacre Quarterly*, May, 1987, pp. 63-72, especially p. 66; *Ethics of Health Care* by Benedict M. Ashley, O.P. and Kevin O'Rourke, O.P. (St. Louis, Mo.: Catholic Health Assoc. 1986),p. 203; "Catholic Positions on Withholding Sustenance for the Terminally Ill, "by Rev. James J. McCartney, O.S.A., PhD, in *Health Progress*, October, 1986, pp. 38-40. Pope Pius XII referred to the perennial Catholic concept of the purpose of life when he stated in his address on euthanasia to the International Union of Catholic Women's Leagues on September 11, 1947: "Is it not false pity which claims to justify euthanasia and to remove from man purifying and

authors who may consider tube feeding to be a medical *treatment* should admit, from a cursory reading of the address, that the Holy Father was not referring to the obligation to provide sustenance. He was speaking of medical treatments;—of "three questions on medical morals treating the subject known as 'resuscitation' [la *réanimation*]" as stated in the opening paragraph of his address.[9]

Another compelling argument that Pope Pius XII was not referring to the withdrawal of nutrition in that address is based on the fact that in the Declaration on Euthanasia as issued by the Congregation for the Doctrine of the Faith in 1980, that particular address of Pope Pius XII on November 24, 1957, is mentioned expressly as one of the previous doctrinal pontifical pronouncements "which retain their full doctrinal force" (" . . . in doctrinae campo, . . . quae vim suam integre servant").[10] Hence the paragraph quoted above from Pope Pius XII's address of November 24, 1957, could not be interpreted as papal approval of withdrawing nutrition and hydration from patients who are in imminent danger of death. Such an interpretation would contradict directly the statement of the Declaration on Euthanasia (1980) as quoted on page 6 of this study. Unfortunately that mis-representation of the thought of Pope Pius XII has been used by the proponents of euthanasia as a statement of the "Catholic teaching" on the subject of withholding or withdrawing nutrition and hydration.

B—Providing Nutrition/Hydration by Artificial Means

The *Declaration on Euthanasia* (1980) makes no distinction between feeding in the natural manner vs. feeding by artificial means when it states that "ordinary cares which are due to the sick person" are not to be interrupted. In accord with a respected Canon Law guideline, "where the law does not distinguish, we should not distinguish" ("ubi lex non distinguit, nec nos distinguere debemus"), this would mean that food and drink are not to be interrupted regardless of the means employed at the time when the patient approaches the imminent-death status. In most cases, the patient who is un-

---

meritorious suffering, not by a charitable and praiseworthy help but by death, as if one were dealing with an irrational animal without immortality?" Address found in *The Human Body* (Boston, Mass: Daughters of St. Paul, 1960), pp. 90, 91.

[9] *The Pope Speaks*, spring, 1958, p. 393.

[10] *Enchiridion Vaticanum* (cf. note 5), n. 347, pp. 334, 335, footnote 2. The text is printed in Latin and in italian, pp. 332-351 (nn. 346-373). English version found in *Origins*, Aug. 14, 1980, pp. 154-157. It is the same as the English version as published by the Vatican Polyglot Press.

able to receive adequate sustenance by way of mouth had already been put on a regimen of tube feeding well in advance of imminent-death status. To say that basic care, such as feeding, can be discontinued automatically if the patient is unable to receive sustenance by way of mouth would be at variance with the precise concept of "euthanasia" as clarified in the Holy See's Declaration on Euthanasia.

With great care and precision, the Declaration on Euthanasia (1980) made a clear distinction between the etymological definition of euthanasia and a more precise and realistic meaning of the word (Latin text, 2nd. paragraph, in brackets):

> Etymologically speaking, in ancient times euthanasia meant an easy death without severe suffering. Today one no longer thinks of this original meaning of the word, but rather of some intervention of medicine whereby the sufferings of sickness or of the final agony are reduced, sometimes also with the danger of suppressing life prematurely. Ultimately, the word euthanasia is used in a more particular sense to mean "mercy killing," for the purpose of putting an end to extreme suffering, or saving abnormal babies, the mentally ill or the incurably sick from the prolongation, perhaps for many years, of a miserable life, which could impose too heavy a burden on their families or on society.

> It is therefore necessary to state clearly in what sense the word is used in the present document. By euthanasia is understood an action or an omission which of itself or by intention causes death, in order that all suffering may in this way be eliminated (". . . actio vel omissio quae suapta natura vel consilio mentis mortem affert, ut hoc modo omnis dolor removeatur") Euthanasia's terms of reference, therefore, are to be found in the intention of the will and in the methods used (" . . . in voluntatis proposito et in procedendi rationibus, quae adhibentur, continetur")[11]

In other words, the crime of euthanasia can be verified not only if a method is used with the intention of bringing about death, but also if the method is of a death-dealing nature ("suapte natura") but is not used with the clearly expressed intention of bringing about death. This conclusion is based on the accepted theological concept of "he who wills the means, wills

---

[11]*Ibid.*, nn. 354, 355; pp. 338 and 340. English version in *Origins*, Aug. 14, 1980, p. 155.

also the end" known as "voluntarium in causa"[12] In the latter instance, the method employed is not merely the *occasion* of death, but the *cause* of death.

In view of the fact that the withdrawal of nutrition and hydration, by its very nature ("suapta natura"), leads to the death of a patient, it is important to consider statements which are made in justification of such an action. Some claim, for example, that no authoritative Church pronouncement states expressly that food and drink must be included as an essential aspect of ordinary nursing care. That statement will be contested in the analysis (cf. section 2.1) of "Pronouncements of Pontifical Agencies" (in 1981 and in 1985). Others claim that feeding by *artificial* means is not to be regarded as nursing care, but rather as a *treatment*, or that it is an aspect of ordinary nursing care which must be considered as an *extraordinary* means of conserving life and hence not obligatory. Since no pontifical document addresses that question expressly, it remains open to discussion among theologians and ethicists. The contention here is that nutrition and hydration by artificial means pertains to nursing care and that, as a general rule, it is an *ordinary* means of conserving human life. As stated in directive 28 of the *Ethical and Religious Directives for Catholic Health Facilities* (to be referred to henceforth as *Hospital Directives*), to deny food and fluids in such cases would be equivalent to euthanasia).

In the Conroy case (1985), the Supreme Court of the State of New Jersey became the first high court in the U.S.A. to rule that there is no legal distinction between artificial feeding and other types of life support (for example, respirators, renal dialysis equipment, etc.). The implication is, therefore, that artificial feeding can be rejected by patients who are in imminent danger of death. The challenge to reverse this trend of thought both in judicial rulings and among ethicists and theologians, is formidable indeed.

C—In Defense of Artificial Feeding as Ordinary Nursing Care

One of the fundamental concepts mentioned by theologians of past centuries in describing the nature of ordinary care is that it involves means which are commonly-used ("media communia"). Bishop Cronin concluded that this element was basic to the concept of "ordinary," and that even when the word

---

[12]Cf.Merkelbach Benedict, O.P., *Summa Theologiae Moralis*, 3 vols., I (Paris: Desclée de Brouwer, 1935), nn. 62-64, pp. 69-71, or any standard manual of Catholic moral theology. In a penetrating article in *By No Extraordinary Means* (Bloomington, Ind.:Indiana University Press, 1986), Alan J. Weisbard, JD, and Mark Seigler, MD, p. 112, state: "Further, unlike withdrawal of respirators or dialysis machines, withdrawal of fluids and nutrition cannot so readily be seen as 'letting nature take its course.' Dehydration or lack of nutrition become the direct cause of death for which moral responsibility cannot be avoided."

"common" is not expressed, "it is presumed, and from the whole context, the reader is aware of the presumption" (cf. p. 92). The word "common," however, should not be limited to means that involve little or even moderate difficulty, so that some difficulty would make such means rate as extraordinary from a theological viewpoint, and as such not obligatory. If such thinking were to prevail, a person with a severe case of pneumonia who cannot control the rising fever with home remedies would be under no obligation to see a physician (presuming that medical help is reasonably available); a woman in an apartment building who accidentally starts a fire, would be under no obligation to sound the fire alarm down the hallway if she were unable to bring the fire under control by using water and other materials conveniently at hand; a nursing mother would have no obligation to switch to bottle-feeding and special formula in feeding her tiny infant if the child were a victim of a serious allergy to mother's milk.

Difficulty and special effort do not necessarily render a means uncommon and hence extraordinary in the usual circumstances of life. What degree of difficulty would render the means extraordinary? Bishop Cronin's extensive survey of theological opinion prompted him to write: " . . . one cannot help but realize that these authors certainly require an *excessive* difficulty before terming a means *extraordinary*" (*Conserving Human Life*, p. 95). Hence in the examples mentioned above, making a date to see a physician, and running down the hallway to sound the fire alarm, and switching to bottle-feeding for the infant would not involve excessive difficulty. As a general rule, the same would apply to tube-feeding for patients in imminent danger of death who are unable to sustain life by oral feeding. For such patients, artificial feeding is a commonly-used means of sustaining life. In most cases, the maintenance of such methods does not involve excessive difficulty.**

The examples given above might be used to illustrate the extent to which the decision on ordinary vs. extraordinary, or proportionate vs. disproportionate (balancing of benefits vs. burdens) depends upon an individual's status (social position, condition, background, etc.). Bishop Cronin introduces this subject when he writes about *relative* factors with regard to "The nature of the ordinary means of conserving life" (*Conserving Human Life*, pp. 85–98). For a person with a possible case of pneumonia and a rising fever who is living alone, without telephone and transportation facilities, the option of bundling up and walking to the house of a nearby neighbor could be viewed as an ordinary and obligatory means of conserving life. The benefits would

---

**A discussion of the precise meaning of the word "excessive" will be presented in the analysis of the phrase "excessive pain and/or burden" ("Primum non nocere"). The reader is referred to section 2.2, B of chapter II of this study.

seem to outweigh the burdens or dangers in most cases. If the sick person is elderly, and in such a weakened condition, however, that only slight hope could be sustained of reaching the neighbor's house or of finding someone "at home," he or she would be justified in passing up such a dubious means as extraordinary, and place his or her hopes and prayers on the chance possibility that some friend or neighbor might drop in before the end of the day (cf. *Ibid.*, pp. 98–111).

With regard to the elderly woman who is unable to control an accidental fire in her apartment, the benefits of leaving her apartment to seek help would involve not only saving her life from a very proximate danger of death, but also of alerting others in the apartment building of the danger to their lives. With such a predominance of benefits over dangers and burdens, she would be obligated to sound the alarm as an *ordinary* means of saving lives. Presuming that she lacks telephone facilities, she could not be excused from making every possible effort to alert others to the danger even if she were handicapped and could get around only with the aid of crutches, or of a walker, or of a wheelchair. Given the urgent circumstances, the relative factors involved would not make "operation alert" an extraordinary means of conserving life for this individual. If this could not be accomplished by screaming or yelling (due to her handicapped condition), she could not escape the obligation of leaving her apartment and either sound the fire alarm or get help from neighboring tenants in the building. Due to the life-threatening danger to others in the building, not even the *virtual* uselessness or *virtual* impossibility of making such an effort (leaving her apartment in search of help) would constitute an *extraordinary* means of conserving life. The commandment "Thou shalt not kill" would require such an elderly and handicapped woman to make *every* possible effort to alert others to the tragic situation.

Applying these concepts to the obligation to conserve life by seeking nutrition and hydration, it is logical to say that if a patient still is able to chew and swallow food and liquids by way of mouth, the installation of a tube-feeding process would be an extraordinary and disproportionate means of conserving life. The burdens would outweigh the anticipated benefits. For a patient who is unable to receive food and drink by way of mouth, however, tube-feeding would be an ordinary and proportionate means of conserving life. Considering that it is a life or death issue, the benefits would far outweigh burdens UNLESS the feeding process itself became useless in terms of conserving the life of the individual, or added excessive pain or burden for the patient. The same exceptional status would apply if (as stated peviously) the installation or the continuation of tube feeding amounted to a virtual impossibility.

It is not difficult to understand why tube feeding might have been viewed as an extraordinary means of conserving life when it was still untried and somewhat risky back in the 1870's when it first came into use. The same might have been a valid moral evaluation of intravenous feeding when first introduced into clinical practice back in the 1890's. In contemporary medical practice, however, both procedures rate as the common or ordinary means of conserving life for patients who cannot receive nutrition and hydration by way of mouth. Just as a bulky life jacket might be viewed as a cumbersome burden for an expert swimmer who is one of a group of good swimmers who are about to swim across a deep river, so it would be a common and ordinary means of survival for a good swimmer who is about to swim across a deep river alone.

In a 1986 publication entitled *By No Extraordinary Means*, Dr. David Major compares the various types of artificial feeding. In his comparison, feeding by gastrostomy (installed through a small surgical opening in the abdomen) as well as feeding by nasogastric tube (inserted through the nasal passages) both receive an "excellent" rating in providing nutrition and fluids, and at a cost which approximates the cost of providing oral feedings. As to "acceptability" for the patient and for others, the gastrostomy process (with a rating of "good") is considerably more acceptable than the nasogastric process.[13] It is generally admitted that the nasogastric installation is irritating to the nose, and can lead to other unpleasant side effects such as causing a gag reflex, tendency to cause bleeding, etc. The gastrostomy process, first used on humans in 1875, is more easily tolerated and more widely used. After installation of the tube in a hospital or clinic, both methods can be administered in the patient's home by a family member or by a visiting volunteer who has received basic instructions from a physician or nurse.[14] Unless there are complicating circumstances, the burdens of tube feeding are far outweighed by the benefit of preserving life and even of enabling such patients to participate in limited social activities.

The difficulty in having recourse to tube feeding to sustain life, as a general rule, is not excessive. Hence what must be done (sustain life) can be

---

[13]"The Medical Procedures for Providing Food and Water: Indications and Effects," in *By No Extraordinary Means* (cf. note 12), p. 22.

[14]*Ibid.*, pp. 23-27. One would like to presume that family members would be less likely to discontinue tube feeding for a loved one in a home setting, than physicians or nurses in a hospital setting. Even in the latter setting, however, one poll of physicians indicated that, for a patient in a persistent vegetative state, 90 percent would discontinue the respirator, but only 50 percent would stop nasogastric feeding. *Ibid.*, pp. 189-193, and footnote 11, p. 194. The article, entitled "Patients With Permanent Loss of Consciousness," was written by Ronald E. Cranford, MD, of the University of Minnesota.

done without departing from ordinary nursing care. This does not become medical treatment just because it is artificial, nor because it involves minor medical assistance to install and slight medical monitoring to maintain. If being "artificial" made feeding a medical treatment, much of the sustenance available to people on scientific expeditions would be by way of medical treatment ("ersatz" nutrition, meatless "meat," etc.) If being installed or administered by medical personnel made feeding a medical treatment, the term might be applied also to spoon-feeding (complete with the monitoring of special supplements and vitamens) for critically ill patients in homes or in health facilities. The distinction between "what must be done," and "how it is done," is of prime importance. The latter does not necessarily cancel out the former.

D—Assessment of Methods of Intravenous (IV) Feeding

Methods of administering food and fluids through the intestines are known as *enteral* techniques. If the mode of provision is through any route other than through the intestines, it is known as a *parenteral* technique. Salt solutions were administered directly into the veins in the 1890s. Over the years, the safety and effectiveness of that approach improved progressively. It is a common practice today to administer fluids into peripheral veins through sharp, sterile and disposable needles. Such conventional intravenous procedures are adequate, however, only on a temporary basis, and only for providing fluids and minerals.[15]

Total parenteral nutrition (TPN) can be provided even for long term therapy by inserting a catheter through a needle into the subclavian vein. This is the large central vein located behind the collarbone. The "catheter through a needle" feature is used for access both to peripheral veins (as above) and to the large subclavian vein. The use of prepackaged plastic catheters that are internal to the needle or that serve as sheaths to the needle allow the needle itself to be withdrawn from the vein, leaving only the catheter in the vein. This decreases considerably the danger of infection or of inflammation. It should be noted that the *peripheral vein* access is a *supplement*, while the *subclavian vein* access can provide a patient with a non-functioning gastrointestinal tract with *total* parenteral nutrition for an unlimited period.[16] This would make TPN through the subclavian vein a *substitute* for a broken-down nutrition-hydration system.

---

[15]*By No Extraordinary Means* (cf. note 12), pp. 22–24. The article, written by David Major, MD, is entitled "The Medical Procedures for Providing Food and Water: Indications and Effects."
[16]*Ibid.*, pp. 23–25.

The distinction between *supplement* and *substitute* is important. The total parenteral nutrition provided by the subclavian entry for a patient with a totally non-functional alimentary system would make it an extraordinary or disproportionate means of providing sustenance. Thus it could be compared to a patient who is hooked up to a mechanical respirator because his or her lungs are totally nonfunctional as far as the capacity to inhale and exhale is concerned. Precisely because of the *assisting or supplementary* role of sustaining nutritional needs through tube-feeding (enteral) or through peripheral-vein intravenous input (parenteral), the patient normally is obligated to allow the process to continue. When the alimentary system as designed by nature is broken down completely, both as to the capacity to ingest and swallow food and also in the capacity to assimilate nutrition, however, there is no obligation to initiate or to continue a *substitute* for that system. Clearly this can be regarded as an extraordinary and non-obligatory means of conserving life.[17]

E—Removal of Tube-Feeding vs. Removal of Respirator

In the noted case of Claire Conroy, an elderly, single woman who was a patient at the Parkland Nursing Home in Bloomfield, N.J., one of the Public Advocates who was active in the case both before the Appellate Division and before the New Jersey Supreme Court, was referring to tube-feeding (as involved in the Conroy case) when he wrote:

> In my view, a humane society must recognize and preserve the basic care which comforts the dying. An ill person is not denied hygienic care. I would include food and fluids in this category of care . . . I believe that food and fluids can be permanently withdrawn only when these two conditions are met:death is imminent and any other course of action would include additional suffering.[18]

Such arguments did not prevail, however, when the nephew and appointed guardian of Miss Conroy petitioned a trial court of the State of New Jersey for a judicial vindication of his right to effect the removal of the nasogastric tube from his long-suffering aunt. On February 2, 1983, after three days of testimony, the trial court declared that the nephew/guardian had that

---

[17]Cf. McFadden, Charles J., O.S.A., *The Dignity of Life* (Huntington, Ind.:Our Sunday Visitor, 1976),pp. 152, 153. Cf. also pp. 147–149 of *Conserving Human Life*.

[18]"The Role of the Public Advocate," by Joseph H. Rodriguez, Jr., JD, in *By No Extraordinary Means* (cf. note 12), pp. 256, 257.

right. He was prevented from exercizing that right, however, when the guardian *ad litem* in the case (an official who is responsible for protecting the rights and interests of an incompetent litigant, etc.) obtained a stay blocking the implementation of the trial court's judgment. Less than two weeks later, the New Jersey Public Advocate intervened in favor of the appeal of the guardian *ad litem*. The subsequent appeal to the Appellate Division reversed the decision of the trial court and severely limited the right of a conscious individual to refuse medical treatment.[19]

Although Miss Conroy died on February 13,1983, just thirteen days after the decision of the trial court that the nasogastric tube could be removed (but was not removed due to the appeal to the Appellate Court), the nephew and guardian of the patient decided to appeal to the Supreme Court of New Jersey "so that others might have less difficulty than he had experienced in caring for his aunt."[20] This appeal was based on the contention that a nasogastric tube is medical treatment, and that the patient has a right to refuse such treatment under the "constitutional right to privacy." As stated on p. 13 of this study, the decision of the Supreme Court of the State of New Jersey on this issue on January 17, 1985 became the first high court decision in the U.S.A. to rule that there is no legal distinction between tube feeding and other types of life support such as respirators. Hence the tube feeding process can be rejected by patients who are in imminent danger of death. The ramifications of this decision for New Jersey and for the entire U.S.A. are bound to be used by the proponents of euthanasia. Claire Conroy was neither brain dead, nor comatose, nor in a vegetative state. This sweeping decision amounted to a "first ever" order of a high court in the U.S.A. to deprive a patient of food and water. Although the decision applies to a limited group (New Jersey citizens residing in nursing homes, incompetent patients, etc.), it could well become a base for a wider interpretation by courts and by ethicists.[21]

Those authors who truly are convinced that tube feeding is a medical *treatment* can point to the *Declaration on Euthanasia* (1980) which states that "it is licit in conscience to decide to renounce *treatments* which can yield only a precarious and painful prolongation of life" (Cf. p. 154 of this study). Those who agree that the feeding/hydration process is an essential aspect of nursing *care* can insist that the process can be renounced if it has to be administered by

---

[19]*Ibid.*, article entitled "The Conroy Case: An Overview, "by William Strasser JD, who represented Miss Conroy's nephew, Thomas Whittemore, in the case. Cf. pp. 245–248.

[20]*Ibid.*, p. 246.

[21]Cf. "In *re* Conroy: History and Setting of the Case," by Jeff Stryker, research analyst, in *By No Extraordinary Means* (cf. note 12), pp. 227–234. Note especially p. 234.

artificial means (tube feeding) because of a sound conviction that such an artificial process automatically becomes an *extraordinary* or disproportionate means of conserving human life. This study is based on the conviction (cf. p. 160 of this study) that providing *food and water to the patient is an essential aspect of nursing care, and that it does not necessarily become either a medical treatment, or an extraordinary means of exercizing patient care when it is administered by artificial means.* Some proponents of the first two opinions above insist that there is no difference, from a moral viewpoint, between removing an artificial feeding process, and removing a respirator. Others admit that there is a difference, but that it is symbolic only (the "deep seated revulsion at the stopping of feeding the dying even under legitimate circumstances.").[22] The real difference goes beyond mere symbolism.

A strong symbolical dimension cannot be denied. It might be called the Good Samaritan dimension. The obligation to feed the hungry and give drink to the thirsty is perceived universally as a duty which transcends the medical context. This popular perception involves not only the "deep seated revulsion at the stopping of feeding" (quotation above), but especially the basic imperative of loving concern for those in need, of sharing sympathetically in the sufferings of others, of response to the golden rule ("do unto others . . . "), etc. Within the medical context, however, there is the physiological fact that "allowing nature to take its course" is far more fraught with human misery and suffering in separating a patient from the source of food and drink, than in separating a patient from the source of air and oxygen. That physiological fact means that in the latter case (respiration), the patient dies within seconds; in the former case (alimentation), the patient continues to live and to breathe in suffering and in indignity for most of a week or more. The fact that painkilling drugs are administered to take the sting out of the suffering does not lessen the abject indignity of the situation.

In line with the observation above, there is the surfacing perception (formerly left unspoken) that it cannot be too wrong to intervene in favor of a more merciful death by helping nature to take its course after the feeding tube has been disconnected. This might be called the psychological argument against equating the removal of artificial feeding with the removal of a respi-

---

[22]Cf. "The Symbolic Significance of Giving to Eat and Drink," by Donald A. Carson, PhD *Ibid.*, pp. 84–88. Cf. also two penetrating articles, as found in the same publication, which challenge the tendency to equate the removal of tube feeding with the removal of a respirator, namely: "On Killing Patients with Kindness: An Appeal to Caution," by Alan J. Weisbard, JD and Mark Seigler, MD, pp. 109–116; and "Terminating Food and Water: Emerging Legal Rules," by Ron M. Landsman, JD., pp. 135–149.

rator. Lawyer Alan J. Weisbard and physician Mark Siegler advance this argument as follows:

> . . . unlike withdrawal of respirators or dialysis machines, withdrawal of fluids and nutrition cannot so readily be seen as "letting nature take its course." Dehydration or lack of nutrition become the direct cause of death for which moral responsibility cannot be avoided. The psychological and social ramifications of bringing death about in this fashion will, in our view, be difficult or impossible to distinguish from those accompanying lethal injections or other modes of active euthanasia"[23]

Any God-fearing individual would recoil at the very concept of helping nature to take its course by smothering a patient with a pillow if the patient continues to breathe after the removal of the respirator. Yet, there seems to be almost a crusading sentiment in favor of helping nature to take its course in situations where, after the removal of tube feeding mechanism, the patient is given a merciful exit by the administration of injection of a lethal drug or a bubble of air. That "crusading sentiment" was given judicial prominence by a high court decision in the U.S.A. in Judge Compton's opinion in the Bouvia case as quoted on the opening page of this study (Introduction).

Today, the practice of allowing nature to take its course by disconnecting the artificial feeding mechanism might be intended only for consenting adults (through "living wills") who are terminal with advanced cases of cancer, heart failure, etc. Tomorrow the practice may well become what ethicist Daniel Callahan calls the "nontreatment of choice" for the "biologically tenacious" patients.[24] This category, sometimes referred to as the "unproductive citizens," would include the retarded, the disabled, the senile, the institutionalized handicapped, etc. The so-called "right to die" could come to be portrayed as the "duty to die." The campaign would be made to look respectable in the media by repeated references to "saddling the young generation with an insupportable burden," or "stopping the destructive spiral of medical costs," or threatening the collapse of the Medicare program," or "loving

---

[23]*Ibid.*, pp. 108–116. Note page 112. Cf. also the *Medical World News*, March 9, 1987, pp. 19, 20, for the report on proposed legislation in California (to constitute, if passed, the *first* of its kind in the Western world) to give physicians the right to "administer aid in dying"—such aid being defined as "any medical procedure that will end the patient's life swiftly, painlessly and humanely."

[24]"On Feeding the Dying," by Daniel Callahan, Director of the Hastings Center, as found in *The Hastings Center Report*, October, 1983, p. 22.

concern for the handicapped," etc. The real consequential hazards of promoting the unwarranted withdrawal of food and drink from the hopeless and the helpless in society can fall upon this generation and generations to come, like a sweeping avalanche. The beginnings seem innocent enough; the consequences can be devastating. Again, in the words of Weisbard and Siegler:

> The line between "allowing to die" by starvation and "active killing" can be elusive, and we are skeptical that any logical or psychological distinction between "allowing to die" by starvation and actively killing, as by lethal injection, will prove viable. If we as a society are to retain the prohibition against active killing, the admittedly wavering line demarcating permissible "allowings to die" must exclude death by avoidable starvation.[25]

From a moral viewpoint, the principal argument against equating the removal of tube feeding with the removal of a respirator (both installed on a long term basis) is based on the fact that in the latter case (respirator) the patient usually is *totally* incapable of breathing on his own. In such a case, there is no obligation to install or to continue using a mechanical *substitute* so as to *prolong* the life of the patient. In the former case (tube feeding), however, the patient is *not totally* incapable of benefitting from the artificial feeding process. The alimentary system still is partially functional; the patient still is able to digest and assimilate food and fluids. The inoperative or dysfunctioning aspect of the alimentary system—that is, the incapacity to ingest and swallow nutrition and fluids—can be bypassed without excessive burden or pain so that digestion and assimilation can continue. When and where such an effective bypass mechanism is available, both as to installation and as to maintenance, there is a moral obligation to use that *supplemental* means so as to *conserve* the life of the individual, (exceptions to this general rule to be discussed in part II of this study).

Because of this moral obligation, the lethal factor in the case of discontinuing an effective *supplemental* aid, should be identified not with the patient's existing and underlying illness or disease, but with a *new and different* pathological condition (starvation and dehydration) as caused by the deliberate deprivation of the staff of life, food and fluids. Almighty God retains dominion over life and over death until the final moment of natural death. To claim that the obligation to continue such supplemental aid and thus conserve the life of the patient ceases "when the decision has been made to allow the patient to

---

[25]Cf. *By no Extraordinary Means* (cf. note 12), Wiesbard and Siegler; p. 113.

die," is to usurp some degree of that divine dominion. To pray that the Good Lord might bring about an end to the pains and burdens of a long-suffering patient is to leave matters in God's hands. To decide when the patient should be allowed to die, and even hasten the process by discontinuing effective life-conserving artificial feeding, however, is to take matters into human hands. In such situations, a definite share of responsibility for contributing to the gradual demise (through starvation and dehydration) of a fellow human being cannot be cast aside by saying: "the patient is not starving to death but is dying of a malfunction of the digestive system and it is time to let nature take its course."[26] Clearly the "malfunction" is man-made. The same "malfunction" follows infallibly when someone who is truly hungry and thirsty (whether sick or healthy) is deprived of food and water on a long term basis.

1.2 TWO PRONOUNCEMENTS OF PONTIFICAL AGENCIES

It is clear from the Code of Canon Law that the term "Apostolic See" or "Holy See" embraces not only the various congregations, secretariates, etc., but also pontifical commissions, councils, etc., "unless the nature of the matter or the context of the words makes the contrary evident" (Can. 361). In other words, agencies such as the Pontifical Academy of Sciences, the Pontifical Commission on Justice and Peace, etc., are all duly organized units which participate in varying degrees in the function of the Roman Curia. The "Roman Curia" (a phrase which dates back to the senate and court of the Roman Empire) might be called the central office of the Catholic Church whereby "the Supreme Pontiff usually conducts affairs of the universal church . . . " (Can. 360).

By the time of the Second Vatican Council, the Roman Curia was in need of reform. The *Decree on the Bishops' Pastoral Office in the Church* of Vatican II stated that the departments of the Roman Curia were to be " . . . reorganized and better adapted to the needs of the times, and of various regions and rites"(n. 9). This call for reform was answered especially in Pope Paul VI's apostolic constitution on the reorganization of the Roman Curia ("Regimini

---

[26]This quotation is found in *Medical Ethics* (St. Louis, Mo.: Catholic Health Association, 1986), by Kevin D. O'Rourke, O.P., JCD, and Dennis Brodeur, PhD Cf. pages 213, 214. These authors state that when the decision is made to allow the patient to die, "the goal is to keep the patient as comfortable as possible" (p. 213). One is constrained to ask: "By denying food and water?" It is important to note that these authors look upon the situation as one of life support (prolongation of life) rather than a matter of conserving human life.

Ecclesiae Universae") as issued on August 15, 1969. One primary regulation of this document, which applies to all agencies of the Roman Curia (from major Congregations to minor commissions, academies, etc.) is that "Above all, nothing important and out of the ordinary is to be done ("hoc in primis solemne sit, ut nihil grave et extraordinarium agatur") unless it has first been made known to the Supreme Pontiff by the head of the Congregation or Department." This "solemn" statement is followed by a regulation that "all decisions require pontifical approval with the exception of those for which special faculties have been given to the Department heads."[27]

Most pronouncements of pontifical agencies (commissions, academies, etc.) would not involve *decisions* (which would require pontifical approval) but rather reports of discussions or conclusions of deliberations depending upon the purpose of the gathering. It could be a regular meeting of the group, or a special meeting with requested agenda from the Holy Father, or an urgent meeting in response to a special scientific or academic challenge, etc. The reports or deliberations of such pontifical groups would not require pontifical approval. By the same token, however, such reports or pronouncements would not be regarded as official. They would not "close" a question which may have been open to theological or scientific discussion and study, for example, unless pontifical approval had been obtained. If the content of such reports or pronouncements is in accord with accepted Church teachings, however, and the publication of same was not followed by adverse comments from an official pontifical source within an appropriate period of time, there is no reason why such reports or pronouncements should not be considered as reliable interpretations or elucidations of the teachings of the Church. They are issued as one aspect of the functioning of the Roman Curia.[28]

---

[27]*Enchiridion Vaticanum*, Vol. II (Bologna, Italy: Edizioni Dehoniane Bologna, 1979), n. 1676, p. 1344. For the English version, cf. *Canon Law Digest*, Vol. VI (New York, N.Y.: Bruce Publishing Co., 1969), pp. 356, 357.

[28]As an example of a report of a pontifical commission which was not approved by the Holy Father, one might mention the commission on the birth control issue which was established by Pope John XXIII in March, 1963, and was confirmed and enlarged by Pope Paul VI. In the words of Paul VI as recorded in *Humanae Vitae* (n. 5), the assigned task of that commission was ". . . the gathering of opinions on the new questions regarding conjugal life, and in particular on the regulation of births, and of furnishing opportune elements of information so that the magisterium could give an adequate reply to the expectation not only of the faithful, but also of world opinion." *Enchiridion Vaticanum, Vol. III* (Bologna, Italy: Edizioni Dehoniane Bologna, 1977), n. 591, pp. 284, 285. English translation from *Love and Sexuality* of the Official Catholic Teachings series (Wilmington, North Carolina: McGrath Publishing Co., 1978), p. 333. As the main reason for not accepting the conclusions of the commission, the Holy father stated: ". . . above all because certain criteria of solutions had emerged which departed from the moral

A—Pontifical Council on Health Affairs, "Cor Unum," June 27, 1981
(Cf. Appendix II of this book)

The Pontifical Council "Cor Unum," established by Pope Paul VI in 1971, became (as of 1975) the Holy See's Council on Health Affairs.[29] From November 12th to 14th, 1976, about 15 persons representing various disciplines (theologians, physicians, religious in hospital work, nurses, chaplains) gathered as a study group to " . . . analyze basic concepts, point out certain distinctions which must be understood clearly, and formulate practical answers to questions brought up by pastoral directives and by the treatment of the dying."[30] The report of this group was not published, however, until *after* the publication of the *Declaration on Euthanasia* of the Congregation for the Doctrine of the Faith (May 5, 1980). The fact that the report of "Cor Unum" was published in 1981, five years after the actual meeting of the group, would seem to justify a presumption that this particular report (group met in 1976) and the *Declaration on Euthanasia* (1980) were viewed as complementing one another.[31] The source or reason for such a request (that is, to publish the "Cor Unum" report) was not indicated.

Of particular interest in the present discussion is the report of this study group with regard to the obligation to continue the administration of nutrition and hydration to patients who are in imminent danger of death. The original French is a bit more forceful than the English translation:

Rest, par contre, l'obligation stricte de poursuivre à tout pris l'application des moyens dits "minimaux," ceux qui sont destinés normalement et dans des conditions habituelle à maintenir la vie (alimentation, transfusions de sang, injections,

On the contrary, there remains the strict obligation to continue by all means those measures which are called "minimal," which are intended normally and customarily for the maintenance of life (alimentation, blood transfusions, injec-

---

teaching on marriage proposed with constant firmness by the teaching authority of the Church." *Ibid.*, p. 333. The purpose of the papal commission was consultative and informative. The members were not authorized in any way to dictate Church doctrine on the subject of birth control.

[29]*Annuario Pontiaficio* (Città del Vaticano: Libreria Editrice Vaticana, 1986), p. 1584.

[30]*Enchiridion Vatiacanum*, Vol. VIII (cf. note 5), p. 1134 (n. 1236), The date of the meeting was June 27, 1981.

[31]*Ibid.*, n. 1238, p. 1134: "L'étude du groupe de travail de 1976 est, elle, d'orde Plutôt pastoral et répond à des questions précises et concrètes posées a Cor unum par des aumôniers, des médecins et des infirmières. A la suite de la Déclaration sur l'euthanasie éditée par la S.C. pour la doctrine de la foi, le conseil pontifical a été sollicité de publier le rapport de son groupe de travail . . . "

ecc.). En interrompre l'administration reviendrait pratiquement à
vouloir mettre fin aux jours du patient.

tions, etc.). To interrupt these
minimal measures would be equivalent, in practice, to wishing to put
an end to the life of the patient.[32]

As of February 11, 1985, the competence of the Pontifical Council "Cor
Unum" in health affairs was transferred to a new commission to be known as
the Pontifical Commission for the Apostolate of Health Care Workers. Pope
John Paul II established this new commission with the publication of his letter
("motu proprio") entitled "Dolentium Hominum."[33] The purpose of the new
commission as stated in the first issue of the official quarterly publication of
that commission (Dolentium Hominum, n. 1, 1986, p. 6) as follows: "To
spread, explain and defend the teachings of the Church on the subject of
health care, and to encourage their penetration into health care practice."

B—Report of the Pontifical Academy of Sciences, October, 1985
(Cf. Appendix III of this book)

The Pontifical Academy of Sciences in its present form dates back to
October 28, 1936, during the pontificate of Pius XI. A similar association
had been founded in Rome in 1603. It was restored under Pius IX in 1847,
and enlarged by Leo XIII in 1887. The present statutes place the Pontifical
Academy of Sciences under the direct guidance of the Holy Father. As of
1986, the required number of members of the academy as chosen from outstanding scientists throughout the world (a total of 70) includes 16 Americans.[34] About twenty members of this prestigious academy met in Rome from
October 19 to 21, 1985, to study "the artificial prolongation of life and the
exact determination of the moment of death." The address of Pope John Paul
II to this group during their deliberations (also found in Appendix III) emphasized that "appropriate care should be provided" for the sick, "whatever
their condition," and included lengthy quotations from the *Declaration on Euthanasia* (1980) *including* the passage about *not interrupting ordinary cares* "when

---

[32]*Ibid.*, n. 1252, pp. 1144–1146. English translation by this writer.

[33]*Annuario Pontificio*, 1986 (cf. note 29), pp. 1584,1585.

[34]*Ibid.*, pp. 1524–1528, and 1630, 1631. As an indication of the high qualifications of the
members of the academy, it might suffice to mention several of the 16 Americans as listed in the
1986 edition of *Annuario Pontificio* in alphabetical order: Christian Anfinsen, professor of bio-
chemistry at Johns Hopkins University, David Baltimore, professor at the Massachusetts Institute of Technology, Christian de Duve, professor of physiological chemistry of the Catholic
University of Louvain (Belgium) and of Rockefeller University of New York, etc.

death is imminent and cannot be prevented by the remedies used" (cf. pp. 154 ff. of this study).[35]

If the message of the Holy Father and his references to the *Declaration on Euthanasia* on general nursing care are kept in mind in reading the following portion of the report of the Pontifical Academy of Sciences, it would seem that an explicit papal approval of the report would not be a pressing issue. The following quotation clearly makes a distinction between *treatment* and *ordinary care*, and mentions explicitly (as found in the "Cor unum" report) that feeding is to be included as an important aspect of *lavish* nursing care (emphasis ours; original Italian in parentheses):

> By the term *treatment* the group understands all those medical interventions available and appropriate in a specific case, whatever the complexity of the techniques involved.

> If the patient is in a permanent coma, irreversible as far as it can be foreseen ("irreversibile, per quanto sia possibile prevederlo"), *treatment* is not required, *but all care should be lavished on him, including feeding* ("non si richiede un trattamento, *ma debbono essergli prodigate le cure, ivi compresa l'alimentazione*") . . . If *treatment* is of no benefit to the patient, it may be interrupted while continuing with the *care* of the patient ("Se il trattamento non può portare alcun beneficio al paziente, può essere interrotto, *continuando le cure*").[36]

Neither of these two reports mentions explicitly that feeding is of obligation only if the patient is able to take sustenance by way of mouth. Surely these experts were mindful of the fact that nutrition and hydration are administered by artificial means in many situations both in homes and in various health facilities. Both of these reports were published *after* the publication of the *Declaration on Euthanasia* (1980), and should be read and interpreted in the light of that major authoritative document as discussed in the first portion of this study.

---

[35]Cf. *Origins* Dec. 5, 1985, pp. 415–417.

[36]*Origins*, Dec. 5, 1985, p. 415. The original Italian of the report is found in *Enchiridion Vaticanum*, IX (Bologna, Italy: Edizioni Dehoniane Bologna, 1987), p. 1727, n. 1768.

1.3 PRONOUNCEMENTS OF THE AMERICAN BISHOPS' CONFERENCE

Vatican II's *Decree on the Bishops' Pastoral Office in the Church* expressed the earnest desire ("exoptat") that synods and councils might flourish with "new vigor" so that "faith will be spread and discipline preserved more fittingly and effectively in the various churches, as the circumstances of the times requires"(n. 36). The decree then proceeds to present guidelines for the formation of episcopal conferences (nn. 37,38) which later were incorporated into the present Code of Canon Law (Cann. 447–459). Another document of Vatican II, *The Dogmatic Constitution on the Church* (n. 25) speaks of the obligation on the part of the faithful to accept and to adhere, "with a religious assent of soul," not only to the authentic teaching authority of the Holy Father, but also to the teaching authority of "Bishops, teaching in communion with the Roman Pontiff . . . in matters of faith and morals." These same sentiments are reflected in Canons 752 and 753 of the Code of Canon Law.

When the bishops of a nation join together as a conference (such as the NCCB; the National Conference of Catholic Bishops) they pursue their objectives not only through plenary meetings of the conference, but also through a permanent council of bishops, a general secretary, and other offices and committees (Cann. 451 and 457, 458). Examples of committees of the NCCB include those on doctrine, on canonical affairs, on liturgy, on pro-life activities, etc. There are many and diverse matters which can be finalized by authoritative decrees of the Catholic conference of a nation, but this would be done only at plenary meetings of the conference.[37] Although the promulgation of such decrees (after review by the Holy See) could indicate a definite power of governance, however, the very concept of a national conference of bishops should be seen as apostolic and pastoral in nature. Thus much of the ongoing concern of the Catholic bishops for orthodox teaching in matters of faith and morals as issued from plenary meetings of the conference would be amplified and clarified, on the apostolic and pastoral level, through established offices and committees of the conference.

The obligation of the faithful to be guided by pronouncements of the national conference of bishops both as issued from plenary meetings and as

---

[37]Cf. *The Code of Canon Law*, text and commentary (Mahwah, N.J.: Paulist Press, 1985), canons 455, 456, pp. 368–373; article "Bishops' Conference Documents:What Doctrinal Authority," by Fr. Avery Dulles, S.J., in *Origins*, Jan.24, 1985, pp. 528–534.

amplified or extended through the committee structure, would depend upon many factors such as the nature of the subject, the preliminary studies, surveys, research, versions, etc. (before final consideration of the subject), the solemnity of the promulgation, etc. Thus pastoral letters or statements of the American Catholic Bishops (NCCB) such as those entitled "Human Life in Our Day" (1968) and "Basic Teachings for Religious Education" (1974) would seem to demand a more profound "religious submission of will and mind" than the pastoral message and letter entitled "Economic Justice for All" (1986). As mentioned in Vatican II's pastoral constitution *The Church Today* (n. 43): "Let the layman not imagine that his pastors are always such experts, that to every problem which arises, however complicated, they can readily give him a concrete solution, or even that such is their mission."

The subject of human dignity stands high on the list of moral concerns of our American Bishops. Through the Committee for Pro-Life Activities of the National Conference of Catholic Bishops, they have issued several statements on the subject of feeding the sick and the helpless which are grounded on the Holy See's *Declaration on Euthanasia* (1980) and which, as such, command the respectful assent the faithful.

A—Bishops' Conference: Guidelines for Legislation on Life-Sustaining Treatment

The American bishops were concerned about the lack of consideration for traditional Catholic moral principles in court decisions and in "living will" legislation on the subject of the treatment of terminally ill patients. On November 10, 1984, they proposed a set of moral principles and legislative guidelines as an expression of the felt obligation of the American Catholic hierarchy to "provide its guidance through participation in the current debate."[38] The document recognizes a clear distinction between *medical treatment* and *nursing care*, and expressly includes nutrition as an aspect of nursing care which "must be maintained." The following are proposed as "legislative guidelines:"

> (g) . . . Medical-treatment legislation may clarify procedures for discontinuing treatment which only secures a precarious and burdensome prolongation of life for the terminally ill patient, but should not condone or authorize any deliberate act or omission designed to cause a person's death.

---

[38]"Guidelines for Legislation on Life-Sustaining Treatment", in *Origins*, January 14, 1985, pp. 526–528.

(h) Recognize the presumption that certain basic measures such as nursing care, hydration, nourishment and the like must be maintained out of respect for the human dignity of every patient.

B—Bishops' Conference: The Rights of the Terminally Ill

Two years later (September 4, 1986), the same U.S. Bishops' Committee for Pro-Life Activities released a statement in commentary on the proposed *Uniform Rights of the Terminally Ill Act* for enactment by state legislatures, as prepared by the National Conference of Commissions on Uniform State Laws. Some of the "living will" enactments by state legislatures could be viewed as "steppingstones to the eventual legalization of euthanasia," and the American bishops issued their statement through the Committee for Pro-Life Activities as an expression of their sense of "responsibility to contribute to this debate."[39]

This statement, like the one of the same committee in 1984 (above), includes both medical treatments and the promotion of comfort and nourishment under the term "measure," but with an implied recognition of a clear distinction between the two. Translating this into the distinction between *medical treatments* and *ordinary care* as emphasized in the Holy See's *Declaration on Euthanasia* (1980), this statement of the pro-life activities committee emphasizes the important distinction between the administration of nutrition and hydration to *promote the comfort* of the patient, and to *sustain the life* of the patient. The latter (sustaining life) is more fundamental and must be continued even in the event when it may not be needed for comfort considerations. Furthermore, the statement (the third paragraph below) emphasizes the immorality of withholding nourishment from "Unconscious or otherwise disabled patients" for "quality of life" considerations. The section entitled "Nutrition and Hydration" reads as follows:

> Because human life has inherent value and dignity regardless of its condition, every patient should be provided with measures which can effectively preserve life without involving too grave a burden. Since food and water are necessities of life for all human beings and can generally be provided without the risks and burdens of more aggressive means for sustaining life, the law should establish a strong presumption in favor of their use.

---

[39]"The Rights of the Terminally Ill," in *Origins*, September 4, 1986, pp. 222–224.

The uniform act states that it will not affect any existing responsibility to provide measures such as nutrition and hydration to promote comfort. But it does not adequately recognize a distinct and more fundamental benefit of such measures—that of sustaining life itself. This is a serious lapse in light of the ambiguous scope of the uniform act, which may include cases in which a patient will live a long time with treatment but die quickly without it. For most patients, measures for providing nourishment are morally obligatory even when other treatment can be withdrawn due to its burdensomeness or ineffectiveness.

Negative judgments about the "quality of life" of unconscious or otherwise disabled patients have led some of our society to propose withholding nourishment precisely in order to end these patients' lives. Society must take special care to protect against such discrimination. Laws dealing with medical treatment may have to take account of exceptional circumstances when even means for providing nourishment may become too ineffective or burdensome to be obligatory. But such laws must establish clear safeguards against intentionally hastening the deaths of vulnerable patients by starvation or dehydration.[40]

That distinction between nutrition and hydration as a means of *promoting the comfort* of the patient and as a means of *sustaining the life* of the patient is of primary importance in understanding the approach of the proponents of euthanasia. Following the recommendation of the Uniform Rights of the Terminally Ill Act (cf. above), organizations such as the Society for the Right to Die would favor a statement on life-sustaining measures which may be withheld (in the declaration of the "living will" signatory) which leaves open the question of whether or not food and fluid would have to be continued if not considered necessary for *comfort care*. In other words, there would be no reference to food and fluids as necessary for *sustaining the life* of the patient. Thus the Society or the Right to Die comments on the "Arizona Medical Treatment Decision Act" as follows:

Arizona's statement on nourishment and hydration reads: "Life-sustaining procedure does not include the administration of medi-

---

[40]*Ibid*, pp. 223,224.

cation, food or fluids or the performance of a medical procedure deemed necessary to provide comfort care," which leaves open the question of whether food and fluids *not* deemed necessary for comfort are life-sustaining procedures that may be withdrawn.[41]

In line with such thinking, it is easy to suspect the verdict for comatose patients in particular, who may be judged by medical personnel as impervious to discomfort and to pain. Appropriately the final paragraph of the statement of the Bishops' Committee for Pro-Life Activities (on "quality of life" judgments) would brand such disregard for sustaining life as "hastening the deaths of vulnerable patients by starvation or dehydration." This second statement of the U.S. Bishops' Pro-Life Committee could hardly have influenced Catholic participation in "living will" legislation in 1985, but the 1984 "Guidelines for Legislation on Life-Sustaining Treatment" (first Pro-Life Committee document as discussed above) must have been welcomed warmly as authentic Church teaching. All 13 of the statutes passed by various states in 1985 prohibit the withdrawal of nutrition and hydration. The Society for the Right to Die stated in their report on the 1985 "living will" acts: "It was at least partly to assuage opposition to living will legislation on the part of the Catholic Conference of Bishops in several states that law drafters specifically excluded this procedure [that is, withdrawing sustenance] from the definition of life support that could be withheld from dying patients."[42] In several states, however, the prohibition against withdrawing nutrition was limited to what is "deemed necessary to provide comfort care" (for example, Arizona and New Hampshire).

Neither of the Bishops' Pro-Life Committee statements specify that prohibitions against withholding food and drink apply only to sustenance administered by way of mouth. Since the distinction between *natural* feeding by way of mouth and *artificial* feeding by intubation is not referred to in either statement, it is only logical to conclude that, as a general rule, and regardless of the mode of administration, feeding and hydration are not to be discontinued.

---

[41]*Handbook of 1985 Living Will Laws* (New York, N.Y.: Society for the Right to Die, 1986), p. 18. The same source mentions that "all 13 of the 1985 statutes make some mention of sustenance in their sections listing definitions," . . . and adds: " . . . it is to be hoped that lawmakers will rethink and amend." p.16.

[42]*Ibid.*, p. 7.

1.4 PRONOUNCEMENT OF THE NEW JERSEY CATHOLIC CONFERENCE

The January 22, 1987 issue of *Origins* published the friend-of-the-court brief of the New Jersey Catholic Conference entitled "Providing Food and Fluids to Severely Brain Damaged Patients." The document was of special urgency in view of the fact that in the Nancy Ellen Jobes case pending before the court, the husband of this 31-year-old brain-damaged woman (she was not terminally ill) had petitioned the court to deny his wife food and fluids. The bishops of New Jersey used the "amicus curiae" approach (speaking for the New Jersey Catholic Conference) as a means "by which the bishops may speak on matters of public policy."[43]

Although this letter of the bishops of the New Jersey Catholic Conference lacks the degree of doctrinal authenticity which would attach to similar pronouncements from the national conference of American Catholic bishops, it is a document which expresses doctrinal reliance on the Holy See's *Declaration on Euthanasia* (1980) and on the two pronouncements of the American bishops (through the Committee for Pro-Life Activities) as discussed above. It might be called a summary of the teachings of the Holy See and of the American bishops on the subject of providing food and fluids for the sick and helpless. The Catholic bishops of New Jersey apparently are presenting their arguments as flowing from the traditional teaching of the Catholic Church on the subject. This statement would seem to be substantiated by the opposition to their arguments as orchestrated by an influential Catholic organization which promoted a special conference on "Ethical Issues Surrounding Nutrition and Hydration" to register viewpoints contrary to the teachings of the Catholic bishops of New Jersey.[44] There is no doubt in the mind of this writer that the letter of the Catholic bishops of New Jersey represents an authentic summary of the traditional teaching of the Catholic Church on the crucial and sensitive subject of feeding the sick and the helpless.

The following selective quotations from the friend-of-the-court brief of the Catholic Bishops of New Jersey are clear regarding the *general rule* that nutrition and hydration should be administered to patients who are in imminent danger of death. In theological language, "general rule" means that something is of obligation *usually*, or *"per se ut in pluribus."* This is not to deny that in particular cases, exceptions to the general rule can and must be made

---

[43]*Origins*, Jan. 22, 1987, pp. 582–584. Quotation on p. 582.

[44]Article entitled "Catholic Health Association, New Jersey Bishops Clash Over Providing Food and Water" by Dave Andrusko, in the *National Right to Life News*, March 19, 1987, pp. 1 and 8 (an article which defends the position of the Bishops of New Jersey).

(the subject of the next section of this discussion). The following quotations also convey the importance of making a distinction between *medical treatments* and *ordinary care*. They also confirm the view that food and fluids constitute an essential aspect of ordinary care. It is also apparent in the following quotations that the obligation to continue nutrition and hydration *usually* applies regardless of whether or not food and drink are administered by way of mouth or by artificial intubation. (quoted from *Origins*, Jan. 22, 1987):

> Our case deals with a most fundamental right, that is, the right to life, and the corresponding duty of society to protect that right. The denial of food and fluids, of nutrition and hydration, ultimately results in starvation, dehydration and death. It is direct. It is unnatural, as unnatural as denying one the air needed to breathe, or murder by asphyxiation.

> Society and society's laws consider the person who starves himself as suicidal. Society and society's laws should oppose the intervention by other parties which may enable or facilitate suicidal starvation, however willing the victim.

> From our Judaeo-Christian heritage, the Catholic Church has developed a distinctive approach to fostering and sustaining human life. Our tradition not only condemns direct attacks on innocent life, but also promotes a general view of life as a sacred trust over which we can claim stewardship but not absolute dominion. A positive duty to preserve life is part of this tradition. Consequently the conference maintains that nutrition and hydration which are basic to human life, and as such distinguished from medical treatment, should always be provided to a patient. Withdrawal of nutrition and hydration introduces a new attack upon human life (p. 582) . . . .

> The conference maintains that nutrition and hydration, being basic to human life, are aspects of normal care, which are not excessively burdensome, that should always be provided to a patient. Nutrition and hydration are clearly distinguished from medical treatment. Medical treatment is aimed at curing a disease. Nutrition and hydration are directed at sustaining life. Medical treatment is therapeutic; nutrition and hydration are not, because they will not cure any disease. For that fundamental reason we insist

that nutrition and hydration must always be maintained . . . (p. 583).

The friend-of-the-court brief also referred to the *Child Abuse Amendments* of
1984 which came to the defense of severely handicapped newborn infants.
According to those amendments, any failure to provide nutrition and hydration for such infants would constitute child abuse. In commentary, the brief of
the Bishops of New Jersey stated:

> We cannot understand why failure to provide nutrition and hydra-
> tion to a handicapped child constitutes actionable child abuse but
> withdrawal of nutrition and hydration from an incompetent adult
> would be permissible (p. 583).

1.5 SUMMARY OF CHURCH PRONOUNCEMENTS ON FEEDING THE HOPELESS AND THE HELPLESS

Man is not the master of his life. Life and "length of days" from birth
until natural death, is in the hand of God. The obligation incumbent upon
every human individual to conserve his life invalidates any claim to a strict
"right to die,"—to say, in effect, "let me starve to death." As stated previously, these truths have been so effectively established and corroborated
("probatae et roboratae") in Bishop Cronin's dissertation that his scholarship
provides the *foundation* of this extended discussion of obligation to feed the
needy and the helpless. God's dominion is universal. Again, to quote St.
Paul's letter to the Romans (14:7): "None of us lives as his own master and
none of us dies as his own master."[45]

In building upon this foundation, three additional questions have been
proposed: (1) whether or not a distinction is to be made between *medical
treatments* and *ordinary care*; (2) whether or not the concept of ordinary care
essentially includes the provision of nutrition and hydration; (3) whether or
not the provision of nutrition and hydration by artificial means remains un-

---

[45]Orthodox Jewish tradition on this subject is surveyed by Michael Nevins, MD, specialist in
internal medicine, cardiology, and geriatrics, in an article entitled "Perspectives of a Jewish
Physician," in *By No Extraordinary Means* (cf. note 12), pp. 99–107. He writes: "Quality of life is
not an issue. Even noncognitive lives have value, if only for others as an object of caring. Our
bodies are not our own—it is as if we are but tenants and have no absolute title. God is the source
of health and sickness and alone decides when life is to end" (p. 100).

der the heading of ordinary care. The first question clearly is answered in the *affirmative* in all of the documents mentioned above: the distinction between medical *treatment* and ordinary *care* is deeply rooted in magisterial documents. The same can be said with regard to the question of whether or not providing nutrition and fluids is an essential aspect of nursing care. In the language of legendary Sherlock Holmes of mystery fame, "elementary, my dear Watson" ("alimentary" for the punster) should apply. Some authors quibble about this. It is true that the major magisterial source, the *Declaration on Euthanasia* (1980) does not make explicit mention of nutrition and hydration as included in ordinary nursing care. That message is implicit, however, in the very nature of the document. At any rate, the two pronouncements from the Roman Curia (the Council on Health Affairs in 1981, and the Pontifical Academy of Sciences in 1985) explicitly mention "alimentation" and "feeding" respectively with reference to ordinary care.

With regard to the third question (alimentation by mouth vs by artificial means), the reader is invited to review the extended discussion as presented earlier (pp. 160 ff.). That discussion warrants the conclusion that, as a general rule, the administration of nutrition and hydration by artificial means is not to be characterized as a medical *treatment*, and that it is an *ordinary* means of conserving life. In addition to the authoritative nature of the two pronouncements of the National Council of Catholic Bishops in 1984 and 1986 (and, for the faithful of the State of New Jersey, the pronouncement of the Catholic Conference of that state in 1987), it is significant that these three documents stand as authentic interpretations of the magisterial teachings of the Church on such a crucial and sensitive subject.

The appropriate answers to the three questions proposed above, therefore, are as follows: (1) The Holy See clearly makes a distinction between medical *treatments* and nursing *care*; (2) nutrition and hydration are included essentially in the very concept of ordinary nursing care; (3) as a general rule, the administration of nutrition and hydration remains a part of ordinary care *even if* the condition of the patient is such that it must be provided by artificial means. Three questions: three affirmative answers. As stated previously, the contention advanced here is that, as a general rule, nutrition and hydration must be administered to all sick and helpless patients. That obligation is all the more humane as the patient becomes more and more defenseless due to the imminent danger of death from natural causes.

CHAPTER II

Possible Exceptions to the Nutrition/Hydration Obligation

The discussion in this section will be limited to patients in a *terminal* condition who are in *imminent danger of death*. The situation of patients who are *not* both terminal and in imminent danger of death merits special attention, and will be discussed in the next section of this study (that is, patients who are diagnosed as permanently unconscious, whether comatose or in a vegetative state). A *terminal condition* is described as an incurable condition caused by injury, disease or illness, which, regardless of the application of life-sustaining procedures, would, within reasonable medical judgment, bring about the death of the patient. In such circumstances, the application of life-sustaining procedures (that is, recourse to mechanical or other artificial means to sustain, restore, or supplant a vital function—a respirator, for example) would serve only to postpone the moment of death of the patient. *Imminent danger of death* means that death probably will occur, in the ordinary course of events, within a period of approximately two weeks (more or less).

Contrary to the views of authors who would remove or relax the obligation to provide nutrition and fluids to a terminal patient who is in imminent danger of death, the contention here is that the obligation remains (as a general rule) *even though* the condition is incurable, and *even though* death is imminent, and *even though* food and fluids must be provided by artificial means. The basic reason is because the *conservation* of life (as opposed to the *prolongation* of life) is still of obligation. Even though the prolongation of life by cure, healing or a "turn for the better" is no longer possible (and not of obligation in the circumstances), the obligation to conserve the ebbing tide of life remains, *unless* circumstances change so that the continued provision of nutrition and/or hydration becomes *extraordinary* (or disproportionate) nursing care and hence non-compulsory. Such exceptional circumstances which would justify the termination of efforts to provide nutrition and/or hydration for terminal patients usually are grouped under three headings: (a) when it is useless in terms of conserving the life of the patient ("nemo ad inutile tenetur"); (b) when it results in excessive pain or burden for the patient ("primum non nocere"), and (c) when the feeding process becomes impossible ("nemo ad impossibile tenetur").

2.1 USELESS IN TERMS OF CONSERVING THE LIFE OF THE PATIENT

> No one is held to what is useless
> ("Nemo ad inutile tenetur . . . ")

Human life must be conserved regardless of the fact that, in particular cases, any hope of a physical cure or even of a temporary improvement in the patient's physical condition must be abandoned. This is one way of saying that human life must be *conserved* even though it cannot be *prolonged* beyond the anticipated life expectancy of each particular individual. Human life, from conception and eventual birth until natural death, is a gift of God. Especially in view of the fact that every individual human life is a probationary prelude to eternal life, no individual human life can be considered as useless. Even the diminished quality of life of a terminal patient who is in imminent danger of death cannot render the conservation of that individual life "not worth the effort." If the feeding process is useless (without effect, futile) in terms of conserving life, however, it may be terminated. When the conservation of human life can no longer be maintained by the hand of fellow men and women, it passes over into the hand of God. In the words of the Book of Wisdom (16:13). " . . . you [O lord] have dominion over life and death."

The following question must be anticipated: "What degree of uselessness would justify the decision to not initiate or to withdraw the feeding process?"

If the phrase *"morally* useless" is used (as in "morally certain," etc.), it must not be interpreted in accord with the primary meaning of "morally" (which is "from the viewpoint of moral rules or principles"), but rather in accord with the secondary meaning of the word "morally" which is, "according to reason or probability: virtually." The word "virtually," in turn, means "almost entirely: for all practical purposes."[46] In other words, the obligation to begin or to continue the feeding process could cease in consideration of reliable clinical evidence that the process is *virtually* or "for all practical purposes" useless in terms of *conserving* the life of the individual. In the *Child Abuse Amendments of 1984*, such a concept of "virtually useless" was applied to the medical *treatment* (not the feeding process) of developmentally-disadvantaged newborn infants. These amendments stated that such treatments would not be required when (among other stipulations),

> . . . in the treating physician's or physicians' reasonable medical judgment . . . the provision of such treatment would be virtually futile in terms of the survival of the infant and the treatment itself under such circumstances would be inhumane.[47]

The requirement of uselessness or futility, therefore, would not mean that the feeding process would have to be entirely or absolutely useless in terms of conserving the life of the individual, but that there is reliable clinical evidence that the feeding process is "for all practical purposes", or virtually useless, to that end. As examples of virtual futility or uselessness in the feeding process, authors mention situations such as the following: a patient with a severe clotting deficiency and a massive body burn (danger of hemorrhage or infection in installing either tube feeding or IV feeding); a patient with severe congestive heart failure who develops cancer of the stomach with a fistula which blocks passage of food from the stomach to the colon (even fluid feeding through IV could be too much for a weakened heart); an infant with an infarction of all but a short segment of bowel (plus the danger of hemorrhage and infection in IV feeding).[48]

In each particular situation, the *judgment* as to the uselessness of the feeding process would be made by the attending physician; but the *decision* to

---

[46]Cf. *Webster's Third International Dictionary*, unabridged (Springfield, Mass.: Merriam-Webster, Inc., 1986).

[47]*Child Abuse Amendments of 1984*, Pub. L., No. 98–457, Oct. 9, 1984. Cf. Conference Report, Title I, Part B, Sec. 121, Section 3.

[48]"Must Patients always be given Good and Water?" by Joanne Lynne, MD, and James F. Childress, PhD, in *By No Extraordinary Means* (cf. note 12), p. 51.

initiate or discontinue an artificial feeding process should be made by the patient after conferring with the physician. If the patient is incompetent, responsibility for decision making would pass to the appointed proxy, family member or relative as the case may be. If the decision is made to not initiate or to discontinue the feeding process on the basis of uselessness (or on the basis of virtual impossibility, or of adding excessive pain or burden to the patient's condition), warranted hydration measures should be maintained and monitored in addition to the meticulous administration of pain-killing drugs and sleep-inducing medications. Moderate hydration measures would include sponging out the mouth, moistening the lips, administering ice chips and/or the "glucose drip," etc. In other words, comfort measures are to be continued.

In an article in *Theological Studies* in June 1950, Father Gerald Kelly, S.J., referred to two examples of "little or nothing" as advanced by the eminent theologian Cardinal De Lugo. One was a man condemned to starvation; another a man to be burned to death. The Cardinal stated that the former would not be obligated to eat if his friends could bring him food only once or twice, and that the latter would not be obligated to put out the fire if he had but a few buckets of water for that purpose. The Cardinal applied the phrase: "a little bit may be reckoned as nothing" ("parum pro nihilo reputatur").[49] Father Kelly saw a close connection, and yet a "slight difference" between that phrase, and the phrase "No one is held to do what is useless."[50] The phrase "a little bit may be reckoned as nothing" was applied in the days when lenten fasting and fasting before receiving Holy Communion were emphasized more consistently. Theologians advised the faithful "not to worry about it" if they accidentally ingested a modicum of food between meals during Lent or with the before-Communion fasting period, because "a little bit is like nothing at all." Naturally the phrase would not apply to the observance of the natural moral law or the divine positive law (ten commandments, etc.). A "little bit" of lying, of blasphemy, of positively "coveting your neighbor's wife," etc. still is morally objectionable. The phrase does illustrate theological thinking, however, with regard to the obligation to feed the hopeless and the helpless.

---

[49] "The Duty of Using Artificial Means of Preserving Life," in *Theological Studies*, June, 1950, p. 208.

[50] *Ibid.*, p. 208. He states: "Furthermore, De Lugo applies his principle even to the taking of food, which is a purely natural means of preserving life, whereas the other authors were speaking only of remedies for illness." This quotation is found also in *Conserving Human Life*, p. 100

Another illustration of theological thinking as applied to the concept of uselessness, is the frequent reference among theologians to the phrase "spes salutis." Although this phrase lends itself to a translation of "hope of welfare or well-being," it appears that leading theologians such as Cardinal De Lugo and Francis Vitoria (and the many who quoted them thereafter) used the expression in the sense of "hope of survival"—that is, the hope of *conserving life (Conserving Human Life,* pp. 85 f.). As a matter of fact, Bishop Cronin discusses "Spes Salutis" under the general title of "The Nature of the Ordinary Means of Conserving Life." In other words, if the nutrition/hydration process, whether natural or artificial, contributes to the *conservation* of life to a "little or nothing" degree, it could be considered a useless means of conserving life. With regard to the positive obligation to conserve human life, "a little bit can be reckoned as nothing." Due to the very slight anticipated benefit (little or nothing), the hope of conserving life simply is not proportionate to the effort involved in initiating or in continuing the feeding process.

2.2   CAUSES EXCESSIVE PAIN OR BURDEN— "PRIMUM NON NOCERE"

The phrase "Primum non nocere" ("above all, do no harm") presumably stands as evidence of the enduring influence of the great physician of antiquity known as Hippocrates (born about 460 B.C.). A portion of the Hippocratic Oath states: " . . . and I will abstain from all intentional wrongdoing and harm." An excellent introduction to the discussion of pain and burden is provided by Gilbert Meilaender as follows:

> The point of medical care is not just to ward off death. That battle
> always will be lost eventually, and to think of medicine's task in
> such a way would be to consign it to futility. Nor is the point of
> medicine just to treat diseases—as if they and not patients con-
> sulted with doctors. Nor is the goal simply to keep blood circulat-
> ing or tissue living when a patient can no longer recover or sustain
> life as a whole, integrated organism. Medicine's point, rather, is
> not so much cure as care—restoration of health when possible,
> continued care when that is not possible. Its subject is the patient
> who may be the bearer of many illnesses but is still "the one flesh

in which . . . diseases inhere." It's focus is the health of the human being, not the isolated functioning of organs or systems.[51]

That "focus on the health of the human being" involves concern for pain and burden both in care and in treatment. Pain and/or burden can be either physical or psychological. The word "physical" refers to the body; the word "psychological" refers to moods of the human mind as varied as debilitating fears, emotional instability, obsessive worries, persistent depression, etc. The scope is so wide that almost any decrease in emotional balance might pass for a "psychological pain and/or burden" unless the term is interpreted from a solidly rational and realistic viewpoint.

Authors commonly speak of "excessive pain or burden" as justification for withdrawing tube feeding in appropriate circumstances. Naturally, the "painful" aspect would apply to the patient only. The same should be said of the "burdensome" aspect unless there are exceptional circumstances in a given situation. This statement is based on the basic principle that there is a limit to the burden that even caring family members and friends can be expected to bear in extremely trying circumstances. This might apply especially in the home care of patients who are victims of advanced dementia. In such circumstances, especially if the caretaker is elderly and alone with the patient, the task of attending to the feeding process could become a *virtual impossibility*. (cf. extended remarks, section 2.3 to follow).

In any Christian context of health care, it is essential to stress that the burden factor, both for the patient and for those who minister to their needs or care for them, cannot be identified with the continued existence of the patient. Regardless of the quality of life of the patient, human life itself cannot be said to be a burden. This conclusion follows from a faith-filled consideration of human dignity and of human destiny in accord with God's plan for mankind. This is not to deny that some aspects of continued survival might be included among the pains and/or burdens which might justify the removal of the tube feeding regimen. The point is that *human life itself* cannot be included as one of those burdens. From the perspective of our Catholic faith with its focus on eternal life, the wide variety of sorrows, sufferings, reverses, which are so endemic to earthly existence (excluding life itself), constitute an ongoing burden, an enduring trial, a probationary period in the pursuit of "an eternal weight of glory." Burdens, suffering, and sorrows are not with-

---

[51]"The Confused, the Voiceless, the Perverse: Shall We Give Them Food and Drink?" by Gilbert Meilaender, PhD, Department Chairman and Associate Professor of Religion, Oberlin College, Ohio, in *Issues in Law and Medicine* September, 1986, pp. 133–48. Quotation on pp. 136, 137.

out purpose and meaning (Cf. St. Paul's Second Letter to the Corinthians, 4:16–18).

A—Caution Required in Considering Possible Psychological Burdens

It is important to emphasize that the focus here is on supportive nursing *care* (with a view to the conservation of life) and not on medical *treatments* (with a view to the prolongation of life). A terminal patient who cannot rely on any hope of a cure or improvement in his condition, and who can continue to breathe only with the help of a mechanical respirator (*a medical treatment*), could be justified in insisting upon the removal of the respirator especially because of the connection between his lingering and "hopeless" condition and burdensome side effects for his family and loved ones. These would be psychological burdens. He may feel, for example, that his lingering condition puts too much strain on his elderly wife who cares for his daily needs, or on loving family members who take turns "around the clock" to lend a hand; or that the money involved in his continued care would deprive a favorite son or daughter, or a grandchild, of the opportunity for higher education; or that his continued care would exhaust most of the savings which he had built up for the support of his wife later on, etc. The *Declaration on Euthanasia* states explicitly that no one is obligated to submit to a type of medical *treatment* ("genus curationis") which, though already in use, is not without risk or is excessively burdensome, and adds:

> This rejection of a remedy is not to be compared to suicide; more accurately ("verius") it is to be regarded as a simple acceptance of the human condition; or of a desire to avoid the burdensome application of a medical technique of unequal value compared to the anticipated results; or, finally, a desire not to impose a heavy burden on the family or on the community.[52]

With regard to *ordinary nursing care* which is central to the very concept of the *conservation of life*, however, the situation is quite the contrary. In the examples of psychological burdens above, the terminal patients who are in imminent danger of death can reject *treatments* which can only *prolong* the moment of death. Once they have exercized voluntarily that option ("discontinue the treatment"), the concerns for the physical welfare or financial welfare of his wife, or for educational opportunities of children or grandchildren, do not

---

[52]Cf. *Enchiridion Vaticanum*, VII (cf. note 5), n. 370. Translation mine. Cf. also *Origins*, August 14, 1980, p. 156.

compete with the patient's right or option for prolonging his life through a medical treatment. That right or option has been passed over voluntarily, and the patient has favored, by his own free will, some other valid and over-riding concern. There is no implication, in the objective analysis of such valid concerns considered in themselves, that the life of the patient is not worth living—that life itself is a burden.

On the basis of *nursing care*, however, concerns such as those mentioned above would compete with the patient's right and *obligation* to reach out for nutrition and fluids as essential for the *conservation* of life. The patient's right and obligation cannot be set aside on moral grounds unless the feeding process (whether natural or artificial) is virtually useless, or unless some aspect of the feeding process adds excessive pain or burden *for the patient*. If concerns which involve burdens for family members or others are allowed to prevail over the right and obligation of the patient to conserve life,—including the obligation of family members and others to aid in that conservation of life,—the implication that the continued life of the patient is in itself a burden could not be denied. There is no doubt, however, that pressing concerns such as financial security for others, the physical welfare of an elderly wife who cares for the patient, etc. could justify the termination of tube feeding in particular cases on the *basis of virtual impossibility* (when the implication mentioned above is not necessarily present), but not on the basis of burdens to others besides the patient. The "virtual impossibility" issue will be discussed at length in the next section of this study.

To say that the life itself of a terminal patient in a lingering and incurable illness cannot be evaluated as a burden is not to deny the anguish of suffering and uncertainty for the patient. Many loyal and devout Christians who are in a lingering terminal illness are inclined to pray as Jesus did: "My Father, if it be possible, let this cup pass me by" (Matthew, 26:39). Yet, such members of the faithful would feel constrained to add, as Jesus did: "Still, let it be as you would have it, not as I." The reality of suffering and sorrows, both present and future, including the inevitability of death itself, cannot justify a member of the Church Militant in saying: "Let me starve to death." That so-called "right to die" which the patient does not have, obviously cannot be exercized by others on the basis of excessive psychological burdens.

In order to be acceptable as a psychological burden for the patient which might justify the removal of the feeding tube, the excusing factor would have to be some excessively burdensome aspect of the nutrition and hydration process itself. One contemporary ethicist refers to a situation of advanced mental illness" . . . when the person is conscious but severely and irreversibly demented, [and] the care in feeding, though not useless, *may* be so burdensome that it should cease."[53] Especially in cases of administering nutrition and hydration by means of a nasogastric tube (which can be quite irritating), the patient may manifest signs of actually being terrified by the repeated efforts to observe the prescribed feeding schedule. In many cases, a resourceful nurse or caretaker might adjust the schedule, and experiment in the process, so as to overcome the patient's reaction. The same author adds: "This requires demonstration during a trial period . . . and the judgment is quite different from concluding that the person's life has become too burdensome to preserve."[54]

The efforts to modify, experiment, and adjust various aspects of the feeding process might involve some temporary decrease in nutritional values until the proper balance and patient-satisfaction have been achieved. If the patient is being fed through a gastrostomy, there is the possibility of night-time feeding as a workable alternative for individuals who object to the regular feeding process. This alternative, known as "cyclic feeding," leaves the patient free of the usual feeding techniques during the day. It involves continuous tube feeding (apparently at a slow rate) during the night hours.[55] Since the patient would be sleeping and perhaps sedated to some extent, during these feeding hours, the potential burden of having the patient "fight" the feeding process during the day would be avoided. If the burden factor for the patient simply could not be eased or avoided by some alternative feeding technique, the nutrition process might have to be curtailed to some extent or even discontinued. In that event, special attention would have to be focused on providing some degree of hydration by moistening the lips, sponging out the mouth, etc.[56] Adequate sedation against pain would also have to be provided.

There are other advantages of reducing the times or the amounts of the feeding process in some cases, and this on the basis of not adding to the pain

---

[53]"Caring for the Permanently Unconscious Patient," by Gilbert Meilaender, PhD, in *By No Extraordinary Means* (cf. note 12), p. 200. See also a discussion of several cases of this type by Ron M. Landsman, JD, *Ibid.*, pp. 135–149. Note especially page 142.

[54]*Ibid.* (Meilaender, p. 200). Cf. also a discussion of "Options for Interventions" in caring for nursing home residents who simply stop eating, by Joanne Lynn, M.D., *Ibid.*, especially pages 164–169. The article is entitled "Elderly Residents of Long-term Care Facilities."

[55]Cf. letter to the editor from K. Sriram, M.D., and Barbara Palac, MS, RD, in the Oct. 5, 1984 issue of the *Journal of the American Medical Association*, p. 1682.

[56]In an article entitled "Observations on Nutrition and Hydration in Dying Cancer Patients," nurses Phyllis Schmitz and Merry O'Brien call the oral cavity the "most frequently neglected part of the alimentary tract." As practical sources of relief for dry mouth, they mention "chewing gum, drinking iced beverages, and sucking on hard candy or popsicles." Found in *By No Extraordinary Means* (cf. note 12), pp. 29–38. Quotation on p. 32.

or burden factor. A reduction in the amounts, even if only on a temporary basis, may reduce the sensations of nausea, vomiting, and of abdominal pain. This might also lessen automatically the added burden of incontinence (hence fewer linen changes), of stuggling with the commode or bedpan, less pulmonary secretions which cause coughing, less congestion, and perhaps less shortness of breath. In this manner, the basic nutrition and hydration process can be continued at least on a curtailed basis, and the patient can be comforted with an improved self image.[57]

The role of the nurse in tailoring the nutritional program to the particular needs of the patient, cannot be minimized in any way. In attending to the needs of terminal patients in particular, the nurses provide those intimate details of individual physical and emotional care which enable them to know each patient as a unique human being. In most institutional settings, the feeding program is based on the physician's prescription for a regular diet or an order for more complicated intravenous or tube-feeding therapy. The implementation and administration of such prescriptions or orders, however, is entrusted to the members of the nursing staff. Even patients in imminent danger of death can experience relief and a renewed sense of autonomy if the nurses strive to tailor the feeding program to the physical and emotional needs of each patient.

If the patient is competent, for example, and can take nutrition by way of mouth, nurses in hospitals and nursing homes can individualize food serving in accord with the preferences and limitations of each patient. This is possible due to the utilization of refrigerators and microwave ovens located near the patient unit. The patient can then be encouraged to work up an appetite by opting for small meals served more frequently, or by having attention paid to passing food-craving episodes, or by requesting treats such as high-caloric drinks, blenderized foods, etc.[58] If such patients can be given nutrition and fluids only through tube-feeding, the social significance of "eating" can still be maintained. Two nurses who care for dying cancer patients explain this approach as follows:

> We prefer to attach the same social significance to artificial feeding as we would to a meal consumed in the natural manner. For example, patients being artificially fed can retain control over their feeding schedule. Controlling "medical" feedings is usually

---

[57]*Ibid.*, pp. 29–31. Cf. also "Terminal Trajectory: Compassion, Comfort, and Dignity," by Sandra S. Bardenilla, Cardiac Care Unit Staff R.N., in *Issues in Law and Medicine*, March, 1987, pp. 391–401.

[58]*Ibid.* (Nurses Schmitz and O'Brien), pp. 36, 37.

a new and enjoyable experience for the patient. Our patients are surprised to learn that such "treats" as coffee, juice, or alcoholic drinks can be put through the enteral tubes, as well as the prescribed nourishment.[59]

If the patient is incompetent, a caring nurse could individualize the feeding program at least to some extent on the basis of the patient's known eating habits and food preferences as manifested previously to family members. If such information is lacking, the feeding process might be designed on the basis of what other terminal patients of similar age and background seem to prefer. For all terminal patients the danger presented by nausea, vomiting, diarrhea, etc., which sometimes accompanies feeding on a regular schedule and could develop into a cause of excessive pain or burden, can be decreased by changing the amount of nourishment (whether articially or orally) in a program of more frequent and smaller servings. These can be scheduled for times when nausea, stomach upsets, intestional motility, etc., are least troublesome.[60] This could well obviate the need of making a decision to discontinue the feeding process altogether.

These observations on "caution required in considering possible psychological burdens" refer to the *maintenance* or continuation of an artificial feeding program. Emphasis has been placed throughout on the responsibility of the attending physician, family members, etc., in maintaining the program. A commentary must be added with regard to the *initiation* of such a process from the viewpoint of the *patient's* obligation to allow the installation of such a process. Let us say that an elderly terminal patient, lady "A," harbors an intense fear and repugnance of the very concept of artificial feeding methods. It is well known among health care workers that the nasogastric method can have the dangerous side effect of causing excessive pain or burden such as pneumonia; and that the gastrostomy method can be associated with very serious and painful infections. Lady "A" had a good friend, now deceased,

---

[59]*Ibid.*, p. 37

[60]*Ibid.* These nurses mention that the good nurse must recognize that "force-feeding or artificial feeding can sometimes be harmful and may thus be contraindicated." P. 37. Situations of this type are discussed by Joyce V. Zerwekh, ARNP MA, in an article entitled "Should Fluid and Nutritional Support be Withheld from Terminally Ill Patients?," in the *American Journal of Hospice Care*, July/August, 1987, pp. 37–38. The article is prefaced with the words "Another Opinion, and does manifest something of a crusading spirit against going too far in respecting what she calls the "myth" that dehydration and electrolyte imbalance "cause suffering in those near death." Cf. p. 38.

who had suffered intense additional pains which had been occasioned by widespread infections associated with the gastrostomy method. Lady "A" felt amply justified in her adamant attitude of "having nothing to do with a gastrostomy hook-up."

Lady "A" presented a real dilemma to her attending physician. She insisted on being transferred to her home in the country, far from hospital facilities, for the remaining days or weeks of her life. Her elderly husband would have to attend to her nursing care. Her physician was concerned about the fact that she was fast losing her ability to ingest food and drink orally. He was convinced that she would be completely unable to eat and drink orally within a few days after arriving at her home. This woman was determined to die at home; and her physician was determined to do whatever medical science could provide to protect this woman from death by starvation and dehydration.

Unless the physician or others could rid lady "A" of her intense sense of fear and repugnance over the prospect of a gastrostomy regimen—either by virtue of his professional experience with many other patients, or by assurances of medical help in the event of a serious infection—her resolute attitude could constitute a valid reason for not putting her on an artificial-feeding regimen. Forcing such a feeding process upon lady "A" would be a clear violation of the guiding rule of "above all, do no harm" ("primum non nocere"). He would be obligated, however, to provide Lady "A" and her elderly husband with adequate information on the administration of sedatives and pain killers, and on simple techniques of proper care of the oral cavity as a minimal means of meeting basic hydration needs. The situation described in this scenario might also be considered as a reason for omitting the installation of an artificial feeding process on the basis of virtual impossibility—which will be discussed at length in the next section of this chapter. On the basis of a excessive psychological burden, the traditional theological term could be translated as "intense emotional fear or repugnance" ("vehemens horror"). Such situations will be discussed in section 2.3, B of this chapter.

B—Proper Interpretation of "Excessive" Pain or Burden

The word "excessive" (from the Latin word, "excedere," which means to "go beyond, to exceed") admits of a wide range of interpretation depending on particular circumstances. Appropriate synonyms for "excessive" range all the way from "immoderate, inordinate, extravagant, exorbitant," to "extreme." According to *Webster's Third New International Dictionary*, "excessive describes whatever notably exceeds the reasonable, usual, proper, necessary, just, or endurable." Pain and/or burden, therefore, depending on the circumstances of each particular case, may be considered as excessive long before it might be characterized as "extreme." In other words, "excessive" is a relative term. Myriad factors such as the individual's personal tolerance of pain and/ or burden, his or her emotional balance, religious outlook, mental attitude, etc., must be evaluated in the light of objective factors such as the severity of the patient's condition, proximity to the moment of death, effectiveness of the administration of pain-killers and analgesics, degree of consciousness, etc.

As an illustration of the relative nature of the word "excessive" with regard to potential pain or burden, this writer remembers well his visit to an elderly friend in his mid 70's who had been hospitalized for a very precarious heart condition. Typical of this gentleman's enviable emotional balance and sense of humor was his remark (made in a weak voice but with an impish grin): "They expect me to die today; but I am going to take my good-natured time." So he did. He died two days later. In all probability, an individual as spiritually prepared and emotionally well balanced as this patient would manifest a high degree of tolerance for pain or burdens, so that the word "excessive" would not apply. He would belong to the category of patients of sturdy spirit who pride themselves in "taking things in stride." In other cases, a terminal patient who is competent may prefer the feeding process to be continued regardless of the pain and/or burden factor. Such a preference must be respected.

As an illustration of a situation when continued nutrition and hydration might not be warranted, some authors refer to the increased burden and some degree of additional pain when the administration of artificial feeding is continued close to the actual time of death. Continuation of the feeding process at such a critical time could be accompanied by terminal pulmonary edema, nausea, and mental confusion.[61] Unless the patient is competent and wants to have the feeding process continued, the situation could warrant a partial or even a total termination of the feeding process. The situation must be monitored professionally and lovingly. If these nutrition needs are less and less an element of sustenance as the moment of death approaches, they can become more and more an element of comfort—knowing that someone loves and cares. This aspect of "primum non nocere" must not be underestimated.

For some patients, the need for artificial nutrition and hydration may arise only after they have been diagnosed as in imminent danger of death. If they can no longer be fed by way of mouth (can no longer swallow, etc.), a temporary peripheral intravenous line may be warranted. It would seem,

---

[61] "Must Patients Always be Given Food and Water?" by Joanne Lynnm MD and James F. Childress, PhD, in *By No Extraordinary Means* (cf. note 15), pp. 52, 53. Cf. also the article by Joyce V. Zerwekh as mentioned in note 60.

however, that any efforts to install tube feeding, either nasogastric or by gastrostomy, when the patient is in such an advanced stage of human debility and suffering, would amount to adding an excessive pain and/or burden factor to the condition of the patient. The very process of installing and maintaining a tube feeding system would be disproportionately painful and burdensome for a conscious patient who is destined to die within a few weeks. The burdens might even include the risk of pneumonia with nasogastric feeding or the risk of infection with the gastrostomy process. In most situations of imminent danger of death, the question of the *usefulness* of the efforts to install and maintain tube feeding would also be open to question. There may be cases, however, when a conscious patient in imminent danger of death requests the installation of a tube feeding process despite the risk of added pain or burden. His or her wishes in the matter should be respected.

2.3 NO OBLIGATION TO DO THE IMPOSSIBLE

Naturally the likelihood of having some type of artificial feeding installed was quite rare earlier in this century when trips to the doctor or to the hospital were personal expenditures. The social obligations of government were promoted during the administration of President Franklin D. Roosevelt (1933–1945) beginning with social security. A wholesome sense of personal responsibility for health care gave way to a rising crescendo for government help and employer insurance coverage. Gone were the "good old days" when elderly parents found care and love by rotating residence among their married sons and daughters, and when doctors were approached only after home care and home remedies had failed. Furthermore, most drugs could be purchased without a prescription. In this age of insurance coverage, HMO's, PPO's, and the expanding wings of Medicare and Medicaid, the recommended first line of defense is "Go, see the doctor."

Another reason for the trend to hospitalization is mentioned in a report of the *President's Commission for the Study of Ethical Problems in Medicine and Biomedical and Behavioral Research* (to be referred to hence forth as *President's Commission*) as follows:

> At the turn of the century, influenza and pneumonia were the leading causes of death, followed by tuberculosis and "gastritis." By 1976, these had been supplanted by heart disease, cancer, and

cerebrovascular disease—illnesses that occur later in life and that are ordinarily progressive for some years before death.[62]

Whereas most people died in their homes around the turn of the century, the fantastic progress in medical technology in response to medical needs on the contemporary scene has increased the trend of patient care in an institutional setting (hospitals, nursing homes, homes for the aged). This explains why the number of deaths in institutional settings rose from 50% of all deaths by 1949, to 61% by 1958, to over 70% by 1977, and perhaps to 80% by the early 1980s.[63]

The number of Americans who would be inclined to seek hospitalization, and thus be put on a tube feeding regimen if warranted, would depend to a considerable extent on the number who can rely on some type of health care coverage. In 1980, according to the Survey of Income and Education (U.S. Dept. of Health and Human Services), 70% of the population (161 million Americans) were insured primarily under private plans (Blue Cross and Blue Shield, prepayment plans such as HMOs); 21% (43 million) were protected under public government financing programs (Medicare for the elderly and the disabled, Medicaid for the poor); 5.2 million were eligible to receive health benefits from the military (the Uniformed Services program and the Veteran's Administration). Three national surveys in 1976, 1977 and 1978, established an estimate of the uninsured as from 22 to 25 million of the population.[64] The total is even higher if the "part-time insured" are also counted. The "part-time" category results from situations such as the fact that many factory workers are not covered when they have been laid off, or that low-income single parents become ineligible for Medicaid once their earnings exceed the state's income cutoff limit. Based on 1977 figures, for example, 18 million people were without insurance coverage for all of 1977 (not insured), and another 16 million lacked insurance coverage for a part of that year. In 1977, 83.9% of the population were always insured, 8.6% were never insured, and 7.5% were part-time insured.[65]

---

[62]Cf. *Deciding to Forego Life-Sustaining Treatment* (Washington D.C.: U.S. Government Printing Office, 1983), p. 16

[63]*Ibid.*, pp. 17, 18.

[64]Cf. another publication of the President's Commission, *Securing Access to Health Care, I* (Washington D.C.: U.S. Government Printing Office, 1983), pp. 91–93.

[65]*Ibid*, pp. 93–95. "National Medical Care Expenditure Survey data show that individuals insured for only part of the year use substantially fewer services when they are uninsured . . . and that these people do indeed forego medical care when they are sick" (p. 93).

These demographic considerations indicate that there must be millions of Americans, especially of the low income and poverty levels, who would be very unlikely candidates for the installation of a tube feeding mechanism if such a supplemental aid is warranted. Without financial coverage for health care, they would look to relatives, friends and neighbors to care for them in time of sickness, and would be among the minority of Americans who die at home. For many if not most individuals of this category, the difficulty of being provided with a tube feeding mechanism could be considered a virtual impossibility (sometimes called a "moral impossibility"). This expression "virtual impossibility" is to be interpreted in the same way as the expression "virtually useless" (pp. 42 ff. of this study). "Virtually impossible" means "for all practical purposes" impossible.

A classic example of virtual impossibility as a justifying reason for not providing nasogastric and gastrostomy installations and pertinent equipment would be the situation of missionaries and health workers in many third world countries. The legendary Mother Theresa of Calcutta, for example, dispenses TLC or "tender loving care" to thousands of off-the-street guests throughout the world. Because of the poverty (and sometimes primitive) conditions, no one would speak of an obligation to provide tube feeding if the sick or infirm person is unable to receive nutrition and fluids by way of mouth. In view of the figures mentioned above, the same would apply to many areas throughout the U.S.A. where poverty is an ever-challenging factor, and where access to hospital and medical facilities is "for all practical purposes," impossible.

The "virtually impossible" response with regard to providing tube feeding could well apply to many Americans who do have private or public insurance coverage, but who reside at a considerable distance from medical facilities. Reaching such medical facilities to have an artificial feeding mechanism installed might be considered "for all practical purposes" impossible because of the distance itself, or because of a lack of transportation facilities (care-taker unable to drive and no alternate driver is reasonably available), or because of the perilous condition of the roads at the time when the medical facilities are needed, etc. Another excusing reason (even though covered by insurance) may be that the patient simply insists on passing his last weeks or months "at home," and the caretaker (wife, husband, relative) is alone with the patient and is incapable of assuming responsibility for the maintenance and functioning of the tube feeding program, etc. "Nemo ad impossibile tenetur."

It should be noted, in passing, that the impossibility with regard to being sustained by artificial means could also be a *physical* (as opposed to a virtual of moral) *impossibility*. It stands to reason that a patient would have no obligation to be sustained by such means if they are simply unavailable, or it they are available but the patient is in no way capable of making use of them.

A—"Conserve Life" as a Positive Precept of the Natural Law

In the section on "The nature of the extraordinary means of conserving life," Bishop Cronin presents the traditional teaching of theologians on the subject of *positive* and *negative* precepts of the natural law (pp. 98, ff.). Negative precepts such as "Thou shalt not lie," and "Thou shalt not kill," are binding always and forever ("semper et pro semper") because they forbid something which is intrinsically evil. The excuse of "virtual impossibility" could not justify the violation of such precepts. Direct abortion, for example, as a violation of "Thou shalt not kill," is wrong "always and forever." Positive precepts such as "Thou shalt honor thy father and mother," and "Thou shalt love the Lord thy God . . . and thy neighbor . . . ", are positive precepts and bind always as a general rule, but not "forever" in the sense of being of obligation in all possible circumstances. If keeping such positive precepts, in particular circumstances, involves a proportionately grave or serious inconvenience, the individual concerned is excused from observing the precept in those particular circumstances.

One of the prime *positive* precepts obligates every individual to conserve his or her life if he or she is physically able to do so, unless it is a "virtually impossible" situation. Bishop Cronin states that an individual is always bound to avoid suicide because it is intrinsically evil: "However, there is a limit to his obligation of conserving his life in a positive manner." This does not mean that a person must use any and all possible means to conserve his life. The obligation is to use means which are considered *reasonable* means which are called *ordinary*. Means which go beyond that reasonable category are called *extraordinary* means. Bishop Cronin's concluding statement to that particular paragraph is of singular importance with regard to the concept of virtual impossibility: "The reason the extraordinary means are not obligatory is the fact that there is a *certain impossibility* connected with either obtaining or using them" (*Conserving Human Life*, pp. 99).

There is a close relationship between the phrase "proportionately serious inconvenience" (as used above) and the phrase "virtual impossibility." It would appear to be the relationship between cause and effect. The "proportionately serious inconvenience" is the cause, and "virtual impossibility" is the effect. It should not be surprising, therefore, to note that theologians seem to equate the one phrase with the other.[66] The word "inconvenience" in En-

---

[66]As mentioned in *Conserving Life*, p. 114, some theologians referred to as certain type of impossibility" (Vitoria, Sayrus, Mazzotta); others use the term "moral impossibility" (Tournely, Mrac-Gertermann, Aertnys-Damen, Kelly); others use the term "grave inconvenience" (Lehmkuhl, Kelly, Pacquin).

glish, however, has a connotation which seems somewhat light and flimsy when compared to the stronger Latin derivative, "incommodum." In *Cassell's Latin Dictionary*, the Latin word "incommodum" is translated as "disadvantage, . . . injury, . . . misfortune." Hence an interpretation of "serious inconvenience" in the stronger sense of "serious disadvantage, injury, or misfortune" would seem to provide a more accurate rendering of the Latin "incommodum" as used by Latin scholars and theologians throughout the centuries.

In answer to the question: "how serious an inconvenience constitutes a virtual impossibility?," the answer should be (as inferred above): "A *proportionately* serious inconvenience" (*burden* aspects) relative to the advantages (*benefit* aspects), with due regard for the gravity of the precept of conserving life. This requires a prudential weighing or balancing of the anticipated *benefits* of submitting to the artificial feeding process as compared to the anticipated *burdens*. This would refer, of course, to *reasonably* anticipated benefits and burdens, all factors and circumstances considered. As emphasized when discussing the interpretation of "causing excessive pain or burden" ("primum non nocere," cf. p. 189 of this study), however, *human life itself* cannot be put in the balance as one of the burdens. To give in to the inclination to regard human life itself as a burden is to open the door to "quality of life" considerations. In line with such thinking, especially with regard to terminal patients who are in imminent danger of death, the "burden" of maintaining the feeble flame of human life often would be seen as disproportionate to the observance of the precept of conserving human life. Human life itself, often for reasons "known to God alone," is always a blessing. From the viewpoint of spiritual salvation, that statement is always a valid and preponderant consideration.

B—Possible Causes of Virtual Impossibility Situations

Throughout the centuries, theologians have discussed various possible situations of virtual impossibility with regard to the precept of conserving life. These theological views not only suggest situations when artificial feeding might be omitted or discontinued, but also illustrate the relativity factor in applying theological theory to practical cases. In other words, much would depend upon the circumstances peculiar to each case. These examples of possible "virtual impossibility" situations might be summarized as follows: excessive *efforts* ("summus labor et media dura"), excessive *suffering* ("quidam cruciatus and ingens dolor"), excessive *cost* ("sumptus extraordinarius, media pretiosa and media exquisita"), and very intense *emotional fear or repugnance* ("vehemens horror"). Bishop Cronin observes that these four elements will not always be present in a given means of conserving life (hence the relative

202

factor), and adds: "If they are present and render a means extraordinary, it is because they have been the cause of moral impossibility" (cf. *Conserving Human Life*, p. 103). "Moral impossibility," as stressed previously, is also known as a "virtual impossibility."

If one or more of the four elements mentioned above apply to the patient in some aspect of the installation or of the maintenance of artificial feeding, it could justify the omission or the termination of the artificial feeding process on the basis of virtual impossibility. This follows from the basic principle that the obligation to conserve human life is based on a *positive* precept of the natural law. Positive precepts of the natural law do not bind or obligate in the presence of a proportionately serious inconvenience.

It would seem that two of the four situations as listed above (excessive suffering, and intense emotional fear or repugnance) would affect primarily the patient. The other two (excessive efforts and excessive costs) would affect primarily family members and loved ones. There should be no moral objections to assigning due weight and pressure to such elements as excessive cost and excessive efforts insofar as they affect others (besides the patient). It would not be a case of competing against the right and obligation of the patient to conserve his life as in similar cases discussed on the *basis of excessive burdens* of a psychological nature (cf. this study, pp. 190 and 191). In such cases, there is a clash between pressing concerns of *others*, and the right and *obligation* of the patient (also incumbent upon others) to conserve his life. In the balancing of the burdens and benefits in the two situations mentioned above (excessive efforts, excessive costs) which involve others besides the patient, there is no implication that the life of the patient is in itself a burden. The prime and formal focus is not on *burden as burden*, but on factors (costs, difficulties, etc.) which combine to constitute a virtual impossibility.

As an example of a situation of virtual impossibility as emerging from *excessive efforts* on the part of others, one might consider the plight of a very elderly immigrant couple who live alone, far away from medical facilities, and who have a very minimal familiarity with the English language. The wife is terminal with cancer of the esophagus, can no longer ingest sufficient nutriment by way of mouth, and is determined to die at home. They also lack transportation facilities, and are not covered by hospital insurance. Even if the wife in her very debilitated condition could be persuaded to make that long trip to a hospital, it is very doubtful that the husband, due to the language difficulty, could be made to understand the basic instructions on the subject of maintaining the tube-feeding process. The best that might be expected would be to summon a physician or nurse who could instruct the husband on the administration of pain killers and analgesics, and on minimal hydration and lubrication for the oral-cavity needs of his wife. Surely these factors would combine to present a "virtual impossibility" situation. Similar situations undoubtedly could be found in rural areas and in secluded areas throughout the nation.

As a example of a similar situation emerging from circumstances of *excessive cost*, many of the factors in the example sketched above (no medical insurance, elderly couple living alone in secluded area, lacking in transportation facilities, etc.), could combine to raise validly the issue of a "for all practical purposes" impossibility. Presuming that such couples often would have very modest savings, and might even lack collateral for negotiating a loan, it would be difficult to imagine how the elderly husband of the patient (who is losing her capacity to obtain nourishment by way of mouth) could even think of obtaining a tube feeding installation for his wife.

C—Withholding vs. Withdrawing Artificial Feeding

It is safe to say that failure to *initiate* a tube feeding process in a warranted situation can be explained and "smoothed over" more easily than a decision to *terminate* such a process which had been effective in the past. The obligation element in both cases can be traced to the traditional teaching that a person can be morally responsible not only for *human actions*, but also for *human omissions*. Based on the wisdom of St. Thomas Aquinas, theologians teach that three conditions are to be verified before it can be established that the effect of an *omitted human act* can be considered *voluntary*. If the omission is voluntary, the individual is responsible (from a moral viewpoint) for the bad effect. In other words, the bad effect can be imputed or ascribed to that particular individual (often called the doctrine of human imputability).[67]

The first of the three conditions is that the bad effect is foreseen at least in a confused manner. The reason is because nothing can be considered voluntary unless it is foreseen to some significant degree. Thus a young lady would not be considered guilty of intoxication if such a condition occurred on a date which featured her first experience with strong "highballs," and she had been led to believe that they were no stronger than a small glass of wine. The second condition is that it is within the power of the individual involved to omit or avoid the action or at least to render it ineffective. The reason for this statement is that an effect cannot be more voluntary than its cause. If a heavy drinker makes no effort to avoid the company of his old cronies who regularly

---

[67]Cf. St. Thomas Aquinas, *Summa Theologica, I–II* (Taurini, Italia: Marietti, 1937), Q. 71, art. 5 corp, and ad 1, 2 and 3. Cf. also Merkelbach, Benedict H., O.P., *Summa Theologiae Moralis*, I (cf. note 12), pp. 67, 68; Jone, Heribert, O.F.M. and Adelman, Urban, O.F.M., *Moral Theology*, first ed. (Westminster, Maryland: Newman Bookshop, 1945), pp. 4, 5.

urge him to join in heavy drinking bouts, he is guilty of the sin of intoxication. The third condition is that the individual must be obligated to prevent the action so that the bad effect does not follow. Thus a man would not be doing wrong if he failed to warn a chance acquaintance at the local bar that he was ordering too many drinks; but he would be obligated to warn his young son in a similar situation.

Let us say that the spouse, or close family member, or guardian of a terminal cancer patient (hence *obligated* to do something about the situation) is told by the attending physician that the patient eventually will starve to death without artificial tube feeding (hence *foresees* the bad effect), and yet does nothing about it. He foresees the bad effect, and is obligated to do something to prevent that bad effect from taking its course, but is it within his power to order or at least urge the installation of the artificial feeding process? If it is not within his power or sphere of influence to instigate tube feeding, or if there are solid reasons to believe that no one will heed his orders or urgent suggestion (for example, more influential relatives who are closer to the patient have joined forces to insist on "no artificial feeding"), he could not be blamed for failing to act, and for the onset of starvation dehydration which would bring about the death of the patient. This scenario is based on the presumption, however, that there are no solid reasons, based on clinical evidence, that the artificial feeding process would be virtually useless, virtually impossible, or that it would add excessive pain and/or burden for the patient.

A person who failed to initiate a feeding process (although *obligated*, able to *foresee* the starvation effects, and in a *position* to do something about it) presumably would be less liable to criticism by family members of the patient than if he had used his position to *terminate* an artificial feeding process which had been in operation for some time. From a moral viewpoint, a *culpable omission* in such circumstances (not initiating the process) is equally as objectionable as the *action* of using personal influence to bring about the termination of an effective feeding process without due cause.

Those who are responsible for initiating a warranted feeding process are also obligated to use their influence to assure the continuation of the process. If artificial feeding loses its effectiveness (becomes virtually useless, or adds excessive pain or burden for the patient), the attending physician or nurse might well incur the suspicions or recriminations of family members if the feeding process is terminated. This emphasizes the importance of providing family members, preliminary to the decision to initiate the artificial feeding process, with clear and frank information on the reasonable expectations of such a feeding process. Even though family members may hold out no hopes whatever of seeing their loved one back in good health, they may get the impression that artificial feeding is almost guaranteed to solve the nutrition/

hydration problem until the very end. Because of such "great expectations" in particular situations, some physicians may be reluctant to initiate a tube feeding regimen if there are indications that it might be of dubious or transient value for the patient.[68] Unless there is another reasonable and available alternative, however (in some cases, for example, a peripheral intravenous procedure), the attending physician remains morally obligated to provide artificial access to nutrition and hydration when warranted.

The difficulty of terminating an artificial feeding process in warranted cases is complicated by what is known as the *symbolic* meaning of administering food and drink. The attending physician cannot simply refuse to take that factor into account in dealing with family members of the patient. Continuation of the artificial feeding process might be contra-indicated due, for example, to complications of incurable renal failure, or pulmonary edema (hence virtually useless, or adding excessive pain or burden), and family members seem adverse to even listening to the explanation of the attending physician as to why the process should be terminated. Some would say that the public must be educated to take control of their emotional reaction to the very concept of denying food and water to dying patients in *any* situation. Daniel Callahan, Director of the Hastings Center, explains why he would vote against such an educational program:

> The feeding of the hungry, whether because they are poor or because they are physically unable to feed themselves, is the most fundamental of all human relationships. It is the perfect symbol of the fact that human life is inescapably social and communal. We cannot live at all unless others are prepared to give us food and water when we need them . . . . It is a most dangerous business to tamper with, or adulterate, so enduring and central a moral emo-

---

[68]Cf. "Must Patients Always be Given Food and Water?." by Joanne Lynn, MD, and James F. Childress, PhD, in *By No Extraordinary Means* (cf. note 12), p. 56. The recent publication of the Hastings Center entitled *Guidelines on the Termination of Life-Sustaining Treatment and the Care of the Dying* (Bloomington and Indianapolis, Ind.: Indiana University Press, 2nd. printing, 1987, to be referred to hereafter as *Hastings Guidelines*) has a brief section entitled "Withholding and Withdrawing Treatment." One helpful paragraph reads as follows (p. 130): "There is actually a strong reason to prefer stopping treatment over not starting it in some cases. Often there is uncertainty about the efficacy of a proposed treatment, or the burdens and benefits it will impose on the patient. It is preferable then to start the treatment and later stop if it is ineffective or overly burdensome from the patient's perspective . . . rather than not to start the treatment for fear that stopping will be impossible or unethical. Not starting in these ciracumstances could deprive the patient of beneficial treatment that the patient might find desirable. "These guidelines list" feeding tubes" as *treatments* (cf. preface, p. IV).

206

tion, one in which the repugnance against starving people to death could be, on occasion, greater than that which a more straitened rationality would call for.[69]

In the scenario sketched above (artificial feeding unwarranted), the attending physician might cushion the shock for family members by maintaining the minimal level of nutrition warranted by the patient's worsening condition (renal failure, pulmonary edema, etc.), or substitute the tube feeding mechanism with a peripheral intravenous line. In many cases, the need for hydration could be met by exercising special care of the oral cavity (ice chips, rinsing with cool water, etc.)

As an indication of how physicians have come to respect the symbolism of food and drink (and perhaps also concern for legal action against professional negligence), a survey of medical staff members and house members in one hospital several years ago revealed that 73% would have ordered adequate amounts of intravenous fluids for a particular comatose cardiac arrest patient who had been resuscitated and put on a respirator. The other 27% indicated that they would write orders for intravenous fluids that could not support life. There was no significant hope of survival for the patient. The account of this survey did mention the possibility of fear of legal liability, as well as the possibility that the 73% who opted for continued adequate IV's may have considered that to be an "ordinary means." The validity of the symbolic factor, however, was expressed as follows: "Perhaps the doctors felt that to stop the intravenous fluids would be seen as abandoning the patient, or perhaps they felt guilty that they just couldn't do any more for this patient."[70]

In a very perceptive article on this delicate subject, Ronald R. Cranford, MD, an expert in neurology at the University of Minnesota, gives due consideration to four factors: (1) respect for the symbolic nature of feeding; (2) the great emotional trauma of family members in seeing their loved one deprived of fluids and nutrition; (3) the inevitability of death if all fluids and nutrition are withdrawn from the patient; and (4) the potential for abuse if stopping nutrition and fluids in certain extreme cases becomes a policy (danger, that is, of extending the policy to the severely retarded, or patients with cerebral palsy). He concludes that health care workers and others ought to be "cautious and sensitive in decision-making practices concerning nutritional support for permanently unconscious patients and to reflect carefully and

---

[69]"On Feeding the Dying, in *The Hastings Center Report*, October, 1983, p. 22.
[70]"An Empirical Study of Physician Attitudes," by Kenneth Micetich, MD, Patricia Steinecker, MD, and David Thomasma, PhD, in *By No Extraordinary Means* (cf. note 12), pp. 39–43. Quotation on page 42.

deliberately before removing what may be the final barrier between life and death."[71] The caring and prudent physician will take all four factors into account before forming a judgment with regard to the termination of an artificial feeding process for dying patients.

Except for passing mention of psychological burdens for patients in the concluding paragraphs of section 2.2, A of this study, the obligation of the *patient* with regard to withholding or withdrawing an artificial feeding process has been discussed only in general terms. The obligation both to allow the tube feeding process to be installed in the first place, and to allow it to remain in effect for the duration of the emergency, has been implied throughout this study. The moral obligation is equally binding in both instances ("starting" and "stopping"). As to the "starting" aspect, the project usually would begin with the explanation of the attending physician that the patient's welfare and even survival requires the addition of some type of tube feeding which, in the vast majority of cases, is effective and free of excessive pain or burden. Aspects of cost (about the same as oral feeding), maintenance (can be done by family members in the home) and imposed limitations on social life (well tolerated by thousands of patients) probably would be explained during the physician-patient-family members discussion period which would follow. On the basis of the contention throughout this study that food and drink, even if administered artificially, are prime aspects of ordinary nursing care, some pastoral counseling should precede the decision of the patient to allow the tube feeding process to be initiated. Emotional issues may torment some patients for a day or two ("why linger on if I cannot be well again?" etc.), but the average practicing Catholic will admit the lack of any personal right to say "let me starve to death."

Once the tube feeding process has been put into operation, however, and is proceeding effectively (sustaining life) and is free of any aspects of excessive pain or burden, the patient is not at liberty to say: "I regret that I ever gave my approval to this artificial type of nursing care. I insist that you discontinue the food and drink service and allow nature to take its course." In the words of the *Declaration on Euthanasia* (last paragraph of section II), when some gravely ill patients beg for death ("pull the plug," or "stop the feeding process"), their words are "not to be understood as implying a true desire for euthanasia; in fact, it is almost always a case of an anguished plea for help and love."

---

[71]"Patients With Permanent Loss of Consciousness," in *By No Extraordinary Means* (cf. note 12), pp. 186–194. Cf. especially pp. 191, 193.

CHAPTER III

The Unique Situation of Permanently Unconscious Patients

Up to this point, the discussion has been focused on the category of patients as included in the quotation from the *Declaration on Euthanasia* (1980): "When death is imminent and cannot be prevented by the remedies used . . . (Cf. p. 6 of this study). In other words, the focus has been on patients who are in a terminal condition and in imminent danger of death. The discussion now shifts to the category of patients as envisioned in the Report of the Pontifical Academy of Sciences (1985): "If the patient is in a permanent coma, irreversible as far as it can be foreseen, *treatment* is not required, but *all care should be lavished on him, including feeding*: (Cf. p. 174 of this study).

In other words, the focus now is on the general classification of *permanently unconscious* (some prefer "persistently unconscious") patients who are *neither in a terminal condition nor in imminent danger of death* in the strict sense of those phrases. They are not dying patients. The general rule is that both categories of patients—the dying (terminal condition plus imminent danger of death) and the permanently unconscious—are entitled to the continued administration of nutrition and hydration. This general imperative is based on the contention throughout this study that feeding, even if administered by artificial means, is an essential aspect of *ordinary care* (and not a *treatment* or *extraordinary care*).

In the interests of clarifying terminology, it should be noted that the *President's Commission* has defined permanently unconscious patients as those who lack all possible components of life—all thought, feeling, sensation, desire, emotion, and awareness of self or environment.[72] Five categories of individuals are mentioned as patients who "might be diagnosed to be permanently unconscious:" . . . (1) patients in a persistent vegetative state (PVS) such as Karen Quinlan; (2) patients who are unresponsive after brain injury or hypoxia and who do not recover sufficient brain-stem function to stabilize in a vegetative state before dying (most of whom die within a few weeks after the brain-damage incident); (3) patients who are end-stage victims of neurologic conditions such as severe Alzheimer's disease; (4) comatose patients with intercranial and untreatable mass lesions such as tumors or vascular masses (death comes within a few days or weeks); (5) patients with congenital underdevelopment of the central nervous system (hypoplasia) such as anencephalic infants (death usually comes within a few days after birth).[73]

Since the persistent vegetative state or condition seems to be the most common and widely discussed form of permanent unconsciousness, it is important to inquire as to the depth of unconsciousness in a PVS (permanent vegetative state) patient. Dr. Ronald E. Cranford M.D. of the University of Minnesota, and Chairman of the Ethics and Humanities Committee of the American Academy of Neurology, provides the following information in an article entitled "Patients With Permanent Loss of Consciousness":

> Such patients perceive neither themselves nor their environment. Neurological examination reveals no neocortical functions. yet these patients do have sleep-wake cycles, and at times their eyes open. From a neurologic standpoint, they simply do not experience pain, suffering, or cognition . . . . Yet in trying to draw a line to separate awareness from unawareness, we cannot decide where exactly to place our pencil: from awareness to unawareness, or consciousness to unconsciousness, is a continuum. While it is very difficult to describe and diagnose many conditions on this continuum, the distinction between complete absense of consciousness and the retention of some slight awareness or thought can ordinarily be accomplished by careful examination by qualified specialists.[74]

---

[72]*Deciding to Forego Life-Sustaining Treatment* (cf.note 62), p. 174

[73]*Ibid.*, pp. 177–181.

[74]*By No Extraordinary Means* (cf.note 12), p. 187. The report (1983) entitled *Deciding to Forego Life-sustaining Treatment* (cf. note 62) as published by the *President's Commission* states that "recovery of consciousness is very unlikely, however, for patients with hypoxia who remain comatose or in

The above quotation introduces only one of the aspects of feeding the permanently unconscious which makes it such an emotional issue—How can we be sure that the individual is *permanently* unconscious? Other emotional aspects of the problem which often are exaggerated unduly by the media might be special emphasis on the exorbitant costs of caring for such patients, or the need of compassion to allow such patients to "die with dignity," or the pitiful scenario of watching such loved ones linger on for months and years "without any hope of return to sentient life," etc. These highly emotional aspects of contining sustenance for permanently unconscious patients often are give exaggerated emphasis in the press and in television and radio programs. Perhaps some of the clouds of misunderstanding can be dissipated by a brief discussion of some of the basic needs in approaching the subject of permanent unconsciousness.

3.1 IMPORTANCE OF A BALANCED CONCEPT OF PERMANENT UNCONSCIOUSNESS

The emotional considerations mentioned above apparently have influenced the general public of some countries to favor active euthanasia for irreversible cases of terminal illness and permanent unconsciousness. In the Netherlands, for example, a series of court decisions has made euthanasia an accepted practice. After a careful screening of patient requests for "doctor assisted" death (by means of "a lethal drink or injection"), 5,000 to 8,000 terminal patients have had their lives terminated through deadly physician-patient cooperation. This type of legal euthanasia is said to be favored by 75 percent of the general public.[75]

A trend in the same direction can be detected in America. According to a poll undertaken for the American Medical Association in the Summer of 1986, approximately two-thirds of U.S. citizens (1,100 out of approximately 1,500 queried) said that they favored "withdrawing life-support systems, including food and water, from hopelessly ill or irreversibly comatose patients if

---

PVS for more than one month. Certainly, extended observation is appropriate before making a diagnosis of permanent unconsciousness, at least for hypoxic injuries in otherwise healthy young people" (pp. 179, 130).

[75]Cf. special article by Gregory E. Pence, PhD, in the January, 1988 issue of *The American Journal of Medicine* entitled "Do Not Go Slowly into That Dark Night: Mercy Killing in Holland," pp. 139–141.

the patients or their families request it."[76] This would be *passive* euthanasia, as recommended by the influential Wanzer Report, and favored by the American Medical Association in many cases.[77] A brief "confession" by a gynecology resident in a large private hospital was published in the Jan. 8, 1988 issue of the Journal of the *American Medical Association* (p. 272). As indicated by the title of the brief article ("It's Over Debbie"), this anonymous physician administered a lethal dose of morphine to a girl of 20 who told him: "Let's get this over with." This shocking evidence of "doctor assisted" death alarmed Americans throughout the land. In the interests of stemming the tide of increased cases of this type in America, it is important to "get the facts straight," and present arguments against such an ungodly and demeaning solution to human suffering.

A—Realistic Estimates of the Number of Permanently-Unconscious Patients

Media reports can leave the reader or listener with the impression that the number of permanently unconscious individuals in the nation is quite large. The *President's Commission* frankly admits their inability to embark "on a large-scale study which would yield national statistics or widely generalizable data" because of limitations of time and of budgeting.[78] The difficulty of assembling reliable data can well be imagined. Many reported cases may not have been carefully studied or adequately described. A later publication of the *President's Commission* in 1983 states that the evidence relevant to the prognosis of permanence is still quite limited, and that the overall number of permanently unconscious patients is small. This report adds:

Furthermore, the number of variables affecting prognosis (for example, the cause of unconsciousness, the patient's age and other

---

[76]Reference found in the *Handbook of Living Will Laws, 1987 Edition* (New York, N.Y.: Society for the Right to Die, 1987), p. 13.

[77]The Wanzer Report was formulated by Sidney H. Wanzer, MD, and nine other physicians from prestigious medical centers throughout the country, from Oct. 28-30, 1982. The meeting was held in Boston, under the auspices of the Society for the Right to Die. The "formulation" proceeded without the imput of any professional ethicist or theologian, and decided (among other things) for patients in a persistent vegetative state (once PVS has been established "with a high degree of certainty") that "it is morally justifiable to withhold antibiotics and artificial nutrition and hydration" from such patients. Cf. *The New England Journal of Medicine*, April 12, 1984, pp. 955-959.

[78]Cf. *Defining Death* (Washington D.C.: U.S. Government Printing Office, 1981) p. 89.

diseases, the length of time the patient has been unconscious, and the kinds of therapy applied) is large and imperfectly understood.[79]

There seems to be a tendency among the general public to generalize when they hear reports of comatose or permanently unconscious individuals, and to include friends or relatives in hospitals, nursing homes, etc., who may lapse into apparent unconsciousness for temporary periods. Noted cases of permanently unconscious patients such as Karen Ann Quinlan of Roxbury Township, New Jersey (1954–1985) and Paul E. Brophy of Easton Massachusetts (1937–1986) died in a persistent vegetative state. Such cases must not be confused with the condition of many men and women in nursing homes and in homes for the aged such as Claire C. Conroy of Belleville, New Jersey (1900–1983) who was neither permanently unconscious nor in a persistent vegetative state,[80] nor with most victims of Alzheimer's disease and other very old and very debilitated individuals who may have intervals of unconsciousness. There is also a tendency to confuse incompetency with unconsciousness. Patients who usually are alert and conscious and competent might have their artificial feeding process terminated in the event that it becomes virtually useless, or adds excessive pain or burden to their condition. As a general rule, such exceptions would not apply to permanently unconscious individuals.

The general "ball park" figure as to the number of permanently unconscious individuals as reported now and then in the press seems to be "5,000–10,000." The 5,000 figure conceivably could come from a footnote in one published report of the *President's Commission* which states that the only "prevalence survey" available estimates that Japan has about 2,000 permanently unconscious patients in long term care. The report adds that such a figure would imply less than 5000 at any one time in the United States "if the prevalence were the same and if differing definitions of terms did not cause substantial error"[81] The 10,000 figure is mentioned in a publication of an organization which could be inclined to over-emphasize the magnitude of the nutrition-termination problem, and that is, the Society for the Right to Die. In their *Handbook of Living Will Laws, 1987 Edition,* a reference is made to the view of the Chairman of the Judicial Council of the American Medical Association to the effect that the opinion of that council recommending the with-

---

[79]*Deciding to Forego Life-Sustaining Treatment* (cf. note 62), p. 177.

[80]"In *re* Conroy: History and Setting of the Case," by Jeff Stryker, in *By No Extraordinary Means* (cf. note 12), pp. 227–235. Reference on p. 230.

[81]*Deciding to Forego Life-Sustaining Treatment* (cf. note 62), p. 176, footnote n. 15.

holding of artificial nutrition and hydration from the irreversibly comatose "could affect at least 10,000 patients who are in 'irreversible coma' ".[82]

Even if the "ball park" figure for the number of permanently-unconscious individuals is considered to be closer to 10,000 than to 5,000, this would average out, at most, as approximately 200 such patients in every state of the union. Add to this the fact that most permanently unconscious patients die within a few weeks after diagnosis (cf. p. 210–211 of this study), and the problem loses much of its numerical magnitude. Especially with regard to long-term-care patients who have lapsed into a persistent vegetative state, however, the social, psychological and emotional aspects present a problem of the first magnitude. A more recent study of patients who became unconscious due to brain hypoxia or ischemia (that is, coma due to the lack of oxygen or lack of blood supply to the brain) revealed that 57% of the 210 patients in the group (all victims of cardiac arrest) died without opening their eyes, 13% regained independent function at some time during the first year following cardiac arrest, and 20% passed over into the vegetative state (PVS).[83]

With regard to the 13% (regained function) and 20% (PVS) categories, the reader is reminded of the notation on page 210 of this study (footnote n. 74) that recovery of consciousness is very unlikely if the patient remains comatose or in a persistent vegetative state for more than one month. Exceptions to this general guideline would depend upon factors mentioned previously; that is, the age and other diseases of the individual, the cause of the unconscious condition (traumatic or non-traumatic), kinds of therapy used, etc. Since most of the long-term survivors are in the PVS category, it is important to note that the basic cause of such a lingering condition usually is a head injury (fights, gunshot, auto accident), or intracranial hypoxia resulting from cardiac arrest, asphyxiation or hypotensive shock, or intracranial hypoglycemia (as from an insulin overdose). In all three situations, the damage to the

---

[82]*Handbook of Living Will Laws, 1987 Edition* (cf. note 76), p. 11. A footnote indicates that the figure of 10,000 is the usual figure ascribed to the permanently unconscious.

[83]Cf. "Predicting Outcome From Hypoxic-Ischemic Coma," by David E. Levy, MD, et al., in the *Journal of the American Medical Association,* March 8, 1985, pp. 1420–1426, and especially the commentary on that study by Peter Black, MD, PhD, in the editorial section of the same periodical, issue of Sept. 6, 1985, pp. 1215 and 1216. The editorial comment is entitled: "Predicting the Outcome From Hypoxic-Ischemic Coma: Medical and Ethical Implications." Dr. Black comments on the suggestion of Dr. Levy and colleagues that "at least in some patients, treatment might be withheld early in the course of coma to facilitate death rather than prolonged coma," by posing the question: "Should 'health care planners' have anything to do with decisions to withhold treatment?"

brain "often initially causes loss of function in areas of the brain that might recover with time and treatment."[84]

A more up-to-date description of unconsciousness such as the persistent vegetative state, was provided in a recent article by a physician in the *New York Times* entitled "When the Mind Dies But the Brain Lives On." He stated that the view that continuous sleep-like comas seldom last more than a month is supported by recent research. He mentioned the use of positron emission tomography (PET) scanning as indicating that PVS is comparable to the deepest stages of anesthesia, and that such patients do not feel pain. They do exert reflex responses, however, when pinched or otherwise stimulated. He also explained that life continues in this state because the brain stem activates the vegetative, or autonomic nervous system, to carry on the vital mechanical functions governing breathing, heart pumping, blood pressure and the elimination of wastes.[85]

Long-term-care PVS patients will be discussed later on in this study. It should be noted that the prognosis for a return to a normal and well-functioning level of life is very poor even for individuals who recover from their comatose or vegetative condition soon after the crucial one-month period. The well publicized case of Jacqueline Cole, wife of Presbyterian Minister Harry Cole of Baltimore, Maryland, may serve as a rather typical example. A cerebral hemorrhage on March 29, 1986, brought on her comatose condition. Her husband waited 41 days for her recovery, and then petitioned the court to allow her to die (in keeping with her expressed sentiments before the hemorrhage). The judge refused to grant the petition. Six days later, Jacqueline Cole awoke, smiled and returned her husband's kiss. Some five months later, her recovery was far from complete. The October 6, 1986 edition of *Time* magazine mentioned that she was "walking with the help of a metal frame, her memory slowly returning."[86] Perhaps future medical technology will provide the basis for more favorable expectations for the families and loved ones of comatose and PVS individuals.

B—Searching for Alternatives to Expensive Hospital Care

There is some validity to the complaint that money and medical resources should not be expended so lavishly in the care of patients who are most unlikely to regain consciousness, when such expenditures of time and

---

[84]*Deciding to Forego Life-Sustaining Treatment* (cf. note 62), pp. 178, 179.
[85]*New York Times,* Nov. 17, 1987, article by Lawrence K. Altman, MD, p. C 3.
[86]*Time* Magazine, October 6, 1986, p. 35.

money could be diverted in part to curable physical needs of others. Once the patient has been diagnosed by qualified experts as permanently unconscious, comfort care including nutrition and hydration must be continued. Aggressive treatment and round-the-clock monitoring (usually in intensive care units), however, would be inappropriate. The obvious burdens would far outweigh reasonably-anticipated benefits in all but truly special cases (for example, drug-related cases, brain injury to children younger than five years, hypothermia cases, etc.).

The report of Dr. Levy and others on the study of comatose patients (cf. footnote 83) referred to 93 poor-prognosis patients, 88 of whom failed even to regain consciousness. To quote from the report: "Continued support of those 88 patients involved a total of 500 hospital days, frequently in intensive care units. Not only was this useless terminal care costly (over $250,000) but the intensive care beds could have been used to treat patients with greater chances of recovery."[87]

Two extremes must be avoided. One extreme would be to subject the unconscious patient to repeated attempts at resuscitation and to advanced and even experimental testing procedures relatively long after qualified experts have reached a definite diagnosis of irreversible coma or persistent vegetative state. That "relatively long" period, depending on each particular case, could be several weeks or even one month. The other extreme, which definitely would be immoral, would be to predict the prognosis of prolonged or even permanent unconsciousness, at least for some patients, on the basis of *predictive* testing procedures on given days (1st day, 3rd day, 7th day, etc) after the onset of coma. Such procedures would include testing of pupillary dilation, spontaneous eye movements, corneal reflex, etc. In other words, objective evidence would be inadequate for a definite prognosis, but the *predictive* outcome would guide physicians, patients' families and health planners in making decisions on treatment, or on non-treatment (for example, terminate all life-support measures). One group which favors this trend emphasizes that those who regain consciousness face incapacitating disabilities, and adds:

The ability to predict outcome could also spare families the emotional and financial burden of prolonged care of patients with hopeless prognoses. The impact on allocation of scarce health re-

---

[87]Cf. footnote 83, article by David E. Levy, MD, et al., *Journal of the American Medical Association*, March 8, 1985, p. 1426.

sources can be appreciated from consideration of the potential effect of confidently identifying poor-prognosis patients.[88]

The spiral of cost can be tempered to a considerable extent not only on the hospital level, when emphasis is shifted from cure to care, but also on more informal levels of health services. A secondary dividend of such a shift in emphasis would involve more generously the TLC (tender loving care) participation of friends and loved ones, as well as the comforting feature for incurable patients of dying at home. In the case of Paul E. Brophy of Easton, Massachusetts (died Oct. 23, 1986), for example, who lingered over three years in a persistent vegetative state, the total cost of care at two hospitals of the Boston metropolitan area (New England Sinai Hospital in Stoughton for over three years, and Emerson Hospital in Concord for approximately one week) must have soared well into six figures. A rough estimate would be in excess of $400,000 for the period (from late March, 1983, until Oct. 23, 1986).[89] Undoubtedly his devoted wife, a registered nurse, had valid reasons for not transferring him to a home care or hospice care setting. But such a transfer would have translated into substantial financial savings.

Contemporary thinking with regard to the prolonged care of incurable and manageable patients seems to be in favor of home care of hospice care, or a combination of both. Even the controversial *Wanzer Report* (cf. footnote 77) states that when the facilities provided by an acute-care hospital are not essential to the comfort and dignity of a dying patient, "care at home or in a less regimented environment, such as a hospice, should be encouraged and facilitated."[90] The same should apply to non-dying patients such as permanently

---

[88]*Ibid.*, p. 1426. Cf. the editorial section of the *Journal of the American Medical Association*, Sept. 6, 1985, p. 1215 for the unfavorable commentary on the above quotation by Dr. Peter Black of the Massachusetts General Hospital, Boston, MA. He would consider the view above as a consequentialist ethical view . . . a view, common to proportionalist ethics, which would base the determination of good and evil on a subjective, rather than an objective foundation. Dr. Black comments as follows: "Levy et al. suggest that, at least in some patients, treatment might be withheld early in the course of coma to facilitate death rather than prolonged coma."

[89]Neurologist Ronald E. Cranford mentions a figure of $10,000 per month as the approximate "cost of maintaining" Paul Brophy in Massachusetts. Multiplying $10,000 times 42 months equals $420,000. Cf. "The Persistent Vegetative State: The Medical Reality (Getting the Facts Straight)," in the *Hastings Center Report*, Feb./March, 1988, pp. 27–32. Reference on pp. 31, 32. This figure would not include the extremely high costs of the first year of care especially for young people (some cases, $200,000 to $250,000 that first year.) *Ibid.*

[90]"The Physician's Responsibility Toward Hopelessly Ill Patients," by Sidney Wanzer, MD, et al., the *New England Journal of Medicine*, April 12, 1984, pp. 955–959. Quotation on p. 958.

unconscious individuals. Blue Cross/Blue Shield, Medicare (since 1983), Medicaid, and most other major third-party payers now provide benefits for hospice care. In the hospice setting (as opposed to traditional home care) the unit of care is the entire family. Mandated services include the services of physicians, nurses, social workers, and other health professionals in the home, hospital, or nursing home. Reimbursement covers both inpatient care and home care, with full reimbursement for inpatient care limited to no more than 20 percent of the patient's total days of hospice care.[91]

Patients with cancer currently constitute 90% of the patients receiving hospice care in the U.S.A. There seems to be no reason why other conditions such as permanently unconscious categories (persistently vegetative, comatose) and AIDS could not be eligible for hospice care. If the basis for such coverage is Medicare (available to individuals 65 or older), four criteria must be met: (1) terminal illness with a life expectancy of 6 months or less; (2) inability to benefit from further aggressive (curative) therapy; (3) ability to receive most of his or her care at home (that is, 80% by law); (4) presence of a care giver (relative or friend) who will assume the responsibility for custodial care and be the decision maker in the event of incompetency.[92] In the wide sense of the term, patients who are permanently unconscious can be considered to be "terminal." No one can predict with accuracy just how long a patient can live once the diagnosis of permanent unconsciousness has been reached and verified. The figures mentioned above indicate that most of the patients so diagnosed would die within six months.

A recent issue of the *Mayo Clinic Health Letter* states that there are approximately 1,700 hospices in the United States, and that they offer services in three general formats: Hospital Hospice (part of a hospital converted into a homelike and informal setting), Home Hospice (patients cared for at home, but are sent to a cooperating hospital in time of crisis); Independent Hospice (founded by a group of volunteers—most of the work done in homes of patients).[93] This "team approach" to the comfort and care of the dying calls for a major commitment from family members especially as the day of death draws near. The dividends both for the patient and for loving family members and friends are of long-range consolation value. As one physician wrote in praise of the hospice concept, "When your patient dies peacefully at home, you know you have not 'lost a case.' You have achieved the aim of medicine at

---

[91]"Rx for Dying: The Case for Hospice," by Wilma Bulkin, M.D. and Herbert Lukashok M.S., in the *New England Journal of Medicine,* Feb. 11, 1988, pp. 376–378.

[92]*Ibid.,* p. 376.

[93]"Hospices, Comfort and Care for the Dying," in the *Mayo Clinic Health Letter,* March, 1988, pp. 6–8.

the end of life." Four years ago, a national study contrasted hospice care with that of nursing homes and hospitals. There were 2 significant finding that patients and their families were more satisified and less anxious in a hospice setting, and that hospice costs were lower and involved fewer medical services.[94] A further dividend is that it dulls the edge of the cost-factor argument of proprponents for euthanasia such as emphasized by the Society for the Right to Die.

3.2 PROMOTING "GREAT EXPECTATIONS" OF MEDICAL TECHNOLOGY

The *President's Commission* sounds a sombre note with regard to repairing neurologic injuries that destroy consciousness. The possibility of regaining consciousness is called "exceedingly remote."[95] As mentioned earlier in this study (Cf. p. 216) some physicians would emphasize the importance of basic *predictive* testing soon after the onset of unconsciousness (before a definitive prognosis is warranted) as a means of providing guidance for physicians and family members with regard to treatment (including whether or not to continue artificial feeding). Even if such individuals are convinced that artificial feeding is to be considered as a medical treatment, their action would be morally wrong because it is based on subjective guessing, instead of on valid, objective evidence. The emphasis rather should be focused on cure instead of on care—that is, to expend every possible effort afforded by contemporary medical technology *as soon as possible after the debilitating disease or injury,* or (if unconscious at the time) *as soon as possible after the onset of coma* to prevent or overcome lapse into an unconscious state. While there is still time, concern for cure rather than care will make all the difference in this world (and perhaps in the next) for the patient.

Admittedly a call for advances in the technology of repairing neurologic injuries borders on the improbable, but it must not be regarded by dedicated men and women of medical science and technology as impossible. Discovering the technological means of preventing the onset of unconsciousness in a victim of cardiac arrest or of terminating its hold on the victim soon after the onset of unconsciousness presumably would not be more spectacular than

---

[94]*Ibid.*, p. 7. Concerned individuals can find out what hospices are available in their particular area by writing to the National Hospice Organization, Suite 307, 1901 North Fort Myer Drive, Arlington, VA 22209 (telephone 703-243-5900).

[95]*Deciding to Forego Life-Sustaining Treatment* (cf. note 62), p. 177.

discovering a vaccine to ward off the transmission of the AIDS infection, or discovering the answers to the neurological mysteries of Alzheimer's disease. With regard to the latter affliction (which often brings on a persistent vegetative state), Dr. Donald Price of Johns Hopkins University and his colleagues have been seeking relief for Alzheimer victims on the basis of preliminary evidence that "the defects in memory of Alzheimer's sufferers probably result from damage to cells of the cerebral cortex, hippocampus and basal forebrain."[96] This is primarily neurological research with hopeful goals in view. In early 1987 the medical world was thrilled with the announcement of the discovery of a group of hormones which "can stimulate the bone marrow to make red or white blood cells in essentially any desired quantity." This discovery gave new impetus to the search for a vaccine against the AIDS infection.[97] With determination and ingenuity, the medical community can advance against the "living death" syndrome known as permanent unconsciousness.

In his enlightening article in the February/March issue of the *Hastings Center Report*, Dr. Ronald E. Cranford states that approximately four to six minutes of complete loss of blood or oxygen to the brain can result in extensive destruction of the cerebral cortex while relatively sparing the brain stem. With reference to such victims of ischemia (lack of blood flow) and hypoxia (lack of oxygen), he continues:

> After experiencing ischemia or hypoxia, the patient often will be in a coma that may persist for a few days or from two to four weeks. This transient coma results from a temporary dysfunction of the brain stem, which is not totally immune to the effects of hypoxic-ischemic injury. After this period, the patient will awaken and evolve into a condition of eyes-open unconsciousness, that is, the vegetative state.[98]

In other words, the completely unconscious patient can be awake, but unaware.

Dr. Cranford does not minimize in any way the difficulty of a diagnosis of PVS beyond the category of "a reasonably high degree of reliability." Comparing a PVS patient with a *brain dead* patient, he states that in the latter, the diagnosis reaches absolute certainty if the accepted criteria are properly ap-

---

[96]"Experts Voice Hope in Alzheimer's Fight," in the *New York Times,* Nov. 17, 1987, pp. C 1 and C 10.

[97]"Clinical Promise with New Hormones," by Gina Kolata, in *Science,* May 1, 1987, pp. 517–519.

[98]Article mentioned in footnote 89. p. 28

plied. With regard to the persistent vegetative state (PVS), however, he adds: ". . . there is no broadly accepted, published set of specific medical criteria with as much clinical detail and certainty as the brain dead criteria. Furthermore, even the generally accepted criteria, when properly applied, are not infallible."[99] Likewise in the efforts to confirm a *clinical diagnosis* of PVS, specific laboratory studies are lacking. He seems to hold out the hope, however, that such studies will be forthcoming due to advanced technological equipment such as magnetic resonance imaging scanning (MRI), computerized axial tomography (CAT), and especially positron emission tomagraphy (PET). He infers a powerful reason for using these tools to discover more about the diagnosis and duration of PVS when he states that the 5,000 to 10,000 PVS patients in the U.S.A. "can be anticipated to significantly increase in the future, especially when coupled with their increased longevity."[100]

If "great expectations" are hopeful but limited regarding the diagnosis, cure and prognosis of permanently unconscious conditions such as PVS, they are hopeful and much less limited with regard to educating the American public on the *preventive* front. The subject is too extensive and too complicated to be assigned more than a modest mention in this study. Just as it is more charitable and prudential to extend self help to poverty-stricken peoples instead of being content with outright grants of food and money, so there is far more wisdom in helping the public to avoid the causes of unconscious conditions and persistent vegetative states instead of being content with efforts to improve or save the life of the victim after tragedy has struck. As just one example of such self help, the *New York Times* recently carried an article on "Recognizing the symptoms of ministrokes and acting on the causes of such transient attacks." Such T.I.A.'s (for transient ischemic attack) may be manifested by brief episodes of double vision, loss of feeling in an arm or leg, difficulty in speaking, etc. It is estimated that 35 to 50 percent of the people who experience such transient attacks can expect to suffer a major stroke within five years unless steps are taken to correct the underlying problem. The article adds: "For most, the stroke occurs within a year of the first attack."[101] There are dozens of other saving guidelines to fore-warn and fore-arm the general public against the threat of passage into the world of unconscious states and conditions. If the preventive approach is promoted with

[99]*Ibid.*, p. 29.

[100]*Ibid.*, pp. 30, 31.

[101]In the *New York Times Health* section, January 28, 1988, p. B 6, by Jane E. Brody. The chief cause of T.I.A.'s is given as the "buildup of fatty material in a blood vessel feeding brain" (vessel, that is, that feeds the brain).

persistence and ingenuity as a first line of defense, there is every reason to hope that the total number of patients diagnosed as permanently unconscious will decrease.

3.3 SHIFTING THE PRIMARY EMPHASIS FROM CURE TO CARE

There are two major categories of permanently unconscious patients; those with eyes-closed unconsciousness (coma) and those with eyes-open unconsciousness (persistent vegetative state). The term "irreversibly comatose" must be used with caution. It is not synonymous with brain death as the word "irreversible" might imply. Furthermore, with regard to the duration of both conditions (coma and PVS), it is important to note that persons in a long-term or permanent coma ("eyes closed" unconsciousness) do not live as long as PVS patients. Dr. Cranford explains that coma patients often have impaired cough, gag, and swallowing reflexes with a resultant inability (involuntary) to clear the passages of the throat and lungs. His conclusion indicates why comatose patients should not be considered as long-term survival patients:

> This impairment leads to frequent, often fatal, respiratory infections—a common cause of death in comatose patients, and one of the major reasons why truly comatose patients typically to not experience the long-term survival period associated with the vegetative state. Thus, in one sense it is reasonable to describe comatose patients as "terminally ill," with death anticipated in six months to a year, unless extremely vigorous therapeutic efforts are made to sustain life.[102]

With regard to patients in a persistent vegetative state, it is false and misleading to project the impression that almost all PVS patients linger on for years and years. The *Guinness Book of World Records* does assign the "longest case of coma" record to a certain Elaine Esposito, who died 37 years and 111 days after she lost consciousness.[103] In view of the information in the paragraph above, it is more likely that she was a PVS patient. Dr. Cranford states that it is not uncommon for patients to survive in this condition for five, ten,

---

[102]The *Hastings Center Report*, Feb./March, 1988, p. 28.
[103]*Deciding to Forego Life-Sustaining Treatment* (cf. note 62), p. 177, footnote 16.

and twenty years. He explains that the duration of PVS is contingent upon several major factors such as: (1) age; the elderly develop more medical complications than younger patients; (2) economic, family and institutional aspects; in general, the wealthy receive better care than indigent patients; (3) the natural resistence of the body to infections and the effectiveness of cough and gag reflexes; (4) the moral view of the appropriateness of providing nutrition and hydration.[104]

A–Dismal Prospects for Long-Term Unconsciousness

Despite occasional news stories of victims of persistent vegetative states who regained consciousness and relative normalcy in society, the sad fact is that medical literature refers to only two patients who recovered consciousness after a year or more in a persistent vegetative state due to hypoxia (lack of oxygen).[105] In one case in the State of New Mexico, which came to the attention of this writer only through a footnote in one of the publications of the *President's Commission*, the patient regained cognitive abilities, but suffered from emotional instability and the paralysis of three limbs, and remained completely dependent upon others for the rest of his life.[106]

A second case, which attracted nationwide attention and publicity, was that of Police Sergeant David Mack, who amazed his doctors in October 1981 by recovering consciousness after having been in an unconscious state for 22 months. As a narcotics officer of the Minneapolis Police Department, he had suffered severe brain damage when he was shot on December 13, 1979, while serving a search warrant with other plainclothes officers. Several months after the tragic event, a team of doctors diagnosed his condition as a persistent vegetative state. Eight months after the shooting (August 1980), the respirator was removed. Like Karen Ann Quinlan of New Jersey a few years earlier,

---

[104]The *Hastings Center Report*, Feb./March, 1988, p. 31.

[105]*NOT of the verified variety* are reported cases such as the following: One found in a weekly paper called the *Weekly World News* in the October 27, 1987 edition. Under a large-print heading, "Coma Mom Awakens While Giving Birth!," readers were told that a woman by the name of Ruth Windrich, wife of a businessman in Durban, South Africa, who had been comatose since an auto accident on Jan. 27, had regained consciousness when her baby was born almost 8 months later. According to the newspaper account, she is "expected to recover and return home to her husband and baby." The *Detroit Free Press* captioned an account in the January 13, 1988 issue (p. 5 C) with the words: "In Coma 5 years, youth suddenly laughs, gives family hope." The young man (20) of Hollywood, Florida, was Chuck Clough. He had been struck by lightning some 5 years earlier, and lost consciousness. The newspaper account projected hope for the young man, but gave no indications of significant improvement in his condition.

[106]*Deciding to Forego Life-Sustaining Treatment* (cf.note 62), p. 179, footnote 22.

however, Sgt. Mack continued to breathe on his own. It was in October 1981 that Sgt. Mack began to show signs that he was aware of what was happening around him. Although he was lucid of mind, he remained paralyzed throughout most of his body, and never regained the ability to speak. He spent the last years of his life at the Northeast Catholic Elder Center, where he communicated with friends and family members with the use of a spelling board. He died in Hennepin County Medical Center on November 2, 1986, five years after his "miracle recovery" in October 1981.[107] In a later newspaper report an article entitled "For Macks, 'Miracle' Meant 7 Years of Pain" tells of the long months of frustration for Sgt. Mack and his family despite the obvious gift of good humor as manifested both by Sgt. Mack and his wife and family.[108]

The above description of the long-term-care case of Sgt. Mack serves as an illustration of the propriety of concentrating on loving care once a confirmation of permanent unconsciousness has been confirmed by professional experts. Such a confirmation should serve as a justification for not pursuing aggressive treatments with a view to the improvement or cure of the neurological condition of the patient. As mentioned above, such a confirmation cannot be absolute with present day technological methods. In such a situation, the medical community must be satisfied with virtual (or "for all practical purposes") certitude. Obviously this is why, in the Report of the *Pontifical Academy of Sciences* of October 30, 1985, the guideline states: "If the patient is in permanent coma, *irreversible as far as it is possible to predict* (emphasis ours) treatment is not required . . . . " The rest of the quotation indicates that primary emphasis in such cases must be on care, not cure: " . . . but care, including feeding, must be provided."[109]

B—Tender Loving Care as the Primary Concern

Surely the very minimal improvement in the condition of Sergeant Mack when he regained consciousness is not an objective which would justify aggressive treatment for a confirmed state of persistent vegetation (PVS). His "improved" condition subjected him to pains, infections and fevers (not to mention emotional sorrows and trials) which escaped him during his unconscious state.[110] Medical authorities have taken a definite position against the

---

[107]*Minneapolis Star and Tribune*, Nov. 3, 1986, pp. 1 A and 7 A.

[108]*Minneapolis Star and Tribune*, Nov. 23, 1986, pp. 1 A, 8 A and 9 A.

[109]Cf. pp. 29 and 30 of this study.

[110]*Minneapolis Star and Tribune*, Nov. 23, 1986, p. 8 A.

claim that patients in a persistent vegetative state might experience pain and suffering. In its *amicus curiae* brief filed in the Brophy case, the American Academy of Neurology stated that no conscious experience of pain and suffering is possible without the integrated functioning of the brainstem and cerebral cortex. Noxious stimuli may activate peripherally located nerves, but only a brain with the capacity for consciousness can translate that neural activity into an experience.[111]

Based on this professional opinion that a patient with a confirmed diagnosis of PVS cannot experience pain or suffering, it must be concluded that such a patient could not be deprived of nutrition and hydration on the grounds that it causes him or her excessive pain and/or burden. The same would apply to the claim that the administration of nutrition and hydration is virtually useless. The answer to such a claim would be the common experience (in the care of comatose and PVS patients) that the patient is thriving on the feeding process whether by way of mouth or by way of tube delivery. There could be an exceptional case when the unconscious patient develops a physical condition which prevents the assimilation of nutrition from food and water (for example, blockage caused by a cancerous growth). Such an exceptional turn of events could justify the removal of the feeding process, and would warrant special attention to the minimal hydration needs of the patient through diligent care of the oral cavity.

Many aspects of previous discussions (2.3) with regard to virtual impossibility ("nemo ad impossibile tenetur"), however, would apply to patients who have been diagnosed as permanently unconscious. Unlike applications of the principles of virtual uselessness or excessive pain/burden which concern effects on the patient only, the principle of virtual impossibility can take into consideration adverse effects for others as well (cost factor, lack of facilities, etc.). The attention of the reader is directed to the discussion of "nemo ad impossibile tenetur" in this study (pp. 198 ff.). Both in the initiation of an artificial feeding process and in the termination of same, factors that combine to present a *virtual-impossibility situation* can constitute an excusing cause (substantial financial problems, lack of medical insurance, significant obstacles in reaching medical facilities, crucial caretaker situations, isolated place of residence, etc.)

Although permanently unconscious patients seem to thrive on the tube-feeding process, they are subject to infections, respiratory diseases, etc. This applies to comatose patients more than to PVS patients. Paul Brophy of Easton, Massachusetts is an example of a PVS patient who was subject to sei-

---

[111]Article by Dr. Cranford, the *Hastings Center Report*, Feb./March, 1988, p. 31.

zures, hemorrhaging and other problems. Although he died on October 23, 1986, eight days after his tube-feeding process was terminated, the cause of death was listed as pneumonia.[112] Since the emphasis now is on care rather than on cure, there would be no moral obligation to administer antibiotics or other treatments to the long-term comatose or PVS patient unless there are clinical indications that such administrations might serve as comfort measures. One valid but non-medical reason for such ministrations might be in consideration of the feelings of family members of the patient, lest they might be confirmed in a premonition that their loved one is being abandoned. If such an opportunistic disease or infection takes on a lethal quality, so that the patient is in imminent danger of death, there may be situations when it would be virtually useless to continue the tube-feeding process. The attending physician would be most qualified to make such a judgment.

One final word must be said about manifestations of tender loving care to comatose and PVS patients right up to the moment of death. In reading the accounts of the dedication of family members to patients such as Karen Quilan, Paul Brophy and Sergeant Mack, there is a sense of a realization of union of soul with the loved one, even though the patient may be unaware to an absolute degree. Parents, wives, children, grandchildren and others actually talked to such PVS patients. The significance was more than merely symbolic (which alone would validate such loving attempts at communication). Since, as the experts admit, it is not possible at the present time to obtain *absolute* assurance that the consciousness is undoubtedly permanent, the slightest possibility exists that the loved one may well be aware of the held hand and of the spoken voice and gentle caresses.

Especially in regard to the care and concern for patients who are permanently unconscious, both the medical and the Church community must realize that it is not merely the patient, but also the family members, who are in need of tender loving care. The very nature of the situation, with all of its emotional frustrations and uncertainties, makes demands of family members which justly might be considered to be beyond the line of duty. Despite the fact that some of the elderly family members are married with duties to their own immediate families, and that some of the younger ones are under pressure to attend to personal planning for employment, education, etc.,—despite all this, it is impressive to note that not only family members and relatives, but even neighbors, want to share the sorrow and the responsibility of participating in the care of the patient.

The sentiments expressed above give meaning to the remark above that it might be appropriate at times to extend comfort measures (such as adminis-

---

[112]The *Boston Globe*, October 24, 1986, pp. 1 and 39.

tering antibiotics) more for the benefit of family members. Especially in the hospice movement, family, relatives and friends of the patient are drawn closely together in a noble venture. That is why many hospices offer support for a family after the death of the patient. This is done through follow-up calls and group meetings which are designed to help the family members cope with bereavement.[113] The greatest need for help and moral support, however, is during the lone period of unknown duration which is lived by patient and by loved ones in anticipation of eventual death. Particularly in reviewing the Karen Quinlan and the Sergeant Mack accounts of that lingering and trying period, the reader is impressed by the balance between deep human frustration and militant emotional stamina on the part of the loved ones of the patient. It should come as no surprise if evidence emerges now and then of family members experiencing such deep valleys of frustration, that thoughts of "taking matters into their own hands", or of requesting the physician to "pull the plug" on nutrition and hydration, might appear as a "respectable" alternative. Yet, the world of faith (world of the unseen) prevails over what St. Paul, in his second letter to the Corinthians (4:17), calls "the present burden of our trial."

Press reports of the Karen Quinlan case and of the Sergeant Mack case provide definite evidence that any conceivable temptations to bring about the termination of the artificial feeding process were resisted by patients (Quinlan) and spouse (Mack) respectively. When the father of Karen Quinlan was asked whether he wanted the artificial feeding apparatus removed from his daughter, he replied: "Oh no, that is her nourishment."[114] The newspaper reports on the Sergeant Mack case reveal that he had asked his wife to have the artificial feeding process terminated. This devoted woman, however, "never considered slipping him a lethal pill or surreptitiously pulling a plug."[115] In both cases, the loved ones undoubtedly regarded the administration of food and drink, even by artificial means, as ordinary care.[116] In other words, they regarded that comfort measure (food and drink) as the least they could and should do for their loved one. Based on that presumption, it can be

---

[113]*Mayo Clinic Health Letter,* March, 1988, article on Hospices, p. 6.

[114]Quoted in an article by Paul Ramsey entitled "Prolonged Dying: Not Medically Indicated," in the Hastings Center Report, February, 1976, p. 16.

[115]Cf. the *Minneapolis Star and Tribune,* Nov. 23, 1986, p. A 8. The account is rich in the human interest aspects of the trials and frustrations as encountered with eminent patients and good humor on the part of Mrs Mack (pp. A, 1, 8 and 9).

[116]On the other hand, if they had regarded the administration of artificial feeding as a *medical treatment* or as an *extraordinary means,* they would have been justified in insisting upon the removal of the artificial feeding apparatus.

said that they were living out, both for themselves and for their loved one, the rest of the quotation from St. Paul's second letter to the Corinthians (4:16-18):

> We do not lose heart, because our inner being is renewed each day even though our body is being destroyed at the same time. The present burden of our trial is light enough, and earns for us an eternal weight of glory beyond all comparison. We do not fix our gaze on what is seen but on what is unseen. What is seen is transitory; what is unseen is forever.

CONCLUSIONS:

(1) Life and death are in the hands of God. No human individual can claim direct dominion over his or her body so as to reserve the right to say: "Let me starve to death," or "help me to end my life." The so-called "right to die" as promoted by euthanasia forces in the world today, has been denied and rejected by Catholic theologians throughout the centuries.

(2) The most authoritative Church pronouncement on the subject of the realities of death and dying, the *Declaration on Euthanasia* (1980), makes a basic distinction between *medical treatments* and *ordinary care*. That same distinction is found in two subsequent and authentic pronouncements of the Roman Curia, namely: the Report of the Pontifical Council on Health Affairs (1981), and the Report of the Pontifical Academy of Sciences (1985). The distinction is also basic in the teachings of the American Bishops as evidenced in two significant pronouncements of the American National Conference of Catholic Bishops (1984 and 1986) on the general subject of euthanasia.

(3) This study is based on the contention that the administration of food and fluids is always a basic component of *ordinary nursing care,* even though it may have to be administered by artificial means to *supplement* a malfunctioning alimentary system. What must be done (conserve human life) does not necessarily become an extraordinary means of conserving life because of how it is done.

(4) Although the *Declaration on Euthanasia* does not state explicitly that food and drink are to be included under the general heading of "ordinary cares" in behalf of the patient, that obvious connection between care and sustenance (basically food and drink) is mentioned explicitly in the other two pronouncements of the Roman Curia as listed above.

(5) The *Declaration on Euthanasia* (1980) indeed justified the rejection of medical *treatments* by the patient "when death is imminent and cannot be

prevented by the remedies used" ("but without interrupting in any way the ordinary cares which are due to the patient in such cases"). When Pope Pius XII addressed the anesthesiologists over 20 years earlier (November 24, 1957), and referred to the patient's "right and duty in case of serious illness to take the necessary treatment for the preservation of life and health" as a right a duty which could be renounced if the *treatment* could be considered as beyond "ordinary means", he simply could not have been speaking of the administration of food and drink by artificial means as a medical treatment, nor of such an artificial process as an extraordinary means of conserving life. Such interpretations would not only be totally out of context (he was speaking of "resuscitation"), but would contradict the doctrinal pronouncements of the *Declaration on Euthanasia* (which approved of the doctrinal content of the address of Pope Pius XII).

(6) The administration of nutrition and fluids by intravenous entry (IV) is to be considered as *ordinary* nursing care if it is administered through what is known as a peripheral line (usually on a temporary basis) as a *supplement* for an alimentary system which still remains functional (still capable of digestion and assimilation of nutrition). It becomes an *extraordinary* means of conserving human life (and may be renounced), however, if it is administered as a *substitute* for a totally non-functional alimentary system (an IV entry known as TPN, or total parenteral nutrition).

(7) The removal of a tube feeding mechanism is not to be equated, from a moral viewpoint, with the removal of a respirator. The respirator usually is installed as a *substitute* for a totally non-functional respiratory system (patient unable to breathe "on his own"). There is no moral obligation to request such a substitute in order to *prolong* human life. An artificial nutrition/hydration mechanism, however, is always a *supplement* or facilitating means for an alimentary system which is not totally dysfunctional. There is a moral obligation to take advantage of such a supplement if possible so as to *conserve* human life. Without that supplement for a patient who is unable to eat and drink by way of mouth, the direct cause of death would not be the patient's underlying illness or disease, but an inevitable process of dehydration and starvation.

(8) The words "ordinary" and "extraordinary" (or "proportionate" and "disproportionate") means are to be understood as relative terms in particular cases. The installation of a tube feeding regimen for a patient who retains the normal capacity to ingest, chew and swallow by natural means, would constitute an *extraordinary* means of conserving life for that patient. For a patient who is unable to receive food and drink orally, however, the tube feeding supplement would be an ordinary and proportionate means of conserving life. Considering that it is a life or death issue, the benefits would far outweigh the burdens of such an artificial process.

(9) The tube feeding process can become an extraordinary or disproportionate means of conserving human life—and hence no longer obligatory—if there is reliable clinical evidence that it has become virtually useless (that is, "for all practical purposes" useless). If the process is effective but only to a very slight degree, it would be appropriate to apply the traditional theological saying, "a little bit is to be reckoned as nothing" ("parum pro nihilo reputatur").

(10) A second source of rendering the tube feeding process an extraordinary means of conserving life—and hence no longer obligatory—would be the presence of reliable clinical evidence that some aspect of the artificial feeding process itself is causing excessive pain and/or burden for the patient. It would be morally wrong, however, to identify the continuation of the patient's life itself as a burden. Emphasis on burdens for others besides the patient can lead to degrading "quality of life" considerations.

(11) Burdens to others may be taken into account by a patient in making a decision *to renounce treatments* "that can only yield a precarious and painful *prolongation* of life" (to which the patient is not obligated). Since the patient renounces his right to a prolonged life in such a situation, the valid concerns of others can be taken into account. With regard to the basic element of *ordinary care* which is dependence on nutrition and fluids, however, the patient is not free to renounce his right and obligation to *conserve* life. Deliberative consideration of burdens to others in such a situation (cost factor, caretaker burdens, etc.) would clash with the right and responsibility of the patient (and of family members and caretakers as well) to conserve life—to project, in effect, that "this life still is worth living."

(12) The word "excessive" in the phrase "excessive pain and/or burden," also is to be interpreted as a relative term. The meaning of "excessive" in a particular case would depend upon the subjective qualities of the patient (religious outlook, tolerance of pain, etc.) as evaluated in the light of objective factors such as proximity to the time of death, degree of alertness and consciousness, etc.

(13) A third source of rendering the tube feeding process an extraordinary means—and hence no longer obligatory—would be a situation of virtual impossibility. In other words, the circumstances are such, as considered in the aggregate, that the installation of a tube feeding process or the continuation of same would be, "for all practical purposes," impossible. This follows from the general prescription of the natural moral law that positive precepts (such as the precept to conserve human life) do not bind *in all possible circumstances*.

(14) The culpable failure to initiate a tube feeding process (that is, withholding artificial feeding) in a warranted case is as much in violation of the natural moral law as the culpable role of an individual in discontinuing an

effective tube feeding process (that is, withdrawing artificial feeding) which is not causing excessive pain or burden for the patient. This follows from the Catholic doctrine on human imputability, whereby individuals are responsible not only for human actions, but also for human omissions under the usual conditions (the individual foresees the evil effect of omission, is obligated and also able to do something about the situation).

(15) Since patients who are permanently unconscious (permanent comatose condition or persistent vegetative state) are considered by professional neurologists to be incapable of experiencing pain or burden, and are sustained by artificially-administered nutrition and hydration (process is not useless), the artificial feeding process could not be considered as an *extraordinary* means of conserving life for such individuals. In many situations, however, adverse circumstances may combine in particular cases (lack of funds and of hospital insurance coverage, far distance from hospital facilities, determination to die at home, unreliable caretaker situation, etc.) so as to constitute justification for not initiating a tube feeding regimen in the first place, or for terminating the artificial feeding process *on the basis of a virtual impossibility.*

(16) The scope and extent of the permanently unconscious situation can be blown far out of due proportion by exaggerated reports in the media and by a lack of factual knowledge of this distressing condition. The argument for euthanasia as based on the exaggeration of the number of such patients can be deflated to some degree by information based on reliable estimates on the limited number of long-term comatose and persistently vegetative patients. The financial fears with regard to the care of such patients can be abated to some extent by promoting the trend to care for such patients in a home-care or hospice-care setting.

(17) There are good reasons for hoping that medical and technological advances in the future will give the medical community the tools to test earlier and more effectively especially accident victims and victims of lack of oxygen or blood to the brain (hypoxia and ischemia) so that they are not in danger of becoming candidates for coma or for a persistent vegetative state. Not only members of the medical community, but all concerned citizens of the nation, should feel obligated to combine forces and abilities to promote preventive measures which are designed to decrease the incidence of encounters with unconsciousness.

(18) Since not only the permanently unconscious but also incurable terminal patients are beyond the boundaries of cure, they are candidates for the speciality which has been the hallmark of the Catholic mission of healing throughout the centuries—*Tender loving care* as emphasized in the second paragraph of the preamble to the *Ethical and Religious Directives for Catholic Health Facilities*: "The total good of the patient, which includes his higher spiritual as

well as his bodily welfare." This would overlook "thou shalt not kill" in favor of hastening the demise of God's children by denying them the staff of life— nutrition and hydration, food and drink.

Conserving Human Life
Part III

THE MORAL OPTION NOT TO CONSERVE LIFE
UNDER CERTAIN CONDITIONS
An Application of the Principles

By
Albert S. Moraczewski, O.P., Ph.D.
Director, Regional Office of Pope John Center, Houston

The Moral Option Not to Conserve Life Under Certain Conditions

Introduction

Families are often torn at a time when they are most vulnerable. A member of the family is very ill, and perhaps dying, and decisions must be made by the patient, or by the family when the patient is incapable of making such vital decisions about initiating or continuing medical treatments. Few problems exist if there is a reasonable hope that the treatment in question truly will be of benefit to the sick or dying member of the family.

Problems arise, however, and not infrequently, when there is some doubt as to whether the initiation or the continuation of the therapeutic procedure will be of benefit relative to the burden anticipated. When the burden associated with the procedure itself is great, the expected benefit has to be all the greater before the procedure may be considered morally obligatory. That burden primarily refers to the extra burden carried by the patient as the result of human intervention. Burden also can apply, *mutatis mutandis,* to that which the family or others including the community, may experience.

Solving ethical conflicts is additionally complex in a pluralistic society because various values may clash and some priority has to be assigned. In recent times, especially since World War II, the Magisterium of the Church has specifically addressed a number of ethical issues arising from the application of technological advances in the biomedical sciences. One of the questions addressed is that dealing with the conditions leading to the moral obligation to use, or to the moral option not to use, technological means to sustain life. The Church's pronouncements on this subject were in response to the earnest and urgent pleas of medical personnel for moral guidance. The present generation had suddenly found itself with powerful instruments in its hands and realized that these can destroy the world if misused. Hence that power must be moderated and directed by ethical principles (see Pope John Paul II, *Redemptor Hominis*, March 4, 1979, Nos. 15 and 16).

Guidance was provided in a great variety of medical concerns by the writings and addresses of Pope Pius XII. Vatican Council II documents and subsequent Magisterial documents have reinforced these teachings. Most recently, the *Congregation for the Doctrine of the Faith* issued several documents on medical-moral issues, e.g., *Declaration on Abortion* (1974), *Declaration on Euthanasia* (1980), *Instruction on Human Life in its Origin and on the Dignity of Procreation* (1987). For the purpose of this article, the most relevant is the *Declaration on Euthanasia* which, in effect, continued the teachings of Pius XII, particularly those contained in his Address to the International Congress of Anesthesiologists (November 24, 1957).

While these Magisterial statements are relatively recent, they did not suddenly appear *ex nihilo*. They are the culmination of a long moral tradition in the Church which has its roots at least as far back as the 13th century. In 1958 Bishop Daniel Cronin (Bishop of Fall River, Massachusetts) as a young priest wrote a doctoral dissertation (at the *Pontificia Universitas Gregoriana*, Rome) which concisely and admirably traced the lineage of the current teaching. In doing so, Bishop Cronin made it clear how the present teaching came to be what it is.

It is essential, in our view, that one needs to know the developmental "embryology" of a particular Church's teaching in order to understand correctly what that teaching is actually stating. Yet, that is not quite enough. One also needs to know the questions and contemporary context which evoked from the Holy See the responses it gave.

The Church is ever mindful that it is striving to apply the gospel to very specific and complex human problems which were not present or foreseen at the time the early Church was preaching the gospel of salvation to all nations. Consequently the Church is always being challenged by our world but at the same time has the assurance that the Holy Spirit will guide it to all truth.

All this having been said, we can now address the question initially raised: what are the moral obligations regarding the use of various technological means to conserve or preserve human life? While there are some ethical problems still associated with the use or non-use of "hi-tech" medicine, the more difficult and more urgent issue has to do with determining the conditions when the provision of water and food by technological means is, or becomes, morally optional. In light of Bishop Cronin's work the question will be considered briefly in three steps: (1) review of the relevant contemporary Magisterial teachings; (2) a condensation of the developmental history of the Church's moral tradition out of which these teachings developed; (3) an overview of the psychosocial milieu in the United States which may influence how these moral teachings are to be applied concretely.

Cronin's work considered life conserving means in general. The present discussion focuses on nutrition and hydration as a means of conserving life.

Contemporary Relevant Magisterial Teachings

One should begin with the principle that generally there is a serious moral obligation to supply food and water to conserve human life. What is being asked here is, whether there are times and under what conditions when the furnishing of artificial nutrition and hydration becomes morally optional. This precise question has not, at the date of this writing, received an official magisterial response. The issue, therefore, is open for legitimate discussion, and that is how the Church's teaching, under the guidance of the Holy Spirit, gradually unfolds to apply to newer and often more complex human problems.

How Church teaching regarding medical means to sustain life is understood to apply to the issue of artifical nutrition and hydration is a matter of current vigorous controversy. This particular conflict appears to have arisen in part because of the inherent ambiguity of certain terms and expressions, and in part because of a well-grounded fear that pro-euthanasia forces will take any carefully nuanced statement of the Magisterium (and of Catholic theologians) and use it as a blunt instrument to further their cause. This fear is reflected in the following remark by a vigorous pro-life attorney, the late Dennis Horan:

> "We will argue that public policy will not be able to preserve the distinction that is drawn by these theologians between deliberate starvation of non-terminal patients, and more direct means of killing patients, and that the Church's moral teaching should take into account the need for clarity in the realm of public policy" (p.33)

> "The nuances and ambiguities which are often acceptable in positions of moral theology, may cause confusion in the arena of public policy." (p. 43). (Dennis J. Horan, Esq. "Hydration, Nutrition

and Euthanasia: Legal Reflections on the Role of the Church teaching" *Linacre Quarterly*, Nov. 1988, pp 32-46).

An example of the inherent ambiguity of certain terms and expressions may be found in the statement of Pope Pius XII:

> But normally one is held to use only ordinary means—according to circumstances of persons, places, times and culture—that is to say, means that do not involve any grave burden for oneself or another. A more strict obligation would be too burdensome for most men and would render the attainment of the higher, more important good too difficult. Life, health, all temporal activities are in fact subordinated to spiritual ends. On the other hand, one is not forbidden to take more than the strictly necessary steps to preserve life and health, as long as he does not fail in some more serious duty (November 24, 1957).

When Pius XII states, "But normally one is held to use only *ordinary means* . . . " [emphasis added], is the expression "ordinary means" referring exclusively to medical treatments? In the preceding paragraph the Pope states " . . . that man . . . has the right and duty in case of serious illness to take the necessary treatment for the preservation of life and health" (ibid). It is not so evident that he is using the term "ordinary means" to include only medical treatment and not food and water. These two sections, in the Pope's address, is prefaced by the statement that " . . . We would like to set forth the principles that will allow formulation of the answer [to three questions asked by Dr. Bruno Haid, chief of Anesthesia Clinic at the University of Insbruck]". Hence, it would appear that the Pope intends to set forth some general principles that would apply to the care of the seriously ill even if he subsequently focuses on the specific questions related to "modern practices of resuscitation" (ibid). It is doubtful that the document itself definitively can resolve the ambiguity in the term "ordinary means" as used in the Pope's statement of principle.

A subsequent Magisterial pronouncement, the *Declaration on Euthanasia* (Vatican Congregation for the Doctrine of the Faith, June 26, 1980), may be of some help. Its focus, as the title declares, is euthanasia defined as:

> An action or an omission which of itself or by intention causes death, in order that all suffering may in this way be eliminated. Euthanasia's terms of reference, therefore, are to be found in the intention of the will and in the methods used (Section II).

The definition notes that there are two components: (1) the intention of the will, namely, to cause death in order to eliminate all suffering; (2) the method used (or not used) which of itself, or by human intention, brings about death. Clearly, there is here no identified distinction between medical procedures or the administration of artificial nutrition and hydration.

Later, in this same Vatican document the question is raised: "However, is it necessary in all circumstances to have recourse to all possible remedies?" In response the *Declaration* states, in part:

> In the past, moralists replied that one is never obliged to use "extraordinary" means. This reply, which as a principle still holds good, is perhaps less clear today, by reason of the inprecision of the term and the rapid progress made in the treatment of sickness. Thus some people prefer to speak of "proportionate" and "disproportionate" means (Section IV).

> It is also permitted, with the patient's consent, to interrupt these means, where the results fall short of expectations. But for such a decision to be made, account will have to be taken of the reasonable wishes of the patient's family, as also of the advice of the doctors who are specially competent in the matter. The latter may in particular judge that the investment in instruments and personnel is disproportionate to the results foreseen; they may also judge that the techniques applied impose on the patient strain or suffering out of proportion with the benefits which he or she may gain from such techniques.

> It is also permissible to make do with the normal means that medicine can offer. Therefore one cannot impose on anyone the obligation to have recourse to a technique which is already in use but which carries a risk or is burdensome. Such a refusal is not the equivalent of suicide; on the contrary, it should be considered as an acceptance of the human condition, or a wish to avoid the application of a medical procedure disproportionate to the results that can be expected, or a desire not to impose excessive expense on the family or the community.

> When inevitable death is imminent in spite of the means used, it is permitted in conscience to make the decision to refuse forms of treatment that would only secure a precarious and burdensome prolongation of life, so long as the normal care due to the sick

person in similar cases is not interrupted. In such circumstances the doctor has no reason to reproach himself with failing to help the person in danger (ibid).

While in these quotations the *Declaration* appears to use "means" as referring to "medical techniques" or procedures, it, however, neither includes or excludes specifically the use of artificial nutrition and hydration.

Unclear, too, is the precise content of the phrase, " . . . so long as the normal care due to the sick person in similar cases is not interrupted." Does "normal care" refer to nursing care? Does that of necessity include artificially provided nutrition and hydration? From the context, it would seem that "normal care" refers not to means that prolong life but to those procedures which make the dying person more comfortable and which recognizes and respect the dignity of the patient. Whether technologically supplied nutrition and hydration are an essential part of such nursing care is not evident, particularly when the patient is in a profound and permanent coma. So, this document does not clarify the matter in any definitive manner.

Two other statements have been invoked to maintain not only that the teachings of the two Magisterial documents mentioned above are to be strictly limited to medical procedures but that the administration of food and water even by technological means is, absolutely required. These statements are contained in two reports made *to* the Pope (but, it should be carefully noted, not officially promulgated by him to date or made part of authoritative teaching).

One report is by a study group prepared under the auspices of the Pontifical Academy of Sciences (which is *not* a part of the Roman Curia as some have erroneously claimed or implied). The relevant passage states:

If the patient is in a permanent, irreversible coma, as far as can be foreseen, treatment is not required, but all care should be lavished on him, including feeding ("The Artificial Prolongation of Life", *Origins,* December 5, 1985, p.415).

It clearly asserts that " . . . all care should be lavished on him, including feeding" (ibid).

There is no doubt here that the report of this study group (of 20 doctors and scientists) clearly distinguishes between treatment and feeding. But it is an *opinion* of a study group reporting to the Pope. To date neither this report nor that distinction has become part of the Magisterial teaching; it is merely one of many reports the Pope receives.

At the time of the meeting of this study group (and another one dealing with parasitic diseases), Pope John Paul II addressed them and noted that "Life is a treasure; death is a natural event . . . the physician is not the lord of life, but neither is he the conqueror of death. Death is an inevitable fact of human life, and the use of means for avoiding it must take into account the human condition." (Pope John Paul II, "The Mystery of Life and Death", *Origins*, Dec 5, 1985, p. 416). The Pope then proceeds to reiterate the relevant principles contained in the 1980 *Declaration on Euthanasia* applicable to determining the obligation to use treatments for sustaining life. But nowhere in that brief address does he specifically allude to the issue of nutrition and hydration, nor does he comment on their report.

The other document which has been erroneously asserted as reflecting authentic teaching is a report of a working group assembled by the Pontifical Council, *Cor num.* The group was composed of 15 persons: "Theologians, doctors, members of Religious Congregations dedicated to the care of the sick, trained nurses, and hospital Chaplains" (*Report of the Pontifical Council on Health Affairs, Cor Unum*, Vatican City, 1981; [Official text in French. See *Enchiridion Vaticanum*, 10 ed., 1982, pp. 1132-1173). Although the report was prepared in 1976, only after the *Declaration on Euthanasia* was the Pontifical Council "requested to publish the report" (Sec. 1.4). The report notes that "our 1976 Working group's reflection is for the most part pastoral. . . " (Sec. 1.4). Hence, it was not composed as a doctrinal study. The report is unsigned and no mention is made as to what ecclesial authority requested its publication.

Although this Pontifical Council is part of the Roman Curia it does not have the authoritative doctrinal status of the Congregations. The same document notes in commentary on the issue of the validity of cerebral death as a criterion for death that "it is for a higher authority than itself [the Working Group] to make such a declaration officially, but has agreed to call attention, by means of this report, to the need for making it" (ibid, Sec. 5.3). Hence, such a report of a working group cannot *ipso facto* be given the doctrinal weight that would settle the matter at hand, namely, what is of strict moral obligation regarding the provision artificial nutrition and hydration to a permanently and profoundly comatose patient. Nonetheless, for the record, only in the 28-page report's brief final paragraph of the section dealing with therapeutic measures is the matter discussed.:

The criteria whereby we can distinguish *extraordinary* measures from *ordinary* measures are very many. They are to be applied according to each concrete case. Some of them are *objective:* such as the nature of the measures proposed, how expensive they are, whether it is just to use them, and what the options of Justice are in the matter of using them. Other criteria are *subjective:* such as not giving certain patients psychological shocks, anxiety, uneasiness, and so on. It will always be a question, when deciding upon measures to be taken, of establishing to what extent the means to be used and the end being sought are proportionate.

Among all the criteria for decision, particular importance must be given to the quality of the life to be saved or kept living by the therapy. The Letter of Cardinal Villot to the Congress of the International Federation of Catholic Medical Associations is very clear on this subject: "It must be emphasized that is the sacred character of life which forbids a physician to kill and makes it a duty for him at the same time to use every resource of his art to fight against death. This does not, however, mean that a physician is under obligation to use all and every one of the life-maintaining techniques offered him by the indefatigable creativity of science. Would it not be a useless torture, in many cases, to impose vegetative reanimation during the last phase of an incurable disease?" (*Documentation Catholique,* 1970, p. 963).

But the criterion of the quality of life is not the only one to be taken into account, since, as we have said above, subjective considerations must enter into a properly cautious judgement as to what therapy to undertake and what therapy not. The fundamental point is that the decision should be made according to rational arguments that have taken well into account the many and various aspects of the situation, including what effect will be had upon the family. The principle to follow is, therefore, that no moral obligation to have recourse to extraordinary measures exists; and that, incidentally, a doctor must follow the wishes of a sick person who refuses such measures.

On the contrary, there remains the strict obligation to apply under all circumstances those therapeutic measures which are called "minimal": that is, those which are normally and customarily used for the maintenance of life: (alimentation, blood transfusions, injections, etc.). To interrupt these minimal measures would, in practice, be equivalent to wishing to put an end to the patient's life (ibid, Secs. 2.4.2 to 2.4.4).

In summary, one can say, that the Church in its official documents has provided the principle (of proportionate [ordinary] and disproportionate [extraordinary] means) for deciding whether there exists, in a particular case, the moral obligation to use, or the moral option not to use, a life sustaining *medical* procedure. But whether this same principle is applicable to the matter of artificially supplied nutrition and hydration is at present an open and present question.

Moral Tradition of the Church Regarding the Means to Conserve Life

The intense current controversy regarding that of a moral obligation always to provide nutrition and hydration even to a comatose person, makes it imperative to review the origin and development of the Church's teaching on the ordinary and extraordinary means of sustaining life. As stated above, Bishop Cronin has done this very well in his dissertation which is reprinted in the first part of this volume. In this section we will sketch the main line of this development with a particular emphasis on the nature of the specific obligation to provide such basic life support as food and water.

Cronin begins his developmental study with the sacred scriptures citing Deuteronomy 32:39 regarding God's absolute dominion over life and death and observing that St. Augustine, and other Church Fathers understood the fifth commandment as also prohibiting suicide (see Cronin, pp. 4–7).

St. Thomas' tract on suicide (*Summa Theologia,* IIa IIac, q.64,1.5), is "the basis for the subsequent theological discussion on the subject down through the years" (Cronin, p.7). Hence, as one bench mark for the discussion on ordinary and extraordinary means there is no doubt about the Church's teaching regarding the malice of suicide (see Cronin, p.13).

Not only is there an obligation not to take one's life (suicide) but also to use the necessary means to maintain one's life:

> A review, therefore, of the foregoing discussions indicates that neither Scripture, the tradition of the teaching Church, nor the nature of man can be cited in support of an argument denying the obligation to conserve one's life. Indeed, the facts reveal the contrary. The reasons demonstrating the malice of suicide and the obligation of self-conservation are intimately related, and the common Catholic teaching has been consistent and constant in regard to both (Cronin, p.19).

After noting that the principles of epikeia and dispensation are not applicable to the natural law precept of self-preservation (ibid, pp. 20–25), Cronin shows how the principle of double effect can be applied (ibid, pp. 26–29) which would permit, under the proper circumstances, indirect suicide.

Next he considers the possibility that moral impossibility might excuse one from the precept of self-conservation. Cronin concludes this inquiry by the following summary:

> Therefore, to summarize the above doctrine and apply it to the problem at hand: an individual is always bound by the affirmative precept of the natural law commanding him to conserve his life. However, the individual is licitly excused from the fulfillment of this precept by circumstances which constitute for him a moral impossibility not commonly experienced by men in general. How grave this difficulty has to be is the question which will occupy a great section of the remainder of this dissertation (ibid, p. 31).

Having shown that since the obligation to conserve one's life is an affirmative precept of the natural law from which moral (or physical) impossibility could excuse, Cronin initiates a historical review of theological opinions in regard to the ordinary and extraordinary means of conserving life (ibid, pp. 33–76).

Cronin notes that there was little theological discussion of the ordinary and extraordinary means of conserving life until the 16th century. St. Thomas' treatment of suicide was the point of departure for a number of theologians. Among the early prominent commentators was Francisco de Vitoria (d. 1546) whose writings on the topic set the tone for subsequent writers.

To shorten and focus this review, we will consider primarily relevant statements regarding the use of food. In brief, the moral tradition of the Church recognized that there were certain conditions when, for a particular individual, the taking of food by mouth by a conscious person was not seriously obligatory. It should be noted, parenthetically, that until this century there was no way of effectively supplying nutrition to an unconscious person. Thus, for example, Cronin comments on de Vitoria (pp. 34–38):

> Therefore, if the conservation of self by food is an obligation, it would seem that a sick person who did not eat because of some disgust for food, would be guilty of mortal sin. Vitoria replies:
>
>> *Regarding the first argument to the contrary—I would say secondly that if a sick man can take food or nourishment with a certain hope of life, he is held to take the food, as he would be*

held to give it to one who is sick. Thirdly, I would say that if the depression of spirit is so low and there is present such consternation in the appetitive power that only with the greatest of effort and as though by means of a certain torture, can the sick man take food, right away that is reckoned a certain impossibility, and therefore he is excused, at least from mortal sin, especially where there is little hope of life, or none at all (cited by Cronin pp,. 35).

Such a "disgust" for food is found in person with anorexia nervosa, or other conditions where, temporarily, such persons may find eating extremely repulsive. Cronin then proceeds to consider another situation.

Later on then, discussing the lawfulness of abstaining perpetually from a certain type of food, even in extreme necessity, Vitoria has this:

Finally, for a solution of the objections, it must be noted: it is one thing not to protect life and it is another to destroy it; for man is not always held to the first and it is enough that he perform that by which regularly a man can live: if a sick man could not have a drug except by giving over his whole means of subsistence, I do not think he would be bound to do so.

Then he adds:

Second conclusion: One is not held to protect his life as much as he can by means of foods. This is clear because one is not held to use foods which are the best, the most delicate and most expensive, even though these foods are most healthful, indeed this is blameworthy. . . Likewise, one is not held to live in the most healthful place, therefore neither must he use the most healthful food. . .

Again:

Third conclusion: If one uses foods which men commonly use and in the quantity which customarily suffices for the conservation of strength, even though from this his life is shortened, even notably and this is noticed, he would not sin. . . From this, the corollary follows that one is not held to use medicines to

245

prolong his life even when the danger of death is probable, for example to take for some years a drug to avoid fevers or anything of this sort.

Vitoria uses the same reasoning in his commentary on St. Thomas:

> *. . . In the second place, I say that one is not held to lengthen his life because he is not held to use always the most delicate foods, that is, hens and chickens, even though he has the ability and the doctors say that if he eats in such a manner, he will live twenty years more, and even if he knew this for certain, he would not be obliged. . . So I say, thirdly, that it is licit to eat common and regular foods. . . Granted that the doctor advises him to eat chickens and partridges, he can eat eggs and other common items* (ibid., pp. 35–37).

Cronin notes as a general preface to the citation of other early moralists that

> In this particular subject, namely, the necessity of using the ordinary means of conserving life and the lawfulness of shunning the extraordinary means, the teaching of Vitoria had tremendous influence. Many of the authors used his speculation as the foundation of their own thinking in the matter. Others were quite content with repeating verbatim his doctrine. (Cronin, p.39).

To explain the apparent repetitiveness of the citations, Cronin remarks that

> To cite, however the same doctrine as each author comes into focus is not just simple repetition, but rather it is an attempt to show the constant tradition that has existed in this matter (Cronin, p.41).

Subsequent moralists continue in this vein, for example, Banez (d.1604):

> *The reason is that, although a man is held to conserve his own life, he is not bound to extraordinary means but to common food and clothing, to common medicines, to a certain common and ordinary pain: not, however, to a certain extraordinary and horrible pain, nor to expenses which are extraordinary in proportion to the status of this man* (cited by Cronin, p.42).

Sanchez (d. 1610) develops the same thesis, namely, that an individual is morally bound only to the kind and quantity of food that the ordinary person uses to maintain life.

> *One must suppose that it is one thing not to prolong life and it is another to shorten life. Let the first conclusion be; no one is held to prolong life, indeed neither is he held to conserve it by using the best and most delicate foods, rather this is reprehensible. This is proved by reason of the fact that one is not bound to live in the most healthful place but can dwell in a region which is harmful due to the cold or heat neither is he held to seek out the most exquisite medicinal remedies etc., therefore. Likewise, he is not bound to abstain from wine in order to live longer. . . Hence the first inference that if one uses foods which men commonly use and in the quantity which customarily is sufficient for conserving strength, although he realizes due to this he will shorten his life considerably, he does not sin. Secondly, it is inferred that one is not obliged to use medicines to prolong life even where there would be the probable danger of death, such as taking a drug for many years to avoid fevers, etc. The second conclusion; one is held however, while sick, to consult doctors and use healthful foods* (cited by Cronin, p.42–43).

Further on Sanchez explains his point and brings out again the distinction between maintaining or conserving life and prolonging it. To the latter, Sanchez asserts, one is not morally bound:

> *It is licit to fast and abstain even from common foods, not only in regard to the plurality of meals but also, in regard to the quantity as long as the food necessary for the nourishment and conservation of the individual is taken. . . This is proved by reason of the fact that this is not to intend to abbreviate life or kill one' self but it is only to use means directed by nature for sustenance and not to prolong life, to which no one is bound, as I said* (cited by Cronin, p. 43).

Cronin notes that De Lugo makes a distinction between (1) an act which positively induces death, and (2) one which fails to take available measures to avoid a perceived threat to death.

Now, in which category should the individual be placed who abstains from food necessary to sustain his life? De Lugo answers that "to abstain from food necessary for the sustenance of life when a person can sustain his life by ordinary means, would pertain to the first genus." Hence, for De Lugo, the refusal to employ the ordinary means (in this case, food) when this can be accomplished easily and in a normal manner is equivalent to performing an act which has positive influence in bringing about one's own death (Cronin, p. 50).

After discussion the difference between natural and necessary causes on the one hand, and on the other, free contingent causes, Cronin underscores De Lugo's insistence on the ordinary means of sustaining one's life.

> For De Lugo, then, the necessity of conserving one's life by ordinary means is beyond dispute. Not to use the ordinary means is the same as to inflict death by one's self.

> > I said, however, that a man must guard his life by ordinary means against dangers and death coming from natural causes. . . because the one who neglects the ordinary means seems to neglect his life and therefore to act negligently in the administration of it, and he who does not employ the ordinary means which nature has provided for the ordinary conservation of life is considered morally to will his death. . . (cited by Cronin, p. 52).

Cronin proceeds to remark:

> Such is not the case however, with the extraordinary means of conserving life. In this paragraph, De Lugo gives a minor discussion on the nature of extraordinary means and the reason why they are not obligatory. However brief this discussion is, his teaching is of great importance and assistance to one trying to determine the nature of the extraordinary means of conserving life. First of all, De Lugo rules out the necessity of any extraordinary diligence in accomplishing the conservation of life. For him, there is a clear distinction between the blameworthy neglect of one's life and the necessary care of it by very extraordinary means. The reason which De Lugo gives is that the "bonum" of a man's life is

not so tremendously important that it demands conservation by all possible means. Perhaps this statement may appear a bit shocking at first. Rightly interpreted, however, its meaning is clear. The affirmative precept of the natural law obliging conservation of one's life does not bind in the presence of a proportionately grave difficulty. Not every possible means must be employed but only those which ordinary diligence requires. If in using ordinary means death occurs, his death nevertheless can not be imputed to the individual as morally culpable (Cronin, p. 52).

In the moral tradition, Cronin notes, an obligatory means involves a procedure in common use for preserving life.

The reader has taken note without doubt, that the theologians cited thus far, when discussing ordinary means, have constantly referred to a comparison with the manner in which men "commonly" live. An interesting application of this principle occurs in De Lugo. He repeats the difference between bringing about one's death in a positive manner and omitting the use of certain means of conserving life. The first is never licit; the second can be licit in certain circumstances. In harmony with this principle therefore, "according to the common opinion of the Doctors, there is no obligation of using choice and costly medicine to avoid death". This omission does not imply a direct killing of one's self but rather, the person concerned permits his death and rests content with using only the ordinary and common means by which men commonly live. Hence, the person does not positively influence his death, but dies on account of old-age or the weakness of his own life (Cronin, p. 55).

De Lugo introduces another element into the obligation to use ordinary means which as Cronin notes is "a teaching of tremendous importance." These must offer some hope of benefit or help to the conservation of life:

> . . . if a man condemned to fire, while he is surrounded by the flames, were to have at hand water with which he could extinguish the fire and prolong his life, while at the same time other wood is being carried forward and burned, he would not be held to use this means to conserve his life for such a brief time because the obligation of conserving life by ordinary means is not an obligation of using means for such a brief

conservation—which is morally considered nothing at all. . . (cited by Cronin, p. 54).

For Cronin, as for the classical moralists, benefit is an important element of ordinary means:

> In other words, here again the element of benefit is introduced. The means and remedies employed, even though in themselves common and ordinary, must offer some hope of benefit or help to the conservation of life before they become obligatory. Furthermore, this benefit must be of some considerable duration—in other words, proportionate. Otherwise, if the profit from using these means is only brief, then for De Lugo, it must be considered of no value morally and thus not obligatory. "Parum pro nihilo reputatur" (Cronin, pp. 54–55).

De Lugo also treats the opinion already reviewed here that a man is not bound to effect a prolongation of his life by using choice and delicate foods. In similar fashion, neither is he bound to abstain from wine in order to live longer. He expresses it as follows:

> *Whence, much less is a man bound to effect a lengthening of his life by choice and delicate food, for just as one is not held to abstain from wine in order to live longer, so neither is he bound to drink wine for the same purpose; because just as a man is not bound to seek a more healthful and wholesome locality and air in order to prolong his life, so neither is he held to eat better or more healthful food* (cited by Cronin, p. 54).

Cronin notes that "Even Vitoria, much earlier, had insinuated the same when he demanded that there be hope of life, which rightly interpreted, would seem to mean hope of recovery" (Cronin, p. 49). That hope of life, then, is not merely the status quo of the sick person but life moving towards recovery of health and consciousness.

The Carmelite Fathers of Salamanca, known as the *Salmanticenses,* have this precise wording of the doctrine on the ordinary and extraordinary means of conserving life:

> *. . . also, in order to conserve his life, one is not bound to use all possible remedies, even extraordinary ones, really choice med-*

icines, costly foods, a transfer to more healthful territory, so that
he will live longer: he is not held to give over all his weath [sic]
in order to avoid death which is threatened by another person,
whether justly or unjustly: neither is a sick individual in des-
perate condition bound to employ very costly remedies, even
though he should know that with these remedies his life would
be extended for some hours, or days or even years (Salmanticenses, cited by Cronin, p. 57).

St. Alphonsus (d.1787) continues the tradition. As Cronin notes there must
be some hope—presumably based on medical experience—of recovery:

> True, the obligation of taking an expensive medicine does not
> exist but if it is an ordinary medication, one would be bound to
> employ this means of conserving his life provided that some hope
> of future health could be foreseen (Cronin, pp. 58–59).

Among others who expressed a similar position was Reiffenstuel (d.1703) as
summarized by Cronin:

> First of all, no one is obliged to conserve his life except
> by means which are ordinary, considering his position
> or status. Secondly, there must be a considerable hope
> of recovery from the illness by using these means.
> Thirdly, Reiffenstuel requires that the individual be
> able to employ the means without tremendous diffi-
> culty. All three of these conditions must be fulfilled
> simultaneously in the same individual, otherwise the
> means is an extraordinary means of conserving life
> (Cronin p. 61).

In answer to the question

> whether a sick man is bound to take means to gain his
> health again. . . [Nicolo] Mazotta (+1746) gives cer-
> tain elements that would render a means extraordi-
> nary and thus not obligatory. First of all, if there is no
> hope of recovery, a means need not be employed
> (Cronin p. 64).

In summarizing the teachings of the moralists since the time of Vitoria, Cronin notes that

> It is clear from the writings of the moralists that a means of conserving life must offer some *hope of a beneficial result* before such means can be termed ordinary and obligatory (Cronin, p. 85).

Cronin goes on to say that

> De Lugo clearly states that any means which is to be employed for the conservation of one's life must give definite hope of being proportionately useful and beneficial before it can be called obligatory. It is noteworthy also that De Lugo applies this doctrine even to the taking of food which is a purely natural means of conserving life (Cronin, p. 88).

It hardly cannot be overemphasized that individually and cumulatively, the teachings of these moralists required that before a means (medical treatment or food) becomes morally obligatory there must be some *proportionate benefit*. This implies that there is some hope of a person regaining, at least, some degree of health. The issue of a person being unconscious or being in a permanent coma does not appear in these earlier discussions. Yet it appears consistent to say that the above principle applied to a person in a coma requires that there is a reasonably founded hope that the person would regain consciousness. This requirement, we maintain, is consistent with the tradition that has been traced briefly here and at greater length in Bishop Cronin's dissertation.

Another specific point to recall is that in the above review of (ethically) ordinary and extraordinary means of sustaining life, the person in question was *conscious*. At that time there was no way to feed a comatose person. Such persons would simply die from starvation if they did not succumb first to some infection, cardiac or respiratory failure, or other injury.

In the earlier moralists reviewed above, a distinction was frequently made between natural and artificial means. The former included food and water, while the latter included surgical procedures and medicines. With regards to their respective moral obligation for using them Cronin notes the following:

> To summarize Vitoria's teaching in this matter, we may say that natural means of conserving life are *per se* intended by nature as the means whereby man is to conserve his life and ordinarily these are strictly obligatory. Furthermore, artificial means of conserving

life *per se* intended by nature as a means whereby man can supplement the natural means of conserving life when these natural means are lacking or insufficient etc. Ordinarily, these artificial means are obligatory too, if they can be obtained and used conveniently and with some certitude of benefit (Cronin, p. 81).

Cronin expands on these words and notes again the need for "some hope of success":

> Hence, we can appreciate that the moral teaching of the older moralists in this matter is quite solid even though in their writings they would seem to confuse principle and practice. *In principle,* artificial means of conserving life are obligatory; but for these authors, *in practice,* these means are not obligatory because of some circumstance which eliminates the duty of using them. For example, the medicines are too costly or they do not provide any serious hope of benefit. This seems to be the reason why in one and the same context an author will require the use of artificial means, and then say that these means are not of obligation.
>
> Actually what these older moralists were saying can be well explained by the terms ordinary and extraordinary means of conserving life. When these moralists were living, artificial means of conserving life were extraordinary means because they were too costly or did not offer any hope of benefit. When, however, medicines became useful and offered some hope of success, these means became ordinary means and the moralists then called them obligatory (Cronin, p. 82).

That artificial means can be viewed also at times as supplementing or aiding a natural means, Cronin points to the example of intravenous feedings:

> As a final point, we may point out that an artificial means of conserving life can be either a cure of the disease, such as a medicine, or it can be a means of supplanting a natural means of sustaining life, such as intravenous feeding. This distinction would not seem to change either in theory or in practice the teaching mentioned here. If the artificial means, whether a cure or a substitution for a natural means of conserving life, is an ordinary means, it is obligatory (Cronin, p. 83).

Common Elements in the Tradition

From the 400-year survey of the writings of moralists on the issue of the moral obligation to conserve life, Cronin identifies some common elements. Among these the most important are the following five identified by Cronin:

Hope of Benefit

It is clear from the writing of the moralists that a means of conserving life must offer *some hope of a beneficial result* before such a means can be termed ordinary and obligatory. Vitoria speaks of the obligation that a sick man has to take food or nourishment if he can take it ". . . with a certain hope of life . . .". Further on in the same writing, he says that a man who has moral certitude that he can regain his health by the use of a drug is bound to use the drug. After Vitoria, this notion of a hope of benefit in the question of the ordinary means of conserving life was repeated by many moral theologians (Cronin, p. 85).

De Lugo clearly states that any means which is to be employed for the conservation of one's life must give definite hope of being proportionately useful and beneficial before it can be called obligatory. It is noteworthy also that De Lugo applies this doctrine even to the taking of food which is a purely natural means of conserving life. In other words, for De Lugo, any means whether natural or artificial, must give proportionate hope of success and benefit, otherwise, it is not an ordinary means and thus not obligatory. G. Kelly, S. J. commenting on these words of De Lugo writes: "It may be that the principle, *parum pro nihilo reputatur*, is really contained in the preceding principle, *nemo ad inutile tenetur*. Yet there seems to be a slight difference. Furthermore, De Lugo applies his principle even to the taking of food, which is a purely natural means of preserving life, whereas the other authors were speaking only of remedies for illness". (Cronin, p. 88).

Cronin also discusses whether there can be an *absolute* norm for ordinary means, i.e., one which holds for all persons and circumstances. He states that even for the matter of food the tradition would hold for some relativity:

The question of an absolute norm in regard to ordinary means, however, is more intricate. It does not seem that one can success-

254

fully establish such a norm because even the older moralists teach that such a purely ordinary and common means of conserving life as food, admits of relative inconvenience and difficulty. Furthermore, they point out that this very common means, food, sometimes can offer no proportionate hope of success relative to a particular individual (Cronin, p. 90).

With regard to the ordinary means, Cronin points out that the hope of benefit is an essential part of ordinary means, which, as pointed out above, also includes food:

> In summary, therefore, we may say that the notion of proportionate hope of success and benefit is an essential part of the nature of ordinary means. Without this hope of benefit, a means is hardly an ordinary means and therefore it is not obligatory. In determining the presence of this hope of success and benefit, one must consider not only the nature of the particular remedy or means involved, but also the relative condition of the person who is to use this means. Then, and then only, can the moral obligation of using such a means be properly determined (Cronin, p. 92).

Sometimes the expression used is a *"reasonable hope* of benefit". The reasonableness of the hope means that prior personal experience of the physician, or of consultants, or the record of similar cases in the medical literature, are the basis of the judgement. It is not a mere wish or desire or even the possibility that God would work a miracle. While we can never absolutely rule out that God will respond to prayer in a dramatic way and work a miraculous cure, this faith cannot be the routine basis for making rational decisions regarding medical treatment or other deliberate human interventions.

Although there may be common agreement that benefit is an important consideration, much less clear is the issue of just what constitutes benefit? In a medical context, a benefit would include: a complete cure or recovery from a lethal disease; a partial cure; a significant relief from severe pain; a notable increase in physical mobility; a return to conscious awareness; an ability to communicate with family and friends. But, in particular, is it of benefit to employ life sustaining means on an individual who is in a permanent and profound coma?

As a point of departure for discussing nutrition and hydration, a case discussed by Cronin in response to the diverse opinions of two moralists regarding intravenous feeding will be helpful:

In his doctoral dissertation, *Catholic Teaching on the Morality of Euthanasia,* Father Sullivan gives the following case. A patient is dying of cancer. He is in extreme pain and drugs no longer offer him any extended relief from the pain because he has developed a "toleration" of any drug given him. Since the disease is incurable, and the patient is slowly dying, the doctor wants to stop the intravenous feeding in order to end the suffering. The doctor believes that otherwise, since the patient has a good heart, he will linger on for several weeks in agony. He therefore stops the intravenous feeding and the patient dies. A similar case is presented by Father Donovan in the *Homiletic and Pastoral Review.* Neither author specifically mentions whether or not the patient is conscious, or whether or not there are relatives who can make the choice. In his reply, Father Sullivan says:

> *Since the cancer patient is beyond all hope of recovery and suffering extreme pain, intravenous feeding should be considered an extraordinary means of prolonging life. The physician was justified in stopping the intravenous feeding. He should make sure first, however, that the patient is spiritually prepared.*

Contrary to this opinion, Father Donovan writes:

> *I fear that to neglect intravenous feedings is a form of mercy killing rather than a means of sustaining life that is morally impossible to use. Here is a cancerous person given three months to live, and he cannot be nourished except by intravenous means, is he therefore to be let starve to death, even if he is willing?*

Father Sullivan has carefully mentioned many conditions in his presentation of the case. It would seem, therefore, that the intravenous feeding is an extraordinary means for the cancerous patient concerned. Even in the situation related by Father Donovan, it would be licit to consider the intravenous feeding an extraordinary means of conserving life. However, recall that we based our definition of ordinary and extraordinary means on the relative norm. In the presumption, therefore, that a doctor alone has the responsibility to make a decision in a particular case, he should consider all the conditions of the patient, because intravenous feeding cannot be called an ordinary means of conserving life, *absolutely speaking*, even though according to a *general norm*, it may be an ordinary means for most men.

If, after due consideration of the particular case before him, the doctor decides that the intravenous feeding is an extraordinary means for the patient concerned, he should then follow out the norms we have given above for the doctor's use of extraordinary means in the treatment of patients. Cases of this nature must be solved in individual instances after prudent consideration of the condition of the patient concerned. General norms are guides and helps, not the definitive solutions of each similar case. The doctor must use great prudence, but he must also feel free to follow out his considered judgment. Euthanasia is illicit and intrinsically evil. However, prolonging a patient's life by an extraordinary means, when all that the doctor can do to cure the person has been done, is not the only morally justifiable alternative. It is licit *per se* to refrain from using an extraordinary means of conserving life (Cronin, p. 132).

Now for the difficult question: is it of benefit that a person be maintained alive in a permanent and profound comatose state? None of the benefits listed above are contained here. What benefit is it to the irreversibly comatose *patient* to be maintained alive? There may be benefit to others, perhaps to society as a witness presumably to the dignity and sanctity of life. But is it? True one may not kill the patient directly, one may not intend directly the patient's death. But if water and nutrition are removed from a patient, is this not a direct killing of the patient? No. Rather it is the concurrent pathology which prevents the patient from chewing and swallowing the food.

The situation is similar to a patient who cannot breath unaided because some part of the respiratory system is not functioning properly. Oxygen, water and food are all necessary elements for maintaining life. If because of some current pathology, the person requires that these be supplied by technological means, then it would seem that the same moral principles can be applied to determime the respective moral obligations to initiate or continue life conserving procedures. By technological means we are circumventing an obstacle that prevents food and water (or oxygen) from entering the body in the normal manner. Hence when we cease by-passing the obstacle, the person dies from a combination of his pathology and the lack of nutrition and hydration (or oxygen).

In each case, then, an *obstacle* is circumvented by technological means. The crucial questions are, under what conditions must these life supportive measure be instituted and when can such measures be forgone or removed? The moral tradition of the Church traced in Bishop Cronin's work, and briefly commented upon in this article with regards to food and water, provides the operative principles. The teachings of Pope Pius XII (1957) and *The Declaration on Euthanasia* (1980) have emerged from that tradition and should be understood and applied in a manner consistent with the tradition.

In Common Use

This element of ordinary or common means may be misleading. Is it restricted to mean those means which humans use ordinarily in daily life, or does the expression refer, also, to those means commonly in use for an individual in that particular circumstance? Cronin's brief discussion of this element does not settle the question entirely.

> Although the moralists use many expressions to describe the nature of ordinary means, the notion of being common seems to be basic. Even when the expression "common" is not used, it is presumed, and from the whole context, the reader is aware of the presumption. For the moralists, the duty of conserving one's life does not demand a diligence or a solicitude that exceeds the usual care that most men normally give their lives. Any means of conserving life that is not the normal or usual course of action adopted by men in general is out of the ordinary—extraordinary—and therefore per se not obligatory. Recall Vander Heeren's phrase that an individual is only bound "to make use of all the ordinary means which are indicated in the usual course of things . . ." (Cronin, p. 92).

Cronin does not address clearly whether "the normal or usual course of action adopted by men in general" refers to the state when they are well and out of the hospital or when they are ill and have available all the contemporary technological aids. Certainly a person who is well and conscious would not use a gastric tube as a means of receiving nourishment (nor a mechanical ventilator for taking in oxygen). But would "men in general" want such technological assistance if they could foresee being in a profound and permanent coma? The evidence is lacking for a definitive answer, but it appears more likely that it would be in the negative. Nonetheless, Cronin suggests that another element is important to make this determination.

Common diligence, therefore, requires the use of common means only. The ordinary conservation of one's life does imply the singular assiduity involved in prolonging life by unusual and uncommon means. In determining, however, whether or not a means is common, it is necessary, of course, to consider relative factors involved. For this reason, the moralists frequently mention in their writings the next element of ordinary means, viz., secundum proportionem status [sic](ibid).

According to One's Status

Basing his remarks on the tradition which considers one's social position and particular status as relevant to the determination of the ordinary means Cronin explains the concept to include an individual's physical condition and psychological status:

It may appear that this element of comparison with one's status is merely the relative norm that we mentioned earlier. The notion of comparison with one's status is contained in that relative norm. Our treatment of it here, however, is no mere repetition of what we have already said. When the authors refer to a comparison with one's status they seem to be implying a relation with one's social or financial condition. Hence, they speak in terms of means being common or ordinary with respect to one's status. They also mention that a means must not be too costly in consideration of an individual's position. The relative norm, however, which we discussed before, is broader than that. It considers not only the financial or social position of an individual but also his physical condition. The relative norm clearly encompasses also the psychological outlook that an individual possesses in regard to the use of a particular means of conserving life. Our task here has been to discuss the elements which the moralists mention and in the light of the discussions which they give. That is the reason that we have allotted separate treatment to the element of comparison with one's status (Cronin, P. 94).

In view of today's overwhelming health care costs, the capacity of an individual or family to pay for long term life support treatment is of paramount importance. Furthermore, hospitals now are much less able to absorb the costs of patients who cannot pay. Even with Medicare, the residual payments are excessive or even prohibitive for most families in the United States. For some conditions such as AIDS, third party payers are increasingly unwilling to cover the expense of treatment. Consequently, the element of cost is a primary consideration. It is not a question of money versus a person's life or health but rather the needs of one person versus the needs of others in the same family or community. How to achieve an equitable solution to such conflicts is a perpetual challenge. Consideration of financial aspect of conserving life will enter into the following discussion of burden.

Not Difficult to Use

In contemporary writings on the subject such terms as "disproportionate burden" or "excessive burden" are used to describe a non-obligatory means. An obligatory means then would involve a procedure or action which does not involve for this individual an excessive burden or difficulty:

> The theologians require that an individual exert definite effort in conserving his life, but they do not demand any endeavor which could not be expected of men in general. Certainly a means whose use, absolutely speaking, entails a difficulty which exceeds the strength of men in general is not an ordinary means. Furthermore, if a means involves great difficulty for a particular individual, even though men in general do not find any great difficulty in its use, it ceases to be ordinary for this individual. In other words, even if the great difficulty is only relative, not absolute, it is still sufficient to render a means extraordinary for a particular individual. We have mentioned earlier in this chapter that Vitoria applied the relative norm even to food, a very common means of conserving life. It will be profitable now, however, to note the words with which he describes this relative difficulty. Vitoria writes: ". . . if the depression of spirit is so low and there is present such consternation of spirit in the appetitive power that only with the greatest of effort and as through by means of a certain torture can the sick man take food, right away that is reckoned a certain impossibility and therefore he is excused . . ." (Cronin, pp. 96–97).

A fifth element identified by Cronin as part of the moral tradition on the issue of conserving life is that the means are reasonable (even if there is some degree of burden) in order for them to be obligatory:

> However, in context, the writings of these authors indicate that they did not intend to require a complete lack of difficulty before terming a means ordinary. They seem to mean that ordinary means must be means that one can employ conveniently—in other words, reasonably.

> To say that an ordinary means must be easy to use is an expression that can be open to misunderstanding. One might easily imagine that the concept of ordinary means must of necessity exclude any type of difficulty. In the light of the discussion given in the previous section, however, it would seem correct to say that the proper expression is *reasonable,* not, easy. Ordinary means are the reasonable means. They are not necessarily easy means because they can entail moderate difficulty (Cronin, p. 98).

Summary of Tradition

In summary, Cronin shows that the contemporary teaching of the Church regarding ethically ordinary (proportionate) and ethically extraordinary (disproportionate) means of conserving life has developed over at least four hundred years. In general, what is judged to be a proportionate means (ethically ordinary) is obligatory and what is deemed to be disproportionate (ethicially extraordinary) is morally optional.

In addition, Cronin also identifies the elements in that tradition which constitutes a particular means as ordinary and therefore obligatory. These elements were: 1) hope of benefit; 2) in common use; 3) proportionate to one's status; 4) not difficult to use; and 5) reasonable for the person in his circumstances.

Of great significance in the tradition was the awareness that there is no absolute norms which would render some means as always ordinary; the norms are relative to the individual person in his particular circumstances. The tradition recognized that food was also a means of conserving life subject to the same principles, namely, in some circumstances, for some individuals the taking of food could be an ethically extraordinary, (and therefore non-obligatory) means of conserving life, even if generally it would be an ordinary means.

The older tradition had not discussed, or anticipated, that nutrition could be supplied by artificial means to an unconscious person. Only in this century has it been possible to provide nutrition and hydration effectively to a comatose person. But the principles developed over 400-years are nonetheless equally applicable.

Although these principles have roots in the deep past, and have evaluated organically under the watchful scrutiny of the Magisterium, there remains the question as to how they are to be applied in the light of today's anti-life ethos dominant in major segments of our society. The task of the next section is to assess that situation.

Psychosocial Milieu in the United States

Those who respect the inherent dignity and sacredness of human life fear that if the artificial provision of nutrition and hydration to a permanently comatose patient is considered morally optional, such as a conclusion would be used by pro-euthanasia forces to further their cause in the legislatures and the courts. That fear on the one hand cannot be simply dismissed, nor on the other hand should one simply allow that concern to override what, I believe, is a valid moral analysis clearly rooted in centuries of moral tradition. In light of that concern it is necessary to consider briefly the current situation in the United States to help define the dimensions of the problem.

One can gather a sense of the medical profession in the United States from a recent statement made by the Council on Ethical and Judicial Affairs of American Medical Association. It should be recalled that not all physicians in the United States belong to this association, nor does the statement by any means necessarily reflect the opinion of all its members. However, it is an official policy statement of the Association. Notable in the statement is that life-prolonging treatment *includes* technologically supplied nutrition and hydration.

> Even if death is not imminent but a patient's coma is beyond doubt irreversible and there are adequate safeguards to confirm the accuracy of the diagnosis and with the concurrence of those who have responsibility for the care of the patient, it is not unethical to discontinue all means of life-prolonging medical treatment.

Life-prolonging medical treatment includes medication and artificially or technologically supplied respiration, nutrition or hydration. In treating a terminally ill or irreversibly comatose patient, the physician should determine whether the benefits of treatment outweigh its burdens. At all times, the dignity of the patient should be maintained *(Current Opinions of the Council on Ethical and Judicial Affairs of the American Medical Association,* 1986, p. 12–13).

The great fear of those who respect life is that in the United States the pro-euthanasia groups (such as the Hemlock Society, Americans Against Human Suffering and Society for the Right to Die) will use every opportunity to obtain legislation which would permit voluntary euthanasia. Thus, one recent publication notes:

Active voluntary euthanasia could soon become legal in California, medical and legal experts tell *Medical Ethics Advisor* (MEA).

Despite strong opposition from most physicians and the state's medical association, momentum is gaining for a public initiative known as the "Humane and Dignified Death Act."

The act won a major victory in September when delegates at the California Bar Association's annual meeting in Los Angeles, by a narrow 282–239 vote, approved a resolution backing physician-assisted suicide for terminally ill patients. *(Medical Ethics Advisor,* Dec. 1987, p. 153).

The same publication observes that "Recent polls indicate that two-thirds of Americans favor the idea of physician assistance in dying"(ibid). In the same vein, the authors of a recent article concludes that:

The withdrawal of basic life support, such as hydration or nutrition by intravenous lines of feeding tubes, is ethically controversial and complex. Although most people eventually feel at peace with stopping more technical medical interventions, these basic measures are regarded more as signs of caring than as treatment. No one is comfortable with the thought that a loved one may "die of thirst" or "starve to death." Indeed, legal sanctions notwithstanding, families feel guilty if these feelings are not explored and resolved.

The three states whose courts have addressed the question of withdrawal of nutrition and hydration from incompetent patients have treated it in the same manner as the withdrawal of advanced life support. As additional cases are adjudicated, broader judicial support is expected for withdrawing these treatments when they are not clearly benefiting patients. (*"Initiating and Withdrawing Life Support,"* John Edward Ruark, M.D., Thomas Alfred Raffin, M.D., and the Stanford University Medical Center Committee on Ethics, *The New England Journal of Medicine,* Jan. 7, 1988, p. 30).

The above quotation reflects a common but by no means universal reaction towards the idea of a loved one dying of thirst or starvation. To say that "no one is comfortable" with that thought is to reduce moral issues of right and wrong to *feelings*. It appears to be a jargon, commonly found in discussions about serious issues, for one to say: "I am comfortable with that," rather than saying, "I believe this to be wrong". While feelings are present on such matters, the feelings follow a moral evaluation even if only vaguely perceived or articulated.

The National Conference of Catholic Bishops' (NCCB) Committee for Pro-Life Activities is very concerned that pro-euthanasia attitudes will dominate the public opinion and legislative enactments. It, accordingly, issued a cautionary statement which, however, did not exclude absolutely the withdrawing of nutrition or hydration:

The Uniform Act [to make uniform the laws in all 50 states on particular issues] states that it will not affect any existing responsibility to provide measures such as nutrition and hydration to promote comfort. But it does not adequately recognize a distinct and more fundamental benefit of such measure—that of sustaining life itself. This is a serious lapse in light of the ambiguous scope of the Uniform Act, which may include cases in which a patient will live a long time with treatment but die quickly without it. From most patients, measures for providing nourishment are morally obligatory even when other treatment can be withdrawn due to its burdensomeness or ineffectiveness.

Negative judgments about the "quality of life" of unconscious or otherwise disabled patients have led some in our society to propose withholding nourishment precisely in order to end these patients' lives. Society must take special care to protect against such discrimination. Laws dealing with medical treatment may have to take account of exceptional circumstances, when even means for providing nourishment may become too ineffective or burdensome to be obligatory. But such laws must establish clear safeguards against intentionally hastening the deaths of vulnerable patients by starvation or dehydration (NCCB, *"Statement on Uniform Rights of the Terminally Ill Act,"* June 1986, p. 3).

A recently published work by a secular ethics group has analyzed carefully the issue of life-sustaining treatment and concluded that

> Among the most effective and widely used methods of sustaining life are medical procedures for supplying nutrition and hydration by tubes, catheters, or needles inserted into the patient's body. Forgoing these procedures is controversial and presents a special ethical problem. On the one hand, they provide food and water, which are often regarded as non-medical means of sustaining life that must be provided in all cases. On the other hand, these methods are also artificial (man-made) means of providing care, requiring the efforts of medical personnel and bodily invasion. They impose burdens as well as provide benefits, and therefore can be considered medical interventions which, like other interventions, may under some circumstances be forgone.

> We have concluded that it is wisest and most plausible to understand these methods as medical interventions that may be forgone in some cases. Therefore, the standards to be used for decisions concerning termination of these procedures are essentially those that apply for the termination of other forms of medical treatment. At the same time, the issue has only recently received widespread attention. It provokes strong feelings, and for some a sense of moral offense. There is also concern about potential abuse. Thus caution is necessary.

> In reaching these conclusions, we have recognized that food and water undeniably have a symbolic and psychological importance. They symbolize our caring for and nuturing of one another, and can be a means for the patient to obtain comfort and satisfaction. In certain circumstances, however, the patient experiences more comfort, caring, and satisfaction from forgoing medical procedures for supplying nutrition and hydration, and instead receiving

supportive care to keep him or her comfortable "Guidelines on Medical Procedures for Supplying Nutrition and Hydration," *(Guidelines on the Termination of Life-Sustaining Treatment and Care of the Dying,* a report of The Hastings Center, Bloomington, The Indiana University Press, 1987, p. 59).

Another study has reviewed the issue of withdrawal of food and water at some length. The book contains a variety of essays, some in favor, some opposed to such withdrawal, and carries out in more detail the arguments pro and con presented above. It is a valuable book to consult: *By No Extraordinary Means: The Choice to Forego Life-Sustaining Food and Water,* Edited by Joanne Lynn, M.D., Bloomington: Indiana University Press, 1986.

A constituent part of the psychosocial milieu of the controversy is the array of slogan-type expressions, which fill the literature. These include "conscious person may be starved to death" *(Missouri Citizens for Life NEWS,* Dec. 1988, p. 8), "The Right to Die", (Society for the Right to Die), and "watering vegetables" *(Discovery,* Dec. 1988, P. 30). While these may state concisely, but often inaccurately, what a person holds, they do not contribute to a clearer understanding of the issue.

What is the Cause of Death?

A major point of misunderstanding, I believe, is whether, in fact, the human agent is morally the *cause* of the comatose patient's death when nutrition and hydration are removed. In this context, to cause a death is to be morally responsible for it. To be responsible for the outcome of an action (or inaction), it is required that the person in question be morally obligated not to act or to act. A living human being is generally obliged by the natural law to breathe, drink, eat, protect himself from environmental threats to life, etc. If he were not to do so he would be responsible for his ill health or death. Should he knowingly and freely consume a lethal poison, he is the cause of his death—through the instrumentality of the poison—and morally responsible for it.

As Cronin points out in his work, while a person is always obliged to negative precepts of the natural law—"you shall not kill," he is not always and everywhere obliged to the affirmative precepts "you shall use the necessary means to maintain your life" (see Cronin, p. 30). If one does not use a necessary means, is that person the cause of his death? Here, a distinction is advisable. If, on the one hand, there is concurrently a lethal pathological condition, eg. cancer, then death is a consequence of the cancer which has lethally injured or impaired a vital function, eg. the respiratory center in the brain stem. If, on the other, one simply refuses to eat and drink, eg. a hunger strike, the proximate cause of death is the bodily injury brought about by the lack of water, calories and essential nutrients which is the consequence of a free choice by the person. he is the morally responsible cause of death by an act of omission.

In the case of the cancer patient, is not the person who withholds treatment morally responsible for the death of the individual? No. A further distinction needs to be made: the *physical* cause of an event and the *morally* responsible cause. The former refers to the biological sequence of events which lead to the individual's death. The latter looks at the knowing and free decisions of a person who initiates or omits a particular physical action which leads ultimately to an individual's death. The *Declaration on Euthanasia's* words are consonant:

"Such a refusal [of a technique which is already in use but which carries a risk or is burdensome] is not the equivalent of suicide; on the contrary, it should be considered an acceptance of the human condition . . . "(Section IV).

In brief, the critical point is not the physical cause of death, but whether a person is morally obligated in light of all the specific circumstances to circumvent an obstacle to continued living by the use of, for example, a mechanical respirator or feeding tube.

For many persons the removal (or the withholding) of a mechanical ventilator to assist a comatose patient who cannot breathe on his own is easier to justify than is the withdrawing (or withholding) of food and water from the same patient. Why this difference?

As has been noted above, the symbolic and emotional content of food and water is closely and visibly connected with everyday life. Any tampering with the responding to that necessity will evoke strong feelings.

Another factor to be considered is that the removal of a respirator from one who is unable to breathe without it will result in death within a few minutes. Removal of food and water results in death usually only after several weeks. The latter process is commonly perceived as a terribly prolonged painful way of dying. But, as a matter of fact, for a comatose or seriously debilitated patient, this is not the case (see, eg., Cox in *Ethics & Medics, September 1987).*

One way to approach the symbolic and emotional content is to realize that both biologically and morally there is no relevant significant difference between the use or non-use of a respirator and of tube feeding. The previously mentioned parallel may help. Oxygen, water and food are all essential for life. For a person whose respiratory system is so impaired that he cannot breathe on his own, that is, he cannot bring air into his lung, a respirator is essential to "push and suck air in and out of our patient's lungs" (Elizabeth Rosenthal, "Crisis in the ICU", *Discovery*, December 1988, p. 30). Once in the lungs the oxygen has to diffuse from the alveoli into the blood stream which then transports it, by means of the hemoglobin molecule in the red blood cells, to every part of the body.

So, too, with food and water. If the digestive system is impaired, eg. the person is unable consciously to chew or swallow, then assistance is required. The obstacle can be by-passed by intravenous feeding, by N-G tubes, or by gastrostomy, for example. Depending on the route of administration, water and nourishment are directly introduced into the blood (IV) or are introduced into the stomach and small intestine and largely absorbed through the villi of the large bowel and then enters the blood stream.

In one case the mechanical ventilator pumps in the oxygen, and in the other, water and food are "pumped" into the body by IV or by stomach tube. Both involve the artful introduction of an essential element for human life; both overcome a serious defect in a fundamental biological system; both would result in death if human intervention had not been introduced to compensate for the dysfunction. One difference is the time scale: removal of the respirator brings about death in a few minutes; removal of the feeding tube brings about death in two or three weeks. But there is no moral difference. The principles applicable to one, are applicable to the other. In a particular case, if one may morally remove the respirator, one also, by the same principles, could morally remove the feeding tubes.

A particular concern of many is that in removing artificially provided nutrition and hydration the intention is lethal. This objection is raised by the late Father John Connery, S.J.:

> It is quite true that an act or omission from which death results is not in itself immoral. It is when this is done precisely to end or shorten the life of the patient that it becomes immoral. Since this is what happens when some means to preserve life is not provided or withdrawn, it is our contention that it constitutes intentional euthanasia by omission.

> Briefly, then, even if one does not place some positive act of violence, but simply omits something necessary to preserve life, he

cannot say that he is just letting death occur, or letting nature take its course. If death results from his failure to do something he can easily do, and this is his intention, he is doing more that just letting it happen. He intends what happens because this is the solution to his problem. And this is immoral ("The Ethics of Withholding/Withdrawing Nutrition and Hydration," *Linacre Quarterly*, February 1987.)

In the withdrawal or withholding of nutrition and hydration *must* one necessarily and always intend the death of the individual? Clearly, this is not the case as John Connery himself explains:

As pointed out, it would obviously not be permissible to forego eating and drinking to bring on death. But if some other reason were present, it could be justified (ibid, p. 19).

Hence, the question: is there present some other reason in the situation of a profound and irreversibly comatose patient? I believe so.

Persons facing the decision whether to continue or discontinue artificially provided nutrition and hydration will ordinarily desire that the patient be restored to full health and consciousness. But if this cannot be, then they may desire that this situation come to an end. They may even pray that the Lord take the beloved if it is His will. And they can do so without desiring or taking steps to terminate directly that person's life.

What the person perceives is the disproportion between the efforts made to sustain life and the resulting condition of the patient. The effort is evaluated as unreasonable relative to the results. The maintenance of the person in an irreversible coma is not perceived as a great good even if clearly life itself is a good. Of course, someone may believe that it is a great good to do so because it witnesses to the high value of human life. Such an individual might find it reasonable and, indeed perhaps, may view it as personally obligatory to expend every effort to maintain life in a permanently comatose individual. But this is not a necessary conclusion from the principles. These moral principles allow for the subjective element, namely, that the individual perceives and experiences the burden to be greater than the anticipated good. The intention is to *stop* the means, the artificial supplying of food and water, which are not bringing about a proportionate benefit. Death is foreseen as the inevitable but not directly intended result. The course of action becomes morally optional.

Possibilities for Misuse of the Principles

Are these principles clear enough and the application sufficiently secure so that they cannot be used legitimately to justify euthanasia?

They cannot be employed to approve morally the *direct* termination of a life, eg, by injecting a lethal dose of morphine, barbituate or other drug. The principle addresses the withholding or withdrawing of a life sustaining measure, not taking positive measures to end a person's life which would have continued if steps had not been taken to stop it.

What about those born who are profoundly handicapped and must be spoon fed? Can the principle of disproportionate (ethically extraordinary) means be applied to them so as to stop nutrition and hydration?

Admittedly, this area is a complex one. If the individual is conscious, the answer is no. The principle that has been under discussion is applicable to the person in a profound and permanent coma. The profoundly mentally retarded person is not in that category.

Another category of persons for whom questions has been raised about withdrawal of nutrition and hydration is that of the persistent vegetative state (PVS). Such persons are not precisely in a permanent and profound coma but nonetheless are unconscious. Their eyes may open and they may go through sleep-awake cycles (as identified by EEG) but at no time are they conscious or aware of their surroundings. After about 12 months in that state, it is very unlikely that such persons will ever regain consciousness. There is no indication that such persons have any kind of deeper, internal mental activity undetectable by outside observers. Although one can raise that conjecture as theoretically possible, moral decisions can only be made on available evidence. To date there is no indication that patients who have been in a profound coma or PVS for at least 12 months have any such internal activity. (The near-death experiences reported by many refers to a different category of patients). In brief, for an ethical analysis of the obligation to conserve life these persons are similar to the permanently comatose patient.

A recent article concisely summarizes the various discussions on the subject of nutrition and hydration for the PVS patient. The authors' summary is a statement of their conclusion which is compatible with the position taken in the above discussion:

> In our judgment, the cumulative effect of our arguments supports the legitimate forgoing or withdrawing of nutrition and hydration to PVS patients. This judgment can properly be reached without supporting any efforts or claims for euthanasia and without making any improper judgments about the worth of a particular life.

270

After carefully considering both the patient's known wishes and the qualitative relation between the patient's medical condition and the pursuit of life's purposes, one may appropriately judge that such a therapy is disproportionate and morally optional. (Thomas A. Shannon and James Walter, "The PVS Patient and the Forgoing/Withdrawing of Medical Nutrition and Hydration," *Theological Studies*, Dec. 1988, p. 640).

One other consideration needs to be brought up albeit briefly. This is the issue of a child born so profoundly retarded that there is no reasonable hope for such a person ever to reach a level of affective-cognitive functioning necessary to reach the purpose of temporal life. There is an abiding concern that such children will be permitted to die by dehydration and starvation as the result of a global decision to forgo or withdraw nutrition and hydration for the entire class.

Will these principles when applied to that situation permit the non-feeding of a very severely handicapped child?

Some years ago, the question was raised about the obligation to treat such a child. The so-called John Hopkins case was made known to a wider public by a documentary film, *Who Shall Live?* This film portrayed a newborn infant with Down's syndrome and duodenal atresia. The parents, after consultation with the parish priest, had refused permission for the necessary surgery to correct the duodenal atresia. The physician and hospital complied. But the ethical community reacted strongly in opposition, even if the debate continues (see Arthur J. Dyck, "Ethical Reflections on Infanticide," in *Infanticide and the Handicapped Newborn*, Dennis J. Horan and Melinda Delahayde, eds., Provo, Utah: Brigham Young University Pres, 1982, pp. 107- 122; Dennis J. Horan and Steven R. Valentine, "The Doctors Dilemma: Euthanasia, Wrongful Life, and the Handicapped Newborn" in *op. cit.* pp.. 33-53).

Horan and Valentine note *(op. cit.)* that one must make the distinction between a treatable and non-treatable condition of the severely handicapped. If treatable, then generally there is an obligation to treat. If not, than at least supportive comfort care is required.

If essentially non-treatable, another writer reached the conclusion that if there was no hope the individual would never attain the potential for human relationships, then the child could be permitted to die:

It [life] is a value to be preserved precisely as a condition for other values, and therefore insofar as these other values are attainable. Since these other values ["higher, more important good"] cluster around and are rooted in human relationships, it seems to follow that life is a value to be preserved only insofar as it contains some potentiality for human relationships (p. 175).

If these reflections are valid, they point in the direction of a guideline that may help in decisions about sustaining the lives of grossly deformed and deprived infants. That guideline is the potential for human relationships associated with the infants condition. If that potential is simply non-existent or would be utterly submerged and undeveloped in the mere struggle to survive, that life has achieved its potential (Richard A. McCormick, S.J. "To Save Let Die: The Dilemma of Modern Medicine," *Journal of the American Medical Association*, 229:175, 1974).

Since then numerous articles and books on the topic have appeared. Both sides of dilemma have been argued. One such book concludes on the basis that the neonate is a person not in the strict sense but in the social sense "because of their role in the moral order."

Parents of severely diseased or defective newborns may reasonably choose not to authorize life-prolonging interventions when one of several conditions obtain: 1) extended life is reasonably judged not to constitute a net benefit to the infant; 2) it is reasonably believed that the infant's condition is such that the capacities sufficient for a minimal independent existence or personhood in a strict sense cannot be attained; or 3) the costs to other persons, especially parents and family, are sufficient to defeat customary duties of beneficence toward a particular human infant (Earl E. Shelp, *Born to Die?*, New York: The Free Press, 1986, p. 203).

While it does not address directly the question of artificial nutrition and hydration, forgoing or withdrawing such would be permitted by Shelp's general argumentation. But his first condition, at least, is much too broad and the withholding of true personhood from the newborn infant is unacceptable.

More recently, Kevin O'Rourke, O.P., considers this topic briefly in the context of the development of the Church's teaching on the obligation to prolong life. He bases his argument on the teaching of Pope Pius XII that temporal life and good are subordinated to the spiritual goal of life (see Kevin O'Rourke, O.P., "Evolution of Church Teaching on Prolonging Life," *Health Progress*, January/February, 1988, p. 32). O'Rourke argues that ethically extraordinary means are

Those means which are optional because they are ineffective or a grave burden in helping a person strive for the spiritual purpose of life (ibid).

He then proceeds to argue that

To pursue the spiritual purpose of life, one needs minimal degree of cognitive-affective function. Therefore, if this function in an adult cannot be restored or if an infant will never develop this function, and if a fatal disease is present, the adult or infant may be allowed to die (ibid, p. 33).

In response to an objection raised (see Albert Moraczewski, O.P., in "Letters to the Editor," *Health Progress,* June 1988, p. 10), O'Rourke clarifies a point regarding an infant who is severely handicapped (mentally and physically) but does not have a fatal illness. He responds that such a child

. . . should receive life-prolonging care and nursing care provided the care is effective and does not involve a great burden (ibid, p. 12).

O'Rourke sums up his position briefly as follows:

From an ethical perspective, the significant questions about any form of care we use are: 1) given the circumstances, is it an effective means enabling the person to strive for the spiritual purpose of life? 2) given the circumstances, does it result in a grave burden for the patient insofar as striving for the spiritual purpose of life is concerned? (ibid).

Presumably, the second condition as stated would only be applicable if the patient had some degree of awareness, sufficient to experience pain and discomfort. If the patient is in an irreversible coma, then the burden would be that which befalls the family or others—as both the teaching of Pope Pius XII (1957) and the 1980 Vatican *Declaration on Euthanasia* assert.

The infant born severely handicapped would be evaluated similarly. According to O'Rourke's principles (stated above), the feeding and hydration of such children morally is not obligatory because these are *not* effective means of "enabling the person to strive for the spiritual purpose of life." Many would find that this conclusion could be definitively rejected or accepted by those who strive to follow the Church's moral teaching.

Recapitulation

Cronin's historical study has clearly shown how the Church's tradition on the moral obligation to preserve life has developed. That tradition recognized that the obligation to conserve life has its limits and conditions. The conditions required to make the obligation optional were identified and included the notion that there must be some reasonable hope of benefit and that the burden is or has become excessive. Applying these principles, to the permanently and profoundly comatose person, one can conclude that the use of means to preserve life is optional. Furthermore, these means include such basic items as food and water technologically supplied (since the person is in a permanent coma or PVS). However, because of the current anti-life attitude rampant in present day society the issue emerges as theologians would be overlooked and their conclusions used as means to press successfully for legislation that would permit voluntary euthanasia. Special concern is present also with regards to the profoundly retarded persons who have some level of awareness. After examining several ethical analyses of the matter, it is clear that more dialogue is required in order to clarify fully and precisely the benefit and burden involved in such situations. Are benefits and burdens for a Christian (or others) to be measured in relationship to the spiritual goal of life? And how is that goal to be defined operationally?

Conclusion

Most, if not all, Catholic scholars writing on the subject of the withholding or withdrawing of nutrition and hydration agree that this may be done when it is clear that:

1. There is no intention to kill the patient.
2. The patient is imminently dying, that is, will die within two or three weeks regardless of treatment according to competent medical judgement.
3. Initiation or continuation of technologically delivered nutrition and hydration in a particular case can be truly futile and/or imposes an excessive burden on the patient.

The principal differences among Catholic scholars appear to be the following:

1. Whether the principles of proportionate or disproportionate means as found in the 1980 Vatican's *Declaration on Euthanasia*

are applicable to the artificial provision of nutrition and hydration.

2. Whether the cessation of artificial nutrition and hydration is equivalent to a statement that the person's life has no longer human value or worth; or whether such cessation is really an acknowledgement of the human condition and that the *benefit* to the individual is truly outweighed by the burden of the *total* effort required to supply nutrition and hydration.

3. Whether in the cases under consideration the forgoing or withdrawing of artificial nutrition is the cause of the person's death such that the decision maker is guilty of murder or assisted suicide, or whether such action is a morally acceptable forgoing or withdrawing of an optional means which results in the patient's death ultimately from a concurrent pathology (the basis for the inability to eat or drink).

4. Whether allowing withholding or withdrawing of artificial nutrition and hydration, even under carefully specified and morally acceptable conditions would in fact be used by pro-euthanasia persons and groups to promote successfully laws which would permit positive or active euthanasia.

All these vexing issues need further non-polemical discussion in order to develop further the Church's moral doctrine on the obligation to conserve life whose origins and earlier development were traced clearly and admirably by Cronin in 1958.

APPENDICES

APPENDIX I—DECLARATION ON EUTHANASIA*

INTRODUCTION

The rights and values pertaining to the human person occupy an important place among the questions discussed today. In this regard, the Second Vatican Ecumenical Council solemnly reaffirmed the lofty dignity of the human person, and in a special way his or her right to life. The Council therefore condemned crimes against life "such as any type of murder, genocide, abortion, euthanasia, or wilful suicide" (Pastoral Constitution *Gaudium et Spes*, 27).

More recently, the Sacred Congregation for the Doctrine of the Faith has reminded all the faithful of Catholic teaching on procured abortion.[1] The Congregation now considers it opportune to set forth the Church's teaching on euthanasia.

It is indeed true that, in this sphere of teaching, the recent Popes have explained the principles, and these retain their full force;[2] but the progress of medical science in recent years has brought to the fore new aspects of the question of euthanasia, and these aspects call for further elucidation on the ethical level.

In modern society, in which even the fundamental values of human life are often called into question, cultural change exercises an influence upon the

*English text in *Origins*, August 14, 1980, Vol. X, n.10, pp. 154–157. Latin and Italian texts in *Enchiridion Vaticanum*, VII, pp. 332–351 (nn.346–373).

[1]*Declaration on Procured Abortion*, 18 November 1974: *AAS* 66 (1974), pp. 730–747.

[2]Pius XII, *Address to those attending the Congress of the International Union of Catholic Women's Leagues*, 11 September 1947: *AAS* 39 (1947), p. 483; *Address to the Italian Catholic Union of Midwives*, 29 October 1951: *AAS* 43 (1951), pp. 835–854; *Speech to the members of the International Office of military medicine documentation*, 19 October 1953: *AAS* 45 (1953), pp. 744–754; *Address to those taking part in*

way of looking at suffering and death; moreover, medicine has increased its capacity to cure and to prolong life in particular circumstances, which sometimes give rise to moral problems. Thus people living in this situation experience no little anxiety about the meaning of advanced old age and death. They also begin to wonder whether they have the right to obtain for themselves or their fellowmen an "easy death", which would shorten suffering and which seems to them more in harmony with human dignity.

A number of Episcopal Conferences have raised questions on this subject with the Sacred Congregation for the Doctrine of the Faith. The Congregation, having sought the opinion of experts on the various aspects of euthanasia, now wishes to respond to the Bishops' questions with the present Declaration, in order to help them to give correct teaching to the faithful entrusted to their care, and to offer them elements for reflection that they can present to the civil authorities with regard to this very serious matter.

The considerations set forth in the present document concern in the first place all those who place their faith and hope in Christ, who, through his life, death and Resurrection, has given a new meaning to existence and especially to the death of the Christian, as Saint Paul says: "If we live, we live to the Lord, and if we die, we die to the Lord" (*Rom* 14:8; cf. *Phil* 1:20).

As for those who profess other religions, many will agree with us that faith in God the Creator, Provider and Lord of life—if they share this belief—confers a lofty dignity upon every human person and guarantees respect for him or her.

It is hoped that this Declaration will meet with the approval of many people of good will, who, philosophical or ideological differences notwithstanding, have nevertheless a lively awareness of the rights of the human person. These rights have often in fact been proclaimed in recent years through declarations issued by International Congresses;[3] and since it is a question here of fundamental rights inherent in every human person, it is obviously wrong to have recourse to arguments from political pluralism or religious freedom in order to deny the universal value of those rights.

---

the IXth Congress of the Italian Anaesthesiological Society, 24 February 1957: AAS 49 (1957), p. 146; cf. also Address on "reanimation" 24 November 1957: AAS 49 (1957), pp. 1027–1033; PAUL VI, Address to the members of the United Nations Special Committee on Apartheid, 22 May 1974: AAS 66 (1974), p. 346; JOHN PAUL II: Address to the Bishops of the United States of America, 5 October 1979: AAS 71 (1979), p. 1225.

[3]One thinks especially of Recommendation 779 (1976) on the rights of the sick and dying, of the Parliamentary Assembly of the Council of Europe at its XXVIIth Ordinary Session; cf. SIPECA, No. 1, March 1977, pp. 14–15.

I
THE VALUE OF HUMAN LIFE

Human life is the basis of all goods, and is the necessary source and condition of every human activity and of all society. Most people regard life as something sacred and hold that no one may dispose of it at will, but believers see in life something greater, namely a gift of God's love, which they are called upon to preserve and make fruitful. And it is this latter consideration that gives rise to the following consequences:

1. No one can make an attempt on the life of an innocent person without opposing God's love for that person, without violating a fundamental right, and therefore without committing a crime of the utmost gravity.[4]

2. Everyone has the duty to lead his of her life in accordance with God's plan. That life is entrusted to the individual as a good that must bear fruit already here on earth, but that finds its full perfection only in eternal life.

3. Intentionally causing one's own death, or suicide, is therefore equally as wrong as murder; such an action on the part of a person is to be considered as a rejection of God's sovereignty and loving plan. Furthermore, suicide is also often a refusal of love for self, the denial of the natural instinct to live, a flight from the duties of justice and charity owed to one's neighbour, to various communities or to the whole of society—although, as is generally recognized, at times there are psychological factors present that can diminish responsibility or even completely remove it.

However, one must clearly distinguish suicide from that sacrifice of one's life whereby for a higher cause, such as God's glory, the salvation of souls or the service of one's brethren, a person offers his or her own life or puts it in danger (cf. *Jn* 15:14).

II
EUTHANASIA

In order that the question of euthanasia can be properly dealt with, it is first necessary to define the words used.

Etymologically speaking, in ancient times *euthanasia* meant an *easy death* without severe suffering. Today one no longer thinks of this original meaning of the word, but rather of some intervention of medicine whereby the sufferings of sickness or of the final agony are reduced, sometimes also with the

---

[4]We leave aside completely the problems of the death penalty and of war, which involve specific considerations that do not concern the present subject.

danger of suppressing life prematurely. Ultimately, the word *euthanasia* is used in a more particular sense to mean "mercy killing", for the purpose of putting an end to extreme suffering, or saving abnormal babies, the mentally ill or the incurably sick from the prolongation, perhaps for many years, of a miserable life, which could impose too heavy a burden on their families or on society.

It is therefore necessary to state clearly in what sense the word is used in the present document.

By euthanasia is understood an action or an omission which of itself or by intention causes death, in order that all suffering may in this way be eliminated. Euthanasia's terms of reference, therefore, are to be found in the intention of the will and in the methods used.

It is necessary to state firmly once more that nothing and no one can in any way permit the killing of an innocent human being, whether a foetus or an embryo, an infant or an adult, an old person, or one suffering from an incurable disease, or a person who is dying. Furthermore, no one is permitted to ask for this act of killing, either for himself or herself or for another person entrusted to his or her care, nor can he or she consent to it, either explicitly or implicitly. Nor can any authority legitimately recommend or permit such an action. For it is a question of the violation of the divine law, an offence against the dignity of the human person, a crime against life, and an attack on humanity.

It may happen that, by reason of prolonged and barely tolerable pain, for deeply personal or other reasons, people may be led to believe that they can legitimately ask for death or obtain it for others. Although in these cases the guilt of the individual may be reduced or completely absent, nevertheless the error of judgment into which the conscience falls, perhaps in good faith, does not change the nature of this act of killing, which will always be in itself something to be rejected. The pleas of gravely ill people who sometimes ask for death are not to be understood as implying a true desire for euthanasia; in fact it is almost always a case of an anguished plea for help and love. What a sick person needs, besides medical care, is love, the human and supernatural warmth with which the sick person can and ought to be surrounded by all those close to him or her, parents and children, doctors and nurses.

III
THE MEANING OF SUFFERING FOR CHRISTIANS AND THE USE OF PAINKILLERS

Death does not always come in dramatic circumstances after barely tolerable sufferings. Nor do we have to think only of extreme cases. Numerous testimonies which confirm one another lead one to the conclusion that nature itself has made provision to render more bearable at the moment of death separations that would be terribly painful to a person in full health. Hence it is that a prolonged illness, advanced old age, or a state of loneliness or neglect can bring about psychological conditions that facilitate the acceptance of death.

Nevertheless the fact remains that death, often preceded or accompanied by severe and prolonged suffering, is something which naturally causes people anguish.

Physical suffering is certainly an unavoidable element of the human condition; on the biological level, it constitutes a warning of which no one denies the usefulness; but, since it affects the human psychological makeup, it often exceeds its own biological usefulness and so can become so severe as to cause the desire to remove it at any cost.

According to Christian teaching, however, suffering, especially suffering during the last moments of life, has a special place in God's saving plan; it is in fact a sharing in Christ's Passion and a union with the redeeming sacrifice which he offered in obedience to the Father's will. Therefore one must not be surprised if some Christians prefer to moderate their use of painkillers, in order to accept voluntarily at least a part of their sufferings and thus associate themselves in a conscious way with the sufferings of Christ crucified (cf. *Mt* 27:34). Nevertheless it would be imprudent to impose a heroic way of acting as a general rule. On the contrary, human and Christian prudence suggest for the majority of sick people the use of medicines capable of alleviating or suppressing pain, even though these may cause as a secondary effect semiconsciousness and reduced lucidity. As for those who are not in a state to express themselves, one can reasonably presume that they wish to take these painkillers, and have them administered according to the doctor's advice.

But the intensive use of painkillers is not without difficulties, because the phenomenon of habituation generally makes it necessary to increase their dosage in order to maintain their efficacy. At this point it is fitting to recall a declaration by Pius XII, which retains its full force; in answer to a group of doctors who had put the question: "Is the suppression of pain and consciousness by the use of narcotics . . . permitted by religion and morality to the doctor and the patient (even at the approach of death and if one foresees that the use of narcotics will shorten life)?", the Pope said: "If no other means exist, and if, in the given circumstances, this does not prevent the carrying out of other religious and moral duties: Yes".[5] In this case, of course, death is

---

[5]Pius XII, *Address* of 24 February 1957: *AAS* 49 (1957), p. 147.

in no way intended or sought, even if the risk of it is reasonably taken; the intention is simply to relieve pain effectively, using for this purpose painkillers available to medicine.

However, painkillers that cause unconsciousness need special consideration. For a person not only has to be able to satisfy his or her moral duties and family obligations; he or she also has to prepare himself or herself with full consciousness for meeting Christ. Thus Pius XII warns: "It is not right to deprive the dying person of consciousness without a serious reason" [6]

IV
DUE PROPORTION IN THE USE OF REMEDIES

Today it is very important to protect, at the moment of death, both the dignity of the human person and the Christian concept of life, against a technological attitude that threatens to become an abuse. Thus, some people speak of a "right to die", which is an expression that does not mean the right to procure death either by one's own hand of by means of someone else, as one pleases, but rather the right to die peacefully with human and Christian dignity. From this point of view, the use of therpeutic means can sometimes pose problems.

In numerous cases, the complexity of the situation can be such as to cause doubts about the way ethical principles should be applied. In the final analysis, it pertains to the conscience either of the sick person, or of those qualified to speak in the sick person's name, or of the doctors, to decide, in the light of moral obligations and of the various aspects of the case.

Everyone has the duty to care for his or her own health or to seek such care from others. Those whose task it is to care for the sick must do so conscientiously and administer the remedies that seem necessary or useful.

However, is it necessary in all circumstances to have recourse to all possible remedies?

In the past, moralists replied that one is never obliged to use "extraordinary" means. This reply, which as a principle still holds good, is perhaps less clear today, by reason of the imprecision of the term and the rapid progress made in the treatment of sickness. Thus some people prefer to speak of "proportionate" and "disproportionate" means. In any care, it will be possible to make a correct judgment as to the means by studying the type of treatment to be used, its degree of complexity or risk, its cost and the possibilities of using

---

[6]Pius XII, *ibid.*, p. 145; cf. *Address* of 9 September 1958: *AAS* 50 (1958), p. 694.

it, and comparing these elements with the result that can be expected, taking into account the state of the sick person and his or her physical and moral resources.

In order to faciliate the application of these general principles, the following clarifications can be added:

—If there are no other sufficient remedies, it is permitted, with the patient's consent, to have recourse to the means provided by the most advanced medical techniques, even if these means are still at the experimental stage and are not without a certain risk. By accepting them, the patient can even show generosity in the service of humanity.

—It is also permitted, with the patient's consent, to interrupt these means, where the results fall short of expectations. But for such a decision to be made, account will have to be taken of the reasonable wishes of the patient and the patient's family, as also of the advice of the doctors who are specially competent in the matter. The latter may in particular judge that the investment in instruments and personnel is disproportionate to the results foreseen; they may also judge that the techniques applied impose on the patient strain or suffering out of proportion with the benefits which he or she may gain from such techniques.

—It is also permissible to make do with the normal means that medicine can offer. Therefore one cannot impose on anyone the obligation to have recourse to a technique which is already in use but which carries a risk or is burdensome. Such a refusal is not the equivalent of suicide; on the contrary, it should be considered as an acceptance of the human condition, or a wish to avoid the application of a medical procedure disproportionate to the results that can be expected, or a desire not to impose excessive expense on the family or the community.

—When inevitable death is imminent in spite of the means used, it is permitted in conscience to take the decision to refuse forms of treatment that would only secure a precarious and burdensome prolongation of life, so long as the normal care due to the sick person in similar cases is not interrupted. In such circumstances the doctor has no reason to reproach himself with failing to help the person in danger.

CONCLUSION

The norms contained in the present Declaration are inspired by a profound desire to serve people in accordance with the plan of the Creator. Life is a gift of God, and on the other hand death is unavoidable; it is necessary therefore that we, without in any way hastening the hour of death, should be able to accept it with full responsibility and dignity. It is true that death marks the end of our earthy existence, but at the same time it opens the door to immortal life. Therefore all must prepare themselves for this event in the light of human values, and Christians even more so in the light of faith.

As for those who work in the medical profession, they ought to neglect no means of making all their skill available to the sick and the dying; but they should also remember how much more necessary it is to provide them with the comfort of boundless kindness and heartfelt charity. Such service to people is also service to Christ the Lord, who said: "As you did it to one of the least of these my brethren, you did it to me" (*Mt* 25: 40).

At the audience granted to the undersigned Prefect, His Holiness Pope John Paul II approved this Declaration, adopted at the ordinary meeting of the Sacred Congregation for the Doctrine of the Faith, and ordered its publication.

Rome, the Sacred Congregation for the Doctrine of the Faith, 5 May 1980.

Franjo Card. Šeper
Prefect

Jérôme Hamer, O.P.
Tit. Archbishop of Lorium
Secretary

APPENDIX II—REPORT OF THE PONTIFICAL COUNCIL ON HEALTH AFFAIRS, "COR UNUM"
"Questions of Ethics Regarding the Fatally Ill and the Dying"*

1. INTRODUCTION

1.1. The Working Group

From the 12th to the 14th of November 1976, in keeping with its mandate of co-ordinating the Activities of the Church in the Health Sector, the Pontifical Council COR UNUM got together a Working Group to study various questions of ethics related to the fatally ill and the dying. The Group was composed of some 15 persons, and was interdisciplinary: there were theologians, doctors, members of Religious Congregations dedicated to the care of the sick, trained nurses, and hospital chaplains.

1.2. The subject discussed by the Working Group

Recent developments in science are influencing medical practice more and more, particularly in the treatment of the fatally ill and the dying. This state of affairs raises problems of a theological and ethical order on which the health professionals are eager to be authoritatively enlightened. Christian

---

*Published by the Pontifical Council Cor Unum, Vatican City. Also published in *Enchiridion Vaticanum,* VII, June 27, 1981, in French and in Italian, pp. 1132–1173 (nn.1234–1281).

members of these professions working in Christian surroundings have long been much concerned about these problems. All the more so are Christians obliged to work in non-Christian surroundings, and who for this reason desire that their work be inspired by their Faith and bear witness to it.

Unfortunately, medical ethics are for many persons a matter of speculation, of more or less accurate information, of erroneous ideas and all this begets great confusion. COR UNUM is not in a position to undertake a vast programme of doctrinal or scientific research: this is for higher and better qualified authorities. The purpose of our Working Group was simply to analyse basic concepts, point out certain distinctions which must be understood clearly, and formulate practical answers to questions brought up by pastoral directives and by the treatment of the dying.

1.3. The Sacred Congregation for the Doctrine of the Faith

On the 5th of May, 1980, this Congregation published a "Declaration on Euthanasia". In it were authoritatively set forth principles of doctrine and morals on this very serious problem, which has attracted and held the interest of large sectors of the public. As a result, mostly, of special cases that have received wide publicity—cases of what has been called "therapeutic obstinacy"—, people's consciences were aroused and much self-questioning had been going on. This important document first recalls to the reader what the value of human life is, and then proceeds to deal with the subject of euthanasia: it provides Christians with principles for making decisions and taking action where suffering and the use of painkillers are concerned and also where the use of one or another therapeutic treatment is possible.

1.4. Publication of the report on COR UNUM's Working Group

Our 1976 Working Group's reflection is for the most part pastoral: it answers precise and concrete questions put to COR UNUM by hospital chaplains, doctors, and trained nurses. As a result of the publication of the "Declaration on Euthanasia" by the S. C. for the Doctrine of the Faith, our Pontifical Council has been requested to publish the report of its Working Group. Let this be the occasion for us to thank all those who, with a competence deriving only from great experience, contributed to its realization.

2. FUNDAMENTAL CONCEPTS

2.1. Life

2.1.1. The Christian meaning of life

Life is given to mankind by our Creator. It is a gift bestowed in order for man to accomplish a mission. Thus, a person's "right to live" is not what is of foremost importance, since this right is not man's but, rather, belongs to God, Who does not give life to human beings as something of which they may dispose as they see fit. Life is directed towards an end toward which it is the responsibility of human beings to direct themselves: toward the perfecting of themselves according to God's plan.

The first corollary of this fundamental concept, is that to give up life of one's own choice is to give up striving towards an end which not we but God has established. Mankind has been called upon to make his life useful; he may not destroy it at will. His duty is to care of his body, its functions, its organs; to do everything he can to render himself capable of attaining to God. This duty implies giving up things which in themselves may be good. This duty sometimes requires that we sacrifice health and life: our concern for them cannot allow us to deny the claim of superior values. All the same, in the matter of cares to be taken for maintaining good health and perserving life, a correct proportion must be arrived at, regarding both the superior goods perhaps at stake and also the concrete conditions in which man lives out his existence on earth.

2.1.2. We cannot freely dispose of the life of someone else

If one may not destroy one's own life at will, this is also true, *a fortiori*, of someone else's life. A sick person cannot simply be made the object of decisions which he himself does not make—or of which, if he is unable to make them, he would not morally approve. Each human individual, as the person principally responsible for his life, must be at the center of all assistance. Others are present in order to help him, *not* substitute him. This does not mean, however, that doctors or members of the family may not at times find themselves in the position of having to take decisions for a sick person, who for various reasons cannot do so himself, concerning therapeutic measure and treatments to be applied to him. But to the doctors and others in this position, more than to anyone else, it is absolutely forbidden to make an attempt on the life of the patient, even out of compassion and pity.

2.1.3. The fundamental rights of the human individual

It is this quintessentially doctrinal subject which the Working Group akes as the basis for its considerations. We are well aware of how immensely difficult it is for those who are not Christians or who have no belief in a life beyond this life on earth, to give meaning to life and to death. Christians will admit, too, that their position is not specific. But what really is at stake is the defense of the fundamental rights of the human individual. We cannot waver where these are concerned. All the less so, because these rights are so very much in the foreground of political and legislative activity. In order to convince people for whom everything ends at death, of what respect is due their own life and the life of others, the surest arguments are those which show what consequences are brought about in a society by the lack of rigid measures taken for the protection of human life.

2.2. Death

2.2.1. The meaning which death has for Christians

The death of a human being is the end of his corporeal existence. It brings to an end that phase of his divine vocation which is his striving, within the compass of time, toward his total perfection. For a Christian, the moment of death is the moment of his finally being united forever to Christ. Today more than ever, it is pertinent to recall this religious and Christological conception of death. It must go hand in hand with a very real perception of the contingency of our living in our body and of the connection between death and our human condition of being sinners. "For . . . whether we live or whether we die, we are the Lord's" (*Romans*, XIV:8) Our attitude toward the dying must be inspired by this conviction, and must not merely be reduced to an effort made by science to put off death as long as possible.

2.2.2. The right to die a human and dignified death

Concerning this topic, the members of the Working Group from the Third World emphasized how important it is, for a human being, to end his days on earth with his personality, as far as possible, whole and entire, both in itself and in its relationships with its milieu, and especially with the family. In countries which are less developed technically and less affected by sophistication, the family gathers round the dying person, and he himself feels a need— almost an essential right—to be thus surrounded. When we observe the conditions required for certain therapies and the total isolation imposed by them upon the sick person, we do not find it out of place to state that the right to die as a human being and *with dignity demands* this social dimension.

2.3. Suffering

2.3.1. The meaning of "suffering" for a Christian

Neither suffering nor pain—between which we must be careful to distinguish—is ever to be considered an end in itself. Scientifically speaking, there is still great uncertainty as to what constitutes pain. As for suffering, Christians see in it only the Love that can be expressed thereby and the purifying effects which it can have. Pius XII pointed out, in his Allocution of the 24th of February 1957, that suffering which is too intense is likely to keep the mind from maintaining the control it ought to have. We are thus not obliged to think that all pain must be endured at any price, or that, stoically, one must not attempt to reduce and calm them. The Working Group feels that we can do no better than to refer the reader to the text of Pius XII.

2.3.2. Effects of suffering and pain

The capacity for suffering varies from person to person. It is for the doctor, the nurses, and the hospital chaplain (let him not be overlooked!) to determine what spiritual and psychological effects suffering and pain are having on a patient, and to decide whether a certain treatment is to be carried out or not. What the patient says must also be carefully listened to, in order to determine what the real nature of his suffering is: for he, after all, is the best judge of it. Of course a doctor may well think that a patient could have more courage and that he can really put up with more suffering than he believes he can; but the ultimate choice is up to the patient.

2.4. Therapeutic measures

2.4.1. Ordinary measures and extraordinary measures

The Working Group considered at some length the distinction between these two kinds of therapies. It is true that the terms are becoming somewhat outmoded in scientific terminology and medical practice, but in theology they are indispensable to the consideration of the validity or invalidity of points of great moral importance. For the theologian applies the term "extraordinary" to measure to which there never exists any obligation to have recourse.

The distinction permits us to draw certain complex realities more closely together. It acts as the "middle term". Life within the compass of time is a basic value but is not an absolute; and we find, consequently, that we must demarcate the limits of the obligation to keep oneself alive. The distinction between "ordinary" and "extraordinary" measures expresses this truth and applies these limits to concrete cases. The use of equivalent terms, particularly the words "care suited to the real needs", perhaps expresses the concept more satisfactorily.

2.4.2. Criteria for distinguishing

The criteria whereby we can distinguish *extraordinary* measures from *ordinary* measures are very many. They are to be applied according to each concrete case. Some of them are *objective:* such as the nature of the measures proposed, how expensive they are, whether it is just to use them, and what the options of Justice are in the matter of using them. Other criteria are *subjective:* such as not giving certain patients psychological shocks, anxiety, uneasiness, and so on. It will always be a question, when deciding upon measures to be taken, of establishing to what extent the means to be used and the end being sought are proportionate.

2.4.3. The criterion of the quality of life: its importance

Among all the criteria for decision, particular importance must be given to the quality of the life to be saved or kept living by the therapy. The Letter of Cardinal Villot to the Congress of the International Federation of Catholic Medical Associations is very clear on this subject: "It must be emphasized that it is the sacred character of life which forbids a physician to kill and makes it a duty for him at the same time to use every resource of his art to fight against death. This does not, however, mean that a physician is under obligation to use all and every one of the life-maintaining techniques offered him by the indefatigable creativity of science. Would it not be a useless torture, in many cases, to impose vegetative reanimation during the last phase of an incurable disease?" (*Documentation Catholique,* 1970, p. 963.)

But the criterion of the quality of life is not the only one to be taken into account, since, as we have said above, subjective considerations must enter into a properly cautious judgement as to what therapy to undertake and what therapy not. The fundamental point is that the decision should be made according to rational arguments that have taken well into account the many and various aspects of the situation, including what effect will be had upon the family. The principle to follow is, therefore, that no moral obligation to have recourse to extraordinary measures exists; and that, incidentally, a doctor must follow the wishes of a sick person who refuses such measures.

2.4.4. Obligatory minimal measures

On the contrary, there remains the strict obligation to apply under all circumstances those therapeutic measures which are called "minimal": that is, those which are normally and customarily used for the maintenance of life (alimentation, blood transfusions, injections, etc.). To interrupt these minimal measures would, in practice, be equivalent to wishing to put an end to the patient's life.

3. EUTHANASIA

3.1. Inaccuracy of the word *"euthanasia"*

Historically and etymologically, the word "euthanasia" means "a peaceful death without suffering and pain". In present-day usage, the word implies performing an action or omitting to perform an action, with the intent of shortening the life of a patient. This common acceptation of the word brings into debates about euthanasia a considerable amount of confusion. It is urgent to clear this up. Documents on the subject, like those which parliamentary assemblies have recently been formulating, show what harmful effects can result from the current lack of precision. Furthermore, present-day progress in medicine has rendered similarly ambiguous—and perhaps also superfluous—the distinction between "active euthanasia" and "passive euthanasia", a distinction that it would be preferable to give up making.

3.2. Actions and decisions which are not a part of euthanasia

Consequently, the Working Group is of the opinion that, at least in Catholic milieux, a terminology should be used which does not include the word "euthanasia" at all:

1) neither to designate the actions involved in *terminal care* which aim at making the last phase of an illness less unbearable (rehydration, nursing care, massage, palliative medication, keeping the dying person company . . .);

2) nor to designate *the decision to stop certain medical therapies* which no longer seem to be required by the condition of the patient. (Traditional language would have expressed this as "the decision to give up extraordinary measures".) It is thus not a matter of deciding to let the patient die but, rather, of using technical resources proportionately following a reasonable course suggested by prudence and good judgement;

3) nor to designate an action taken to relieve the suffering of the patient at the risk of perhaps shortening his life. This sort of action is part of a

doctor's calling: his vocation is not only that of curing diseases or prolonging life but—much more generally—also that of taking care of a sick person and relieving his suffering.

3.3. The strict meaning of the word

"Euthanasia" must be used only to mean "to put an end to a patient's life by a specific act". Pius XII makes it abundantly clear that, understood in this meaning, euthanasia can never be sanctioned. (Allocution of the 24th of November 1957, *Documentation Catholique,* p. 1609.)

Despite the fact that, in practice, the distinctions stated above are sometimes difficult to make, they are nonetheless capable of giving to the word "euthanasia" a meaning free of ambiguities. They can thus be points of reference for the attending physician, who, after consultation with the other doctors and the nurses on the case, with the hospital chaplain, and with the family, will then make his decision.

It will be a decision based upon the principle that neither moral values nor values inherent to the human individual, are to be meddled with; that the best judgment concerning what must or must not be done, continued, stopped, or undertaken, will be based upon these values according to each case, and can never be arbitrary.

4. THE USE OF PAINKILLERS IN TERMINAL CASES

4.1. There are various ways to ease suffering

The use of painkillers affecting the central nervous system, involves the risk of secondary effects: they can affect respiratory functions, alter the state of consciousness, cause dependency, and, losing their effect, necessitate larger and larger doses. This is why it is always better not to use them so long as the patient's suffering can be relieved by other means.

These latter are not few in number: remedies such as aspirin, the immobilization of certains parts of the body, various radiation therapies, even surgical operations . . . and, above all, combatting the solitude and anguish of the patient simply with the presence of another human being. There are also quite new methods coming into use, which enable the patient to acquire a certain mastery of his own body.

4.2. The use of painkillers acting on the central nervous system

In many cases, however, the relief of sometimes truly unbearable suffering does require the use of painkillers acting on the central nervous system (for example, morphine along with other narcotics) at least at the present state of medical knowledge and techniques.

There exists no reason to refuse to make use of such drugs, especially as their side effects can be greatly reduced if they are used judiciously: that is, in appropriate dosages and at accurately determined intervals. For the using of drugs against pain while still keeping the patient as conscious as possible, requires a perfect knowledge of these products: the ways to give them, their secondary effects, and their contra-indications. When decisions are being made concerning them, it becomes important for the pharmacologist to be consulted and, even, actually to be with the patient.

4.3. The necessity of a human presence

When speaking of the narcotics, we must warn against the temptation of believing that they are a sufficient remedy for suffering. Human suffering very frequently contains an element of anguish, of fear in the face of the unknown, brought out by severe illness and the nearness of death. Drugs can diminish anguish but, more often than not, are powerless to relieve it completely. It is *only a human presence,* discreet and attentive, that can procure the relief so much needed, by allowing the sick person to express his thoughts and by giving him human and spiritual comfort.

4.4. Is it permissible to put the sick person into a state of unconsciousness?

We can now approach the question of whether it is right, when death is very near, to use narcotics to put the patient into a state of unconsciousness. In certain cases, the use of them for this purpose is necessary, and Pope Pius XII has recognized the moral rightness of doing so *under certain conditions.* (Allocution of the 24th of February 1957.)

The problem is, however, that there exists a great temptation to have recourse to narcosis as a general practice, doubtless, at times, out of pity, but often more or less deliberately, in order to save the doctors, nurses, family, and others around the patient, the emotional wear and tear of being with a person on the verge of death. This clearly indicates that it is not the good of the patient which is being sought; rather, it is the protection of people who are perfectly well but who are members of a society that is afraid of death, that flees death by any means at its disposal.

Yet systematic narcosis deprives the dying patient of the possibility of "living out his death". It deprives him of arriving at a serene acceptance of it, of achieving a state of peace; of sharing, perhaps, a last intense relationship between a person reduced to that last of human poverties and another person who will have been privileged by thus knowing him. And, if the dying person is a Christian, he is being deprived of experiencing his death in communion with Christ.

What is therefore important, is to protest vigorously against any systematic plunging into unconsciousness of the fatally ill, and to demand, on the contrary, that medical and nursing personnel learn how to listen to the dying. They must learn how to create relationships among themselves which will sustain them through their days and nights with dying, and which can help them to help families be with their near and dear one during the last phase of life.

4.5. Narcosis and the decision of the patient

The fundamental principle has been laid down, in this entire question, by Pius XII: it must be left to the patient to make decision. "It would be clearly unpermissible to narcotize the dying patient against his express wish (when he is *sui juris*). If there are serious reasons in favour of deep narcosis, then it must be remembered that the dying person cannot submit to it morally, if he has not yet discharged all the duties that are so urgent when life draws to a close". (See below, Section 6.1.1.). If the doctor is requested by the patient to give him deep narcosis, "the doctor will not do so—especially if he is Christian—without first having asked the patient, or better, still, having had an intermediary ask him, to fulfill all his duties beforehand". Pius XII goes on to state that, if the dying person refuses to fulfill his duties but still insists upon being narcotized, the doctor may do so: "He may consent to it without making himself guilty of formal collaboration in the sin committed. This sin does not derive from the act of narcotization, but rather, from the immoral wish of the patient: for whether he is given narcosis or not, his behaviour will not have changed: he will not have discharged his duties".

5. CEREBRAL DEATH

5.1. It is for the science of medicine to define this

In his Allocution of the 24th of November 1957, Pius XII states that "it is for the physician . . . to give a clear and precise definition of 'death' and 'the moment of death' ". Naturally, we cannot ask of medical science any more than a detailing of criteria whereby it can be established that death has taken place. But what Pius XII means, is that it is for medical science and not for the Church to establish these criteria. To the reasons he gives as practical illustrations of his point, can today be added requests for organ transplants, and the resultant necessity of precisely establishing the donor's moment of death before proceeding to remove the organ to be transplanted.

5.2. The difficulties involved in arriving at this definition

Setting up a medical definition of death is complicated by the fact that, at the present state of our knowledge, death apparently does not take place all at once. It is not an instantaneous cessation of all the functions of the body but, rather, a series of cessations of our various life processes, one after the other. It seems that what stops first is the mechanism that regulates the functioning together of all the organs of the body. This mechanism is situated in the brain. After it stops, necrosis then begins to spread to the various systems: the nervous system, the cardio-vascular, respiratory, digestive, urogenital, and locomotor systems. And last of all, necrosis reaches the cellular and subcellular components. Yet even today, one cannot be too cautious in this matter, for many uncertainties still exist concerning the "medical definition of death".

There is, however, a growing consensus of opinion that considers a human being dead in whom a total and irreversible absence of life activity in the brain has been established. This is known as "cerebral death". Various authoritative groups have drawn up lists of criteria concerning it. These criteria may not be completely identical, but there is sufficient correspondence among them to make up a list of symptoms of death whose accuracy can be taken as very highly probable. Conventional agreements and administrative procedure are already in effect or are being arrived at, which, if all the required criteria can be demonstrated, permit or will permit the release of death certificates and, thereafter, the removal of the organs to be used in transplant operations.

5.3. The Church has been asked for a declaration

On the other hand, families are showing increased reticence in the matter of giving permission for the removal of organs for transplant. The Working Group was informed that this is why certain highly authoritative medical groups have requested the Chruch to make an official declaration on the validity or non-validity of taking cerebral death, duly established, as the "moment of death" of the human being.

The Working Group feels that it is for a higher authority than itself to make such a declaration officially, but has agreed to call attention, by means of this report, to the need for making it. However, the theologians in the

Group point out that, even though the proper ecclesiastical authority complied with the request, the Church would not be able to answer the question merely by making its own any scientific assertion or, still less, by issuing a list of criteria whereby cerebral death is to be determined. The very most the Church could do, would be to reiterate the conditions that would make it legitimate to accept the better judgement of those to whose specific competence has been entrusted the determination of the moment of death.

5.4. Measures to be taken in cases of apparent death

As Pius XII states, it is the physician's duty, in cases of apparent death, to do everything he can do, by every ordinary means, to restore life activity. Nonetheless, a moment always comes when death can be considered as having taken place, and when reanimation measures can be stopped without committing either a professional or a moral error. (Pius XII, Allocution of the 24th November 1957).

6. COMMUNICATING WITH DYING PEOPLE

6.1. The right to know the truth

The communication with dying patients brings up the moral question of their right to know the truth. The clergy, pastorally, and doctors and nurses, professionally, must consider what sort of behaviour a dying person has a right to expect from those around him. The dying, and, more generally, anyone with an incurable disease, have a right to be told the truth. Death is too essential an event for the envisioning of it to be avoided. In the case of a believer, its approach requires preparation and specific actions made in full consciousness. In the case of any human being, dying brings the responsibility of fulfilling certain duties towards one's family, of putting order to business affairs, bringing accounts up to date, settling debts, etc. In any case, preparation for dying should begin long before the approach of death and while a person is still in good health.

6.1.2. The responsibility of those surrounding a dying person

Whoever is nearest the patient must inform him of the possibility of his dying. The family, the chaplain, and the group providing medical care, must assume their share in this duty. Each case is different, depending on the sensitivities and capabilities of all concerned, and on the condition of the patient and his ability to relate to others. How he will react to the truth—by rebellion, depression, resignation, and so on—is what those surrounding him must try to foresee, in order to be able to behave with tact and calm. A ray of hope may licitly be held out to the patient; death may even be presented as not 100% certain—but only provided that doing this does not totally conceal the possibility of dying, the serious probability.

6.1.3. The mission of the hospital chaplain

Here is where the continuous assistance of the chaplain during the illness has its utmost importance. His mission confers upon him a privileged role in preparing a patient little by little for death. Of course the duty to believe, right to the very end, in the efficacy *ex opere operato* of the sacraments (Confession, Viaticum, and Extreme Unction) and when necessary, of giving them conditionally according to canon law, remains untouched. And yet we must point out that the unexpected appearance of the priest at the last moment, makes the performance of his ministry very difficult and, at times, impossible. The hospital chaplain will try, therefore, to create, through continual contacts, a relationship of confidence with the patients, especially in milieux where there are lax or indifferent Catholics. He must be careful not to talk of the nearness of death too soon, while at the same time not concealing the truth. The Working Group does not consider it superfluous, furthermore, to insist that, at least in Catholic hospitals and by Catholic doctors and nurses, the chaplain be granted his rightful position, both in consultations about the patient and as one of the persons having access to him at all times.

6.2. Society's attitude toward death

6.2.1. In the Western World

Western Society, today, is going through what can only be called "flight in the face of death". Medical and hospital personnel are experiencing this phenomenon, and families too. The representatives of the Committee for the Family who took part in our Working Group, reported to us some very discomforting examples of the change in attitude toward death within the same families over the course of only 30 years. One case was that of a family which, around 1930, fully took on the death of the mother—even the youngest members; and which, in the 1960's, fled from death, did not even speak of it to the children, totally abandonned a dying wife.

We find that, while the medical personnel is trying to put off as long as possible the moment of physiological death, under the pretense of calming pain, they are really causing by these very measures the greatest anguish and moral suffering in the patient, who, in most cases, is more aware of the seriousness of his condition than those around him affect to think that he is. The dying person feels sadness, guilt, anxiety, fear, and depression, and all of that along with physical pain. Worst of all for him, is the isolation, the loneliness, which seriously influence him psychosomatically. The present-day tendency of cutting a dying person off, first from society, then from family, and finally from the other patients in the hospital, deprives him, in his distress, of any and every possibility of communicating with someone else. And there are so many ways to relieve his loneliness without even taxing him physically: the expression of a human face, a hand to hold! Often merely a silent presence is all he needs, but he needs it with every fibre of his being.

Thus, the practice of Western hospitals in these cases must be revised completely. Even the hospital personnel, for reasons not totally without cause, now tend to protect themselves against what seems a nerve-racking contact: they avoid being with dying patients, whose distress requires the very comfort their presence might give. Once again, it should be a matter for group work—teamwork—to keep the dying from being deprived of this moral support. And doctors, nurses, and chaplains alike, must share in this teamwork.

6.2.2. In other parts of the world

In other societies, quite to the contrary, we find respect of the patient's right to be assisted by his near and dear, and of the family's right to be with their dying loved ones. Often the family even prefers to remove the dying person from the hospital so that he may be sure to have their presence, and, if they are believers, so as to communicate with him through prayer. It is true that sometimes, in the real interest of the patient, doctors must know how to curtail the demands of the family and their insistence upon having the right of decision in the matter of what treatment is to be followed—unless, that is, the patient is a child and thus under parental responsibility. And yet this curtailment should in no way risk fostering the all too real Western tendency of ignoring the family, their presence, and, particularly, their just demands to know the truth.

7. THE RESPONSIBILITIES OF DOCTORS AND NURSES

7.1. Necessary knowledge of the medical deontology

It is becoming clearer and clearer that the scientific aspects and the ethical aspects of the medical profession cannot easily be considered separately. If progress in knowledge and technics is providing a doctor with new instruments and new therapies, the immediate result is that he is often being confronted by ever more complex moral questions.

We have spoken earlier of the fact that it is for the physician, in the last analysis, to make his decision by referring to objective moral criteria. This means, however, that he must have been taught what these criteria are and must have been trained to apply them to specific individual cases. The teaching of moral theory and of codes of medical ethics is rightly, therefore, an essential part of the training of doctors and nurses.

Professors and students must in no way consider such courses as supplementary or "extra"—only for those who wish to take them out of curiosity. In countries where there exists a tradition of common law, future physicians are at least encouraged to look into the requirements of moral theory and practice, by the very fact that their breaking an ethical and legal precedent would subject them to penal sanctions. But no future physician anywhere should avoid considering the essential interests of patients whom moral law defends and for whom codes of medical ethics have been evolved.

As to the best way to impart these teachings, it can be carried out, on the one hand, in special courses and, on the other, the moral aspects of scientific questions will be treated along with the scientific teaching itself, and thereby illustrated and insisted upon.

7.2. The choice of one therapy or another

As a general rule, and despite what the press leads people to believe, a doctor does not ask himself whether to allow or not allow a patient to die. He decides upon a certain medical treatment: what are its indications, what are its contra-indications? These all require him to consider various factors. He does so in the light of moral principles as well as of scientific knowledge; This is how it becomes of great value to a doctor to consider them while he reflects: what must or must not be undertaken? when should extraordinary measures be recurred to and when not? and if so, for what reasons and for how long? Too often, a doctor may come to question himself as to the advisability of continuing a certain treatment, and the question he may put to himself is:

"Was it wise to have begun the treatment in the first place?". For, if there exist moral reasons for prolonging life, there also exist moral reasons for not opposing death with what is known as "therapeutic obstinacy".

7.3. Massive therapy and choosing the persons to receive it

Among the ethical questions brought up by "massive therapies" requiring very highly evolved and expensive equipment and techniques, is to be considered the selection of patients to whom to apply a therapy that cannot be applied to everyone with the same malady. Is it legitimate to use the resources of refined medical technics for the benefit of only one patient, while others are still not receiving the most elementary treatment? One has a right to ask. If certain persons believe that such a question is "going against progress", Christians, at least, should bear it in mind in their valuation.

7.4. Trained nurses, male and female

7.4.1. The importance of their responsibilies

Despite the fact that many doctors tend to look upon them as purely auxiliary, nurses have a fundamental role of mediation between doctors and patients. Although nurses are, it is true, by no means free of the danger of avoiding the patient during the final stages of his illness, they are nevertheless responsible for actions that can often be of crucial importance. They must decide, for example, whether or not to call the doctor when they find that the patient has suddenly become worse; or must decide whether or not to give the patient a calming substance the doctor has left it up to their judgement to use at the appropriate moment, etc. Fortunately, in many hospitals today, a true feeling of teamwork between doctors and nurses is beginning to prevail. Their close collaboration is essential to the relief and proper care of each patient.

7.4.2. Co-operation and conscience

At times, especially when she or he works in non-Christian hospitals or for non-Christian doctors, the nurse is brought up against a moral dilemma posed by an order given by the doctor, the execution of which would gravely endanger, if not actually put an end to, the patient's life.

First and foremost, the nurse must adhere to the absolute prohibition against performing an act whose only purpose is to kill. Neither the doctor's order, nor the request of the family, nor even the plea of the patient, can free the nurse from responsibility for such an act. Where actions are concerned which in themselves are not toward killing (even though the nurse knows that an unpermissible result is being aimed at), the case is different *if* the nurse performs these actions by order of the doctor. Examples of this are: doing something which will shorten the life of the patient, suspending a treatment which is not "extraordinary", depriving of consciousness a patient who has not been able to fulfill his obligations. The nurse may not take the initiative for such actions. The only possible way to look at a nurse's performing them, is as their being a "material co-operation" excusable only by necessity when examined in the light: 1) of the gravity of the action; 2) of the nurse's participation in the whole process and the obtaining of the immoral goal; 3) and of reasons which might have led the nurse to obey the order: fear of something personal being done to her or to him if the order is not carried out; an important personal good be protected by not exposing oneself to the risk of being dismissed. Insofar as her or his status permits, the nurse who finds her or himself involved in practices of which one's conscience cannot approve, will make every effort possible to bear witness to her or his personal convictions.

Catholic chaplains and physicians are in duty bound to help nurses face up to such difficult situations, in every way they can.

7.4.3. Ethical training in nursing schools

All that we have reported in Section 7.1. concerning the necessity of ethical training for doctors, pharmacologists, *et alii,* holds true in the case of nursing schools as well. Catholic nursing schools have the right and the duty to defend, through their teaching, the ethical principles of the Church's Magisterium, particularly in courses which treat of the exercise of the nurse's profession: the value of each human individual, respect for life, morality and marriage, and so on. It is the duty of Catholic nursing schools to make this ethical orientation clear to all students applying for entrance. The schools further have the right to demand of all students their acceptance of these principles and their attendance at courses specializing in the teaching of professional ethics. The students must arrive at the conviction that here is an essential element, a condition *sine qua non,* of the proper training of a responsible nurse. Nor should this teaching be limited to a casuistical presentation of the subject. Rather, the professors will in every way seek to inculcate a profound familiarity with such fundamental notions as life, death, the personal vocation which a nurse has, and so on.

7.4.4. Training for the nursing of the incurably ill

The familiarization of hospital personnel with the demands made by death and by the care of the dying, does not take place only at the intellectual level. The actual face-to-face encounter with suffering, with a patient's anxiety, with death, can be a source of great anguish. Here is one of the main reasons why many professional people today are beginning to avoid having anything personal to do with the incurably ill, and are abandonning them to their loneliness. Thus must be added to the teaching of the theory and study of professional ethics, an education in how to relate to people, and especially to the incurably ill. If this is not taught, then any teaching of ethics is in danger, in the long run, of not being applied to the real situations encountered professionally.

8. THE RESPONSIBILITIES OF FAMILY AND SOCIETY

8.1. Education for suffering and death

The ties between life and death have become so very much loosened, at least in our Western society, that death has little by little lost its significance.

The family and the society by which it is surrounded have each their own part in this situation, which can only be considered highly destructive. It is urgent that education about suffering and death be undertaken. This would perhaps be the solution to the numerous problems existing today concerning death and the dying.

8.2. Questions we must ask ourselves

The family must begin to question itself on this subject;

1) in order to see whether suffering, death, failure, etc., are present or absent in its child-education habits, beginning with the earliest ages of life;

2) in order to determine what place it accords to sick persons, the handicapped, people who have failed in life, old people, and the dying.

If it is found that this education and this sharing are not a part of the family ways; if there is no family attitude and habit which are signs of love and of faith in the value of each and every human being—then how can we hope to create the communication so greatly desired between the dying person and his family during the last moments of earthly life?

8.3.   Society and the family. Legislation

Society, too, must also ask itself what it is bringing of any value to the family where this educative mission is concerned, whether it be to the family's habitat, to the various kinds of work its members perform, to its health, or to its problems with the sick and the aged.

Above all, we have every cause to be apprehensive lest the family's solidarity with its members who are suffering—and solidarity in every sort of suffering—be gravely threatened by certain sorts of present-day legislation: for example, laws "regulating" divorce, contraception, and abortion. Tomorrow, there will perhaps be laws "regulating" euthanasia . . .

APPENDIX III—REPORT OF THE PONTIFICAL ACADEMY OF SCIENCES ON THE ARTIFICIAL PROLONGATION OF LIFE*

On the invitation of the Pontifical Academy of Sciences, a study group met October 19–21, 1985, to study "the artificial prolongation of life and the exact determination of the moment of death."

After having noted the recent progress of the techniques of resuscitation and the immediate and long-term effects of brain damage, the study group discussed the objective criteria of death and of the rules of conduct in the fact of a persistent state of apparent death. On the one hand, experiments carried out reveal that brain resistance to the absence of cerebral circulation can permit recoveries otherwise deemed impossible.

On the other hand, it has been found that when the entire brain has suffered irreversible damage (cerebral death), all possibility of sensitive and cognitive life is definitely ruled out, while a brief vegetative survival can be maintained by artificial prolongation of respiration and circulation.

1. Definition of Death

A person is dead when he has irreversibly lost all capacity to integrate and coordinate the physical and mental functions of the body.

Death occurs when:

a) The spontaneous cardiac and respiratory functions have definitely ceased; or

b) If an irreversible cessation of every brain function is verified.

*Published in *Origins*, Dec. 5, 1985, as it appeared in the English edition of *L'Osservatore Romano*. Italian version found in *Enchiridion Vaticanum*, IX, pp. 1726, 1727.

From the debate it emerged that cerebral death is the true criterion of death, since the definitive arrest of the cardio-respiratory functions leads very quickly to cerebral death.

The group then analysed the different clinical and instrumental methods that enable one to ascertain the irreversible arrest of the cerebral functions. To be certain—by means of the electroencephalogram—that the brain has become flat, that is to say, that it no longer displays electric activity, it is necessary that the examination be carried out at least twice at a distance of six hours (in the Italian version: " . . . è necessario che l'esame sia effettuato almeno due volte a distanza di sei ore").

2. Medical Guidelines

By the term treatment the group understands all those medical interventions available and appropriate in a specific case, whatever the complexity of the techniques involved.

If the patient is in a permanent, irreversible coma, as far as can be foreseen,* treatment is not required, but all care should be lavished on him, including feeding.

If it is clinically established that there is a possibility of recovery, treatment is required.

If treatment is of no benefit to the patient, it may be interrupted while continuing with the care of the patient.

By the term care the group understands ordinary help due to sick patients, such as compassion and spiritual and affective support due to every human being in danger.

3. Artificial Prolongation of Vegetative Functions

In the case of cerebral death, artificial respiration can prolong the cardiac function for a limited time. This induced survival of the organs is indicated in the case of a foreseen removal of organs for transplant.

This eventually is possible only in the case of total and irreversible brain damage occurring is a young person, essentially as a result of a very severe injury.

---

*A more precise translation would be: "If the patient is in a permanent coma, irreversible as far as it can be foreseen . . . " The Italian text reads as follows: "Se il paziente è in coma permanente, irreversibile, per quanto sia possibile prevederlo . . . " The phrase "per quanto sia possibile prevederlo" qualifies the irreversibility of the condition, but not the permanency. Cf. page 82 of this study. Italian text found in *Enchiridion Vaticanum*, IX, p. 1727 (n. 1768).

Taking into consideration the important advances made in surgical techniques and in the means to increase tolerance of transplants, the group holds that transplants deserve the support of the medical profession, of the law and of people in general.

The donation of organs should, in all circumstances, respect the last will of the donor or the consent of the family, if present.

ADDRESS OF POPE JOHN PAUL II to "two study groups of physicians and scientists convened by the Pontifical Academy of Sciences to discuss the artificial prolongation of life and parasitic diseases."

Published in the December 5, 1985 issue of *Origins* under the title of "The Mystery of Life and Death"*

1. I extend a most cordial welcome to all of you. And I rejoice with the Pontifical Academy of Sciences and its illustrious present, Professor Carlos Chagas, for having succeeded in bringing together two groups of such distinguished scientists to reflect on the themes: "The Artificial Prolongation of Life and the Determination of the Exact Moment of Death," and "The Interaction of Parasitic Diseases and Nutrition."

In the specialized areas encompassed by these themes, the men and women of science and medicine give yet another proof of their desire to work for the good of humanity. The Church joins with you in this task, for it too seeks to be the servant of humanity. As I said in my first encyclical, *Redemptor Hominis,* "The Church cannot abandon man, for his destiny, that is to say, his election, calling, birth, death, salvation or perdition, is so closely and unbreakably linked with Christ"(n/14).

---

*This address, presented as "The text of his English-language address," was published in the Dec. 5, 1985 issue of *Origins* directly after the Report of the Pontifical Academy of Sciences as above (pages 415–417).

2. Your presence reminds me of the gospel parable of the Good Samaritan, the one who cared for an unnamed person who had been stripped of everything by robbers and left wounded at the side of the road. The figure of the Good Samaritan I see reflected in each one of you, who by means of science and medicine offer your care to nameless sufferers, both among peoples in full development and among the hosts of those individuals afflicted by diseases caused by malnutrition.

For Christians, life and death, health and sickness, are given fresh meaning in the words of St. Paul: "None of us lives to himself, and none of us dies to himself. If we live, we live to the Lord and if we die, we die to the Lord; so then, whether we live or whether we die, we are the Lord's" (Rom. 14:7-8).

These words offer great meaning and hope to us who believe in Christ; non-Christians, too, whom the Church esteems and with whom it wishes to collaborate, understand that within the mystery of life and death are values which transcend all earthly treasures.

3. When we approach the theme which you have dealt with in your first group, "The Artificial Prolongation of Life and the Determination of the Exact Moment of Death," we do so with two fundamental convictions, namely: Life is a treasure; death is a natural event.

Since life is indeed a treasure, it is appropriate that scientists promote research which can enhance and prolong human life and that physicians be well informed of the most advanced scientific means available to them in the field of medicine.

Scientists and physicians are called to place their skill and energy at the service of life. They can never, for any reason or in any case, suppress it. For all who have a keen sense of the supreme value of the human person, believers and non-believers alike, euthanasia is a crime in which one must in no way cooperate or even consent to. Scientists and physicians must not regard themselves as the lords of life but as its skilled and generous servants. Only God, who created the human person with an immortal soul and saved the human body with the gift of resurrection, is the Lord of life.

4. It is the task of doctors and medical workers to give the sick the treatment which will help to cure them and which will aid them to bear their sufferings with dignity. Even when the sick are incurable they are never untreatable; whatever their condition, appropriate care should be provided for them.

Among the useful and licit forms of treatment is the use of painkillers. Although some people may be able to accept suffering without alleviation, for the majority pain diminishes their moral strength. Nevertheless, when considering the use of these, it is necessary to observe the teaching contained in the declaration issued June 26, 1980, by the Congregation for the Doctrine of the Faith:

Painkillers that cause unconsciousness need special consideration. For a person not only has to be able to satisfy his or her moral duties and family obligations; he or she also has to prepare himself or herself with full consciousness for meeting Christ.

5. The physician is not the lord of life, but neither is he the conqueror of death. Death is an inevitable fact of human life, and the use of means for avoiding it must take into account the human condition. With regard to the use of ordinary and extraordinary means the church expressed herself in the following terms in the declaration which I have just mentioned:

If there are no other sufficient remedies, it is permitted, with the patient's consent, to have recourse to the means provided by the most advanced medical techniques, even if these means are still at the experimental stage and are not without a certain risk . . . . It is also permitted, with the patient's consent, to interrupt these means where the results fall short of expectations. But for such a decision to be made, account will have to be taken of the reasonable wishes of the patient and the patient's family, as also of the advice of the doctors who are specially competent in the matter . . . . It is also permissible to make do with normal means that medicine can offer. Therefore one cannot impose on anyone the obligation to have recourse to a technique which is already in use but which carries a risk or is burdensome . . . . When inevitable death is imminent in spite of the means used, it is permitted in conscience to take the decision to refuse forms of treatment that would only secure a precarious and burdensome prolongation of life, so long as the normal care due to the sick person in similar cases is not interrupted.

6. We are grateful to you, ladies and gentlemen, for having studied in detail the scientific problems connected with attempting to define the moment of death. A knowledge of these problems is essential for deciding with a sincere moral conscience the choice of ordinary or extraordinary forms of treatment and for dealing with the important moral and legal aspects of transplants. It also helps us in the further consideration of whether the home or the hospital is the more suitable place for treatment of the sick and especially of the incurable.

The right to receive good treatment and the right to be able to die with dignity demand human and material resources at home and in hospital which ensure the comfort and dignity of the sick. Those who are sick and above all the dying must not lack the affection of their families, the care of doctors and nurses and the support of their friends.

Over and above all human comforts, no one can fail to see the enormous help given to the dying and their families by faith in God and by hope in eternal life. I would therefore ask hospitals, doctors and above all relatives, especially in the present climate of secularization, to make it easy for the sick to come to God, since in their illness they experience new questions and anxieties which can find an answer only in God.

7. In many areas of the world the matter which you have began to study in your second working group has immense importance, namely the question of malnutrition. Here the problem is not merely that of a scarcity of food, but also the quality of food, whether it is suitable or not for the healthy development of the whole person. Malnutrition gives rise to diseases which hinder the development of the body and likewise impede the growth of maturity in intellect and will.

The research which has been completed so far and which you are now examining in greater detail in this colloquium aims at identifying and treating the diseases associated with malnutrition. At the same time, it points to the need of adapting and improving methods of cultivation, methods which are capable of producing food with all the elements that can ensure proper human subsistence and the full physical and mental development of the person.

It is my fervent hope and prayer that your deliberations will encourage the governments and peoples of the economically more advanced countries to help the populations more severely affected by malnutrition.

8. Ladies and gentlemen, the Catholic Church, which in the coming world Synod of Bishops will celebrate the 20th. anniversary of the Second Vatican Council, reconfirms the words which the council fathers addressed to the men and women of thought and science:

> Our paths could not fail to cross. Your road is ours. Your paths are never foreign to ours. We are the friends of your vocation as researchers, companions in your labors, admirers of your successes and, if necessary, consolers in your discouragement and your failures.

It is with these sentiments that I invoke the blessings of God, and Lord of life, upon the Pontifical Academy of Sciences, upon all the members of the two present working groups and upon your families.

APPENDIX IV—THE PROLONGATION OF LIFE

An Address of Pope Pius XII to an International Congress of Anesthesiologists*
November 24, 1957

DR. BRUNO HAID, chief of the anesthesia section at the surgery clinic of the University of Innsbruck, has submitted to Us three questions on medical morals treating the subject known as "resuscitation" [*la réanimation*].

We are pleased, gentlemen, to grant this request, which shows your great awareness of professional duties, and your will to solve in the light of the principles of the Gospel the delicate problems that confront you.

Problems of anesthesiology

According to Dr. Haid's statement, modern anesthesiology deals not only with problems of analgesia and anesthesia properly so-called, but also with those of "resuscitation." This is the name given in medicine, and especially in anesthesiology, to the technique which makes possible the remedying of certain occurrences which seriously threaten human life, especially asphyxia, which formerly, when modern anesthetizing equipment was not yet available, would stop the heart-beat and bring about death in a few minutes. The task of the anesthesiologist has therefore extended to acute respiratory difficulties, provoked by strangulation or by open wounds of the chest. The anesthesiologist intervenes to prevent asphyxia resulting from the internal obstruction of breathing passages by the contents of the stomach or by drowning, to remedy total or partial

---

*This English version, as pubished in *The Pope Speaks,* Vol. IV, n.4 (Spring, 1958), included the following footnote: "Reported in Osservatore Romano, November 25–26, 1957. French text. Translation based on one released by N.C.W.C. News Service. This is a response to three

respiratory paralysis in cases of serious tetanus, of poliomyelitis, of poisoning by gas, sedatives, or alcoholic intoxication, or even in cases of paralysis of the central respiratory apparatus caused by serious trauma of the brain.

The practice of "resuscitation"

In the practice of resuscitation and in the treatment of persons who have suffered headwounds, and sometimes in the case of persons who have undergone brain surgery or of those who have suffered trauma of the brain through anoxia and remain in a state of deep unconsciousness, there arise a number of questions that concern medical morality and involve the principles of the philosophy of nature even more than those of analgesia.

It happens at times—as in the aforementioned cases of accidents and illnesses, the treatment of which offers reasonable hope of success—that the anesthesiologist can improve the general condition of patients who suffer from a serious lesion of the brain and whose situation at first might seem desperate. He restores breathing either through manual intervention or with the help of special instruments, clears the breathing passages, and provides for the artificial feeding of the patient.

Thanks to this treatment, and especially through the administration of oxygen by means of artificial respiration, a failing blood circulation picks up again and the appearance of the patient improves, sometimes very quickly, to such an extent that the anesthesiologist himself, or any other doctor who, trusting his experience, would have given up all hope, maintains a slight hope that spontaneous breathing will be restored. The family usually considers this improvement an astonishing result and is grateful to the doctor.

If the lesion of the brain is so serious that the patient will very probably, and even most certainly, not survive, the anesthesiologist is then led to ask himself the distressing question as to the value and meaning of the resuscitation processes. As an immediate measure he will apply artificial respiration by intubation and by aspiration of the respiratory tract; he is then in a safer position and has more time to decide what further must be done. But he can find himself in a delicate position, if the family considers that the efforts he has taken are improper and opposes them. In most cases this situation arises, not at the beginning of resuscitation attempts, but when the patient's condition, after a slight improvement at first, remains stationary and it becomes clear that

questions submitted to the Holy Father by Dr. Bruno Haid, chief of the anesthesia section of the surgery clinic of the University of Innsbruck. It was delivered during an audience granted delegates to an International Congress of Anesthesiologists, meeting at Rome's Mendel Institute."

only automatic artificial respiration is keeping him alive. The question then arises if one must, or if one can, continue the resuscitation process despite the fact that the soul may already have left the body.

The solution to this problem, already difficult in itself, becomes even more difficult when the family—themselves Catholic perhaps—insist that the doctor in charge, especially the anesthesiologist, remove the artificial respiration apparatus in order to allow the patient, who is already virtually dead, to pass away in peace.

A fundamental problem

Out of this situation there arises a question that is fundamental from the point of view of religion and the philosophy of nature. When, according to Christian faith, has death occurred in patients on whom modern methods of resuscitation have been used? Is Extreme Unction valid, at least as long as one can perceive heartbeats, even if the vital functions properly so-called have already disappeared, and if life depends only on the functioning of the artificial-respiration apparatus?

Three questions

The problems that arise in the modern practice of resuscitation can therefore be formulated in three questions:

First, does one have the right, or is one even under the obligation, to use modern artificial-respiration equip-

ment in all cases, even those which, in the doctor's judgment, are completely hopeless?

Second, does one have the right, or is one under obligation, to remove the artificial-respiration apparatus when, after several days, the state of deep unconsciousness does not improve if, when it is removed, blood circulation will stop within a few minutes? What must be done in this case if the family of the patient, who has already received the last sacraments, urges the doctor to remove the apparatus? Is Extreme Unction still valid at this time?

Third, must a patient plunged into unconsciousness through central paralysis, but whose life—that is to say, blood circulation—is maintained through artificial respiration, and in whom there is no improvement after several days, be considered *"de facto"* or even *"de jure"* dead? Must one not wait for blood circulation to stop, in spite of the artificial respiration, before considering him dead?

Basic principles

We shall willingly answer these three questions. But before examining them We would like to set forth the principles that will allow formulation of the answer.

Natural reason and Christian morals say that man (and whoever is entrusted with the task of taking care of his fellowman) has the right and the duty in case of serious illness to take the necessary treatment for the preservation of life and health. This duty that one has toward himself, toward God, toward the human community, and in most cases toward certain determined persons, derives from well ordered charity, from submission to the Creator, from social justice and even from strict justice, as well as from devotion toward one's family.

But normally one is held to use only ordinary means—according to circumstances of persons, places, times, and culture—that is to say, means that do not involve any grave burden for oneself or another. A more strict obligation would be too burdensome for most men and would render the attainment of the higher, more important good too difficult. Life, health, all temporal activities are in fact subordinated to spiritual ends. On the other hand, one is not forbidden to take more than the strictly necessary steps to preserve life and health, as long as he does not fail in some more serious duty.

Administration of the sacraments

Where the administration of sacraments to an unconscious man is concerned, the answer is drawn from the doctrine and practice of the Church which, for its part, follows the Lord's will as its rule of action. Sacraments are meant, by virtue of divine institution, for men of this world who are in the course of their earthly life, and, except for baptism itself, presupposed prior baptism of the recipient. He who is not a man, who is not yet a man, or is no longer a man, cannot receive the sacraments. Furthermore, if someone expresses his refusal, the sacraments cannot be administered to him against his will. God compels no one to accept sacramental grace.

When it is not known whether a person fulfills the necessary conditions for valid reception of the sacraments, an effort must be made to solve the doubt. If this effort fails, the sacrament will be conferred under at least a tacit condition (with the phrase *"Si capax est,"* "If you are capable,"—which is the broadest condition). Sacraments are instituted by Christ for men in order to save their souls. Therefore, in cases of extreme necessity, the Church tries extreme solutions in order to give man sacramental grace and assistance.

The fact of death

The question of the fact of death and that of verifying the fact itself *("de facto")* or its legal authenticity *("de jure")* have, because of their consequences, even in the field of morals and of religion, an even greater importance. What We have just said about the presupposed essential elements for the valid reception of a sacrament has shown this. But the importance of the question extends also to effects in matters of inheritance, marriage and matrimonial processes, benefices (vacancy of a benefice), and to many other questions of private and social life.

It remains for the doctor, and especially the anesthesiologist, to give a clear and precise definition of "death" and the "moment of death" of a patient who passes away in a state of unconsciousness. Here one can accept the usual concept of complete and final separation of the soul from the body; but in practice one must take into account the lack of precision of the terms "body" and "separation." One can put aside the possibility of a person being buried alive, for removal of the artificial respiration apparatus must necessarily bring about stoppage of blood circulation and therefore death within a few minutes.

In case of insoluble doubt, one can resort to presumptions of law and of fact. In general, it will be necessary to presume that life remains, because there is involved here a fundamental right received from the Creator, and it is necessary to prove with certainty that it has been lost.

We shall now pass to the solution of the particular questions.

A doctor's rights and duties

1. Does the anesthesiologist have the right, or is he bound, in all cases of deep unconsciousness, even in those that are considered to be completely hopeless in the opinion of the competent doctor, to use modern artificial respiration apparatus, even against the will of the family?

In ordinary cases one will grant that the anesthesiologist has the right to act in this manner, but he is not bound to do so, unless this becomes the only way of fulfilling another certain moral duty.

The rights and duties of the doctor are correlative to those of the patient. The doctor, in fact, has no separate or independent right where the patient is concerned. In general he can take action only if the patient explicitly or implicitly, directly or indirectly, gives him permission. The technique of resuscitation which concerns us here does not contain anything immoral in itself. Therefore the patient, if he were capable of making a personal decision, could lawfully use it and, consequently, give the doctor permission to use it. On the other hand, since these forms of treatment go beyond the ordinary means to which one is bound, it cannot be held that there is an obligation to use them nor, consequently, that one is bound to give the doctor permission to use them.

The rights and duties of the family depend in general upon the presummed will of the unconscious patient if he is of age and *"sui juris."* Where the proper and independent duty of the family is concerned, they are usually bound only to the use of ordinary means.

Consequently, if it appears that the attempt at resuscitation constitutes in reality such a burden for the family that one cannot in all conscience impose it upon them, they can lawfully insist that the doctor should discontinue these attempts, and the doctor can lawfully comply. There is not involved here a case of direct disposal of the life of the patient, nor of euthanasia in any way: this would never be licit. Even when it causes the arrest of circulation, the interruption of attempts at resuscitation is never more than an indirect cause of the cessation of life, and one must apply in this case the principle of double effect and of *"voluntarium in causa."*

Extreme unction

2. We have, therefore, already answered the second question in essence: "Can the doctor remove the artificial respiration apparatus before the blood circulation has come to a complete stop? Can he do this, at least, when the patient has already received Extreme Unction? Is this Extreme Unction valid when it is administered at the moment when circulation ceases, or even after?"

We must give an affirmative answer to the first part of this question, as We have already explained. If Extreme Unction has not yet been administered, one must seek to prolong respiration until this has been done. But as far as concerns the validity of Extreme Unction at the moment when blood circulation stops completely or even after this moment, it is impossible to answer "yes" or "no."

If, as in the opinion of doctors, this complete cessation of circulation means a sure separation of the soul from the body, even if particular organs go on functioning, Extreme Unction would certainly not be valid, for the recipient would certainly not be a man anymore. And this is an indispensable condition for the reception of the sacraments.

If, on the other hand, doctors are of the opinion that the separation of the soul from the body is doubtful, and that this doubt cannot be solved, the validity of Extreme Unction is also doubtful. But, applying her usual rules: "The sacraments are for men" and "In case of extreme measures," the Church allows the sacrament to be administered conditionally in respect to the sacramental sign.

When is one "dead"?

3. "When the blood circulation and the life of a patient who is deeply unconscious because of a central paralysis are maintained only through artificial respiration, and no improvement is noted after a few days, at what time does the Catholic Church consider the patient "dead," or when must he be declared dead according to natural law (questions *'de facto'* and 'de jure')?"

(Has death already occurred after grave trauma of the brain, which has provoked deep unconsciousness and central breathing paralysis, the fatal consequences of which have nevertheless been retarded by artificial respiration? Or does it occur, according to the present opinion of doctors, only when there is complete arrest of circulation despite prolonged artificial respiration?)

Where the verification of the fact in particular cases in concerned, the answer cannot be deduced from any religious and moral principle and, under this aspect, does not fall within the competence of the Church. Until an answer can be given, the question must remain open. But considerations of a general nature allow us to believe that human life continues for as long as its vital functions—distinguished from the simple life of organs—manifest themselves spontaneously or even with the help of artificial processes. A great number of these cases are the object of insoluble doubt, and must be dealt with according to the presumptions of law and of fact of which We have spoken.

May these explanations guide you and enlightened you when you must solve delicate questions arising in the practice of your profession. As a token of divine favors which We call upon you and all those who are dear to you, We heartily grant you Our Apostolic Blessing.

BIBLIOGRAPHY

BIBLIOGRAPHY

SOURCES

Acta Apostolicae Sedis, Commentarium Officiale, Romae, 1909.

Acta Leonis XIII, Pontificis Maximi, Romae: Typ. Vaticana, 1881–1902.

Annuario Pontificio, Cittá del Vaticano: Libreria Editrice Vaticana, 1986.

Codex Juris Canonici Pii X Pontificis Maximi Jussu Digestus Benedicti Papae XV Auctoritate Promulgatus, Typis Polyglottis Vaticanis, 1947.

Code of Canon Law, Latin-English Edition, Washington, D.C.: Canon Law Society of America, 1983.

Denzinger H., Bannwart, C., Umberg, J., *Enchiridion Symbolorum Definitionum et Declarationum de Rebus Fidei et Morum,* ed. 24–25, Friburgi Brisgoviae: Herder and Co., 1942.

Documents of Vatican II, Walter M. Abbot, S.J., ed., Piscataway, New Jersey: New Century Publishers, 1966.

Enchiridion Vaticanum, 9 vols. as of 1987, Bologna, Italy: Edizioni Dehoniane Bologna. II, 1979; III, 1977; IX, 1987.

Mansi, Joannes, *Sacrorum Conciliorum Nova et Amplissima Collectio,* ed. novissima, Phil. Labbeus-Cossaritius-Coleti, vols. 1–21, Florentiae-Venetiis, 1759–1798.

Mansi, Joannes, *Sacrorum Conciliorum Nova et Ampliora Collectio,* vols. Supplementum ad vol. 31–53, Parisiis-Arnhem-Lipsiae, 1901–1927

Migne, J. P., *Patrologiae Cursus Completus, Series Latina,* 211 vols., Parisiis, 1844–1864.

REFERENCE WORKS

Abaelardus, Petrus, *Theologica et Philosophica,* MPL, CLXXVIII.

Aertnys, Joseph, *Theologia Moralis,* recognitum, auctum et accommodatum a C.Damen, ed. 16, 2 vols., Taurini: Marietti, 1950.

Alphonsus M. de Ligorio, S., *Homo Apostolicus,* Torino, 1848

————, Theologia Moralis, ed. Gaudé, 4 vols., Romae, 1905-1912.

Antonius, S., *Theologia Moralis,* Veronae, 1740.

Aquinas, S. Thomas, *Summa Theologica,* Taurini: Marietti, 1950.

————, *De Coelo et Mundo,* Taurini: Marietti, 1952.

————, *Super Epistolas S. Pauli,* Taurini: Marietti, 1953.

————, *Somme Theologique,* ed. de la Revue des Jeunes, Paris: Desclée, 1934.

Arregui, Antonius, *Summarium Theologiae Moralis,* ed. 18, Bilbao, 1948.

Ashley, Benedict, O.P. and O'Rourke, Kevin, O.P., *Ethics in Health Care,* St. Louis, Missouri: Catholic Health Association, 1986.

Augustine, S., *The City of God,* Modern Library Edition, New York: Random House Inc., 1950.

————, *De Civitate Dei,* MPL, XLI.

Ballerini, Antonius, *Opus Morale in Busenbaum Medullam,* absolvit et edidit Dominicus Palmieri, 7 vols., Prati, 1899.

Banez, Dominicus, *Scholastica Commentaria in partem Angelici Doctoris S. Thomae,* 4 vols., Duaci, 1614-1615.

————, *Decisiones de Jure et Justitia,* Vol. IV.

Bertke, Stanley, *The Possibility of Invincible Ignorance of the Natural Law,* The Catholic University of America Studies in Sacred Theology, No. 58, Washington, D.C.: The Catholic University of America Press, 1941.

Billuart, Carolus, *Summa Sancti Thomae,* 8 vols., Parisiis, 1852.

Bonacina, Martinus, *Moralis Theologia,* Venetiis, 1721.

Bonnar, A., *The Catholic Doctor,* ed. 6, London: Burns, Oates and Washbourne Ltd., 1952.

Bucceroni, Januarius, *Institutiones Theologiae Moralis,* ed. 6, 4 vols., Romae: Typis Instituti Pii IX, 1914-1915.

Busenbaum, Hermannus, *Medulla Theologiae Moralis,* 3 vols, Romae, 1757.

Canon Law Digest, 10 vols as of 1986; VI, New York, N.Y.: Bruce Publishing Co., 1969.

Capellmann, C., *Medicina Pastoralis,* ed. 13, Aquisgrana, 1901.

Cathrein, Victor, *Philosophia Moralis,* ed. 20, Friburgi Brisgoviae: Herder, 1955.

Catholic Encyclopedia, The, Herbermann, C., Pace, E., *et al.* editors, 16 vols., New York: Appelton Co., 1907-1914.

Code of Canon Law: A Text and Commentary, The, Coriden, James A., Green, Thomas J., Heintschel, Donald E., editors, New York: Paulist Press, 1985.

Code of Ethical and Religious Directives for Catholic Hospitals, St. Louis: The Catholic Hospital Association of the United States and Canada, 1949.

Connell, Francis J., *Morals in Politics and Professions,* Westminster: The Newman Press, 1951.

Costa-Rossetti, Julius, *Philosophia Moralis seu Institutiones Ethicae et Juris Naturae*, editio altera, Oeniponte: Rauch, 1886.

Cronin, Michael, *The Science of Ethics*, 2 vols., Dublin: Gill and Son Ltd., 1917.

Cunningham, Bert J., *The Morality of Organic Transplantation*, The Catholic University of America Studies in Sacred Theology, No. 86, Washington, D.C.: The Catholic University of America Press, 1944.

Cunningham, R., *The Story of Blue Shield*, The Public Affairs Committee, 1954.

Curran, Charles E., and McCormick, Richard A., S.J., eds., *Readings in Moral Theology, N.3*, New York, N.Y.: Paulist Press, 1982.

Davis, Henry, *Moral and Pastoral Theology*, ed. 3, 4 vols., London: Sheed and Ward, 1938.

Deciding to Forego Life-Sustaining Treatment, Report of the President's Commission for the Study of Ethical Problems in Medicine and Biomedical and Behavioral Research, Washington, D.C.: U.S. Government Printing Office, 1983.

Diana, Antonius, *Coordinatus*, per R. P. Martinum de Alcolea, Lugdini, 1667.

Elbel, Benjamin, *Theologia Moralis per Modum Conferentiarum*, ed. I. Bierbaum, 3 vols., Paderbornae, 1891–1892.

Escobar, Antonius de, *Universae Theologiae Moralis, Receptiores absque Lite Sententiae necnon Controversae*, 7 vols., Lugdini, 1652–1663.

Ethical and Religious Directives for Catholic Health Facilities, St. Louis, Missouri: Catholic Health Association, 1983.

Fanfani, Ludovicus, *Manuale Theorico-Practicum Theologiae Moralis*, 4 vols., Romae: Libraria Ferrari, 1950–1951.

Ferreres, Joannes, *Compendium Theologiae Moralis*, ed. 16, 2 vols., Barcinonae: Subirana, 1940.

Gabrielis a S. Vincentio, *Summa Moralis*, Romae, 1663.

————, *Tractatus de Justitia et Jure.*

Gannon, Timothy J., *Psychology—The Unity of Human Behavior*, Boston: Ginn and Co., 1954.

Genicot, Eduardus—Salsmans, Joseph, *Institutiones Theologiae Moralis*, ed. 17, 2 vols, Bruxelles: L'Edition Universelle, S.A., 1951.

Guidelines on the Termination of Life-Sustaining Treatment and the Care of the Dying, A Report of the Hastings Center, Bloomington, Indiana: Indiana University Press, 1987.

Gury, Joannes, *Compendium Theologiae Moralis*, ab auctore recognita et Antonii Ballerini adnotationibus locupletata, 2 vols., Romae, 1866.

————, *Compendium Theologiae Moralis,* adnotationibus locupletatum Antonii Ballerini, textus identidem emendato a Dominico Palmieri, 2 vols., Romae, 1907.

————, *Compendium Theologiae Moralis,* cura Raphaelis Tummolo, ed. 4, 2 vols., Neapoli: Ufficio Succursale della Civiltà Cattolica, 1928.

Gustavson, Gustav, *The Theory of Natural Appetency in the Philosophy of St. Thomas,* Washington, D.C.: The Catholic University of America Press, 1944.

Guthrie, Douglas, *A History of Medicine,* London: Nelson and Sons, 1947.

Handbook of 1985 Living Will Laws, New York, N.Y.: Society for the Right to Die, 1986.

Handbook of Living Will Laws, 1987 Edition, New York, N.Y.: Society for the Right to Die, 1987.

Healy, Edwin, S.J., *Moral Guidance,* Chicago: Illinois: Loyola University Press, 1942.

————, *Medical Ethics,* Chicago, Illinois, Loyola University Press, 1956.

Hieronymus, S., *Commentaria in Jonam,* MPL, XXV.

Holzmann, Apollonius, *Theologia Moralis,* 2 vols., Beneventi, 1743.

Human Body, The, Boston, Massachusetts: Daughters of St. Paul, 1960.

Hürth, Franciscus, *De Statibus,* Romae: Pont. Univ. Gregoriana, 1946.

Hürth, Franciscus-Abellan, Petrus, *De Principiis,* Romae: Pont. Univ. Gregoriana, 1948.

————, *De Praeceptis,* Romae: Pont. Univ. Gregoriana, 1948.

Iorio, Thomas, *Theologia Moralis,* ed. 4, 3 vols., Neapoli: D'Auria, 1953–1954.

Jone, Heribert, O.F.M. and Adelman, Urban, O.F.M., *Moral Theology,* first ed., Westminster, Maryland: Newman Bookshop, 1945.

Kelly, Gerald, S.J., *Medico-Moral Problems,* St. Louis, Missouri: The Catholic Hospital Association of the United States and Canada, 1958.

La Croix, Claudius, *Theologia Moralis,* Ravennae-Venetiis, 1761.

Lactantius, *Divinae Institutiones,* MPL, VI.

Lanza, Antonius-Palazzini, Petrus, *Theologia Moralis,* Taurini Romae: Marietti, 1949.

Laymann, Paulus, *Theologia Moralis,* 2 vols, Venetiis, 1719.

Leclercq, Jacques, *Lecons de Droit Naturel,* Namur: Maison d'Edition Ad. Wesmael-Charlier, 1937. IV—*Les Droit et Devoirs Individuels.*

Lehmkuhl, Augustinus, *Theologia Moralis,* ed. 10, Friburgi Brisgoviae: Herder, 1902.

Leo XIII, "Pastoralis oficii," epistola and episcopos Germ. et Austr., Sept. 12, 1891, Al., XI (1892), 283–289.

————, "Rerum Novarum," Ency. letter of May 15, 1891, AL., XI (1892), 97-144.

Lessius, Leonardus, *De Justitia et Jure Ceterisque Virtutibus Cardinalibus,* Lugduni, 1622.

Liebard, Odile M., ed., *Love and Sexuality,* Consortium Series, Official Catholic Teachings, Wilmington, N. Carolina: McGrath Publishing Co., 1978.

Lugo, Joannes de, *Disputationes Scholasticae et Morales,* 8 vols., Parisiis: Vivès, 1868-1869.

————, *De Justitia et Jure,* Vol. VI.

Lynn, Joanne, MD, ed., *By No Extraordinary Means,* Bloomington, Indiana: Indiana University Press, 1986.

Marc. Clemens-Gestermann, F.X., *Institutiones Morales Alphonsianae,* recog. a J. Raus, ed. 18, 2 vols, Lugduni: Typ. E. Vitte, 1927.

Mazzotta, Nicolò, *Theologia Moralis,* 5 vols, Venetiis, 1760.

McFadden, Charles, O.S.A., *Medical Ethics,* ed. 3, Philadelphia: Davis Co., 1955

————, *The Dignity of Life,* Huntington, Indiana: Our Sunday Visitor, 1976.

Merkelbach, Benedict H., O.P., *Summa Theologiae Moralis,* ed. 2, 3 vols., Parisiis: Desclée de Brouwer et Soc., 1935-1936.

Meyer, Theodorus, *Institutiones Juris Naturalis,* 2 vols., Friburgi Brisgoviae: Herder, 1885-1900.

Molina, Ludovicus, *De Justitia et Jure,* Coloniae Agrippinae, 1614.

Noldin, H., *Summa Theologiae Moralis,* recog. et emendat. ab A. Schmitt, ed. 27, 3 vols., Oeniponte: Rauch, 1940-1941.

O'Rourke, Kevin, O.P., JCD and Brodeur, Dennis, Ph D, *Medical Ethics,* St. Louis, Missouri: Catholic Health Association, 1986.

Paquin, Jules, *Morale et Médicine,* Montreal: L'Immaculée-Conception, 1955.

Patuzzi, Joannes, *Ethica Christiana sive Theologia Moralis,* 6 vols., Bassani, 1770.

Payen, Georges, *Déontologie Médicale D'Après Le Droit Naturel* (Résumé), Zi-ka-wei: Imprimerie de la Mission Catholique, 1928.

Philosophiae Scholasticae Summa, 3 vols., Matriti: Biblioteca de Autores Cristianos, 1952-1955.

Pighi, Joannes, *Cursus Theologiae Moralis,* 4 vols., Veronae, 1901.

Pius XI, "Casti connubii," Ency. letter of Dec. 31, 1930, AAS, XXII (1930), 539-392.

Pius XII, "Discourse to the First International Congress on the Histopathology of the Nervous System," Sept. 13, 1952—(found in: *Discorsi e Radiomessaggi di Sua Santita Pii XII,* Typographia Polyglotta Vatican, XIV,

1952-1953, 317-330).

Prümmer, Dominicus, *Manuale Theologiae Moralis*, ed. 2 et 3, 3 vols., Friburgi Brisgoviae: Herder, 1933.

Rabanus Maurus, *Commentaria in libros Machabaeorum*, MPL, CIX.

Regatillo, Eduardus et Zalba, Marcellinus, *Theologiae Moralis Summa*, 3 vols., Matriti: Biblioteca de Autores Cristiahos, 1952-1954.

Reiffenstuel, Anacletus, *Theologia Moralis*, 2 vols, Mutinae, 1740.

Riley, Lawrence J., *The History, Nature and Use of Epikeia, In Moral Theology*, The Catholic University of America Studies in Sacred Theology, Second Series, No. 17, Washington, D.C.: The Catholic University of America Press, 1948.

Roberti, Francesco Cardinal, Director, Msgr. Pietro Palazzini, editor, *Dictionary of Moral Theology*, Westminster, Maryland: The Newman Press, 1962.

Rodrigo, Lucius, *Praelectiones Theologico-Morales Comillenses*, Series I, *Theologia Moralis Fundamentalis*, Vol. II, *Tractatus de Legibus*, Santander: Sal Terrae, 1944.

Roncaglia, Constantinus, *Theologia Moralis*, Lucae, 1730.

Salmanticenses, *Cursus Theologiae Moralis*, 6 vols., Ventiis, 1734.

Sanchez, Thomas, *Consilia seu Opuscula Moralia*, 2 vols., Lugduni, 1634.

Sayrus, Gregorius, *Clavis Regia Casuum Conscientiae*, Venetiis, 1625.

Scavini, Petrus, *Theologia Moralis*, ed. 12, 4 vols., Mediolani, 1874.

Schuster, Joannes, *Philosophia Moralis*, Friburgi Brisgoviae: Herder, 1950.

Securing Access to Health Care, Vol. I, Report of the President's Commission for the Study of Ethical Problems in Medicine and Biomedical and Behavioral Research, Washington, D.C.: U.S. Government Printing Office, 1983.

Sertillanges, Antoine Gilbert, *La Philosophie Morale de Saint Thomas d'Aquin*, Paris: Aubier—Editions Montaigne, 1946.

Soto, Dominicus, *Theologia Moralis*, Lugduni, 1582.

————, *Tractatus de Justitia et Jure.*

Sporer, Patricius, *Theologia Moralis*, 2 vols., Venetiis, 1726.

Suarez, Franciscus, *Opera Omnia*, 28 vols., Paris: Vivès, 1856-1878.

————, *De Virtutibus Theologicis—Vol. XII*, ed. Berton.

Sullivan, Joseph, *Catholic Teaching on the Morality of Euthanasia*, The Catholic University of America Studies in Sacred Theology, Second Series, No. 22, Washington, D.C.: The Catholic University of America Press, 1949.

Tamburini, Thomas, *Explicatio Decalogi*, Venetiis, 1719.

Tanquerey, Adolph, *Synopsis Theologiae Moralis et Pastoralis*, Parisiis: Desclée et Soc., 1953.

Tournely, Honoratus, *Theologia Moralis*, Venetiis, 1756.

Ubach, Joseph, *Theologia Moralis*, ed. 2, 2 vols., Bonis Auris: Sociedad San Miguel, 1935.

Vermeersch, Arthurus, *Quaestiones de Virtutibus Religionis et Pietatis*, Brugis, 1912.

————, *Theologiae Moralis Principia-Responsa-Consilia*, Vols. I,III,IV, ed. 4; Vol.II, ed. 3; Romae: Pont. Univ. Gregoriana, 1945–1954.

Victoria, Franciscus, a. *Relectiones Theologicae*, Lugduni, 1587.

————, *Relectio IX*—De Temperantia.

————, *Relectio X*—De Homicidio.

————, *Commentarios a la Secunda Secundae de Santo Tomas*, Salamanca: ed. de Heredia, O.P., 1952.

Vives, Joseph, *Compendium Theologiae Moralis*, ed. 9, Romae: Puster, 1909.

Waffelaert, Gustav, *Tractatus de Virtutibus Cardinalibus*, Brugis: Beyaert-Storie, 1885–1886.

————, *De Justitia*—Vol. II.

ARTICLES

Altman, Lawrence, K., MD, "When the Mind Dies but the Brain Lives On,"—*New York Times Nov. 17, 1987, C 3.*

Andrusko, David, *"Catholic Health Association, New Jersey Bishops, Clash Over Providing Food and Water,"—National Right to Life News*, March 19, 1987, 1 and 8.

"The Artificial Prolongation of Life, "Report of the Pontifical Academy of Sciences—*Origins*, Dec. 5, 1985, 415–417 (includes address of Pope John Paul II to assembled scientists).

Bardenilla, Sandra S., RN, "Terminal Trajectory: Compassion, Comfort, and Dignity"—*Issues in Law and Medicine*, March, 1987, 391–401.

Bender, L., "Organorum humanorum transplantatio,"—*Angelicum*, XXXI (1954), 139–160.

Boyle, Philip, O.P., King, Larry, MD, O'Rourke, Kevin, O.P., "The Brophy Case: The Use of Artificial Hydration and Nutrition,"—*Linacre Quarterly*, May, 1987, 63–72.

Bulkin, Wilma, MD and Lukashok, Herbert, MS, "Rx for Dying: The Case for Hospice,"—*New England Journal of Medicine*, Feb. 11, 1988, 376–378.

Callahan, Daniel, "On Feeding the Dying,"—*Hastings Center Report*, Oct. 1983, 22–23.

Carson, Donald A., "The Symbolic Significance of Giving to Eat and Drink,"—*By No Extraordinary Means* (cf. Reference Works, Lynn, Joanne, MD), 84–88.

"Il caso del Sindaco di Cork e una discussa questione morale,"—*La Civiltá Cattolica*, IV, 1920, 521–531.

Clark-Kennedy, A. E., "Medicine in Relation to Society,"—*British Medical Journal*, 1955, 619-623.

Connery, J., "Notes on Moral Theology,"—*Theological Studies*, XVI (1955), 558-590.

Cranford, Ronald E., MD, "Patients With Permanent Loss of Consciousness,"—*By No Extraordinary Means*, 186-194 (cf. Carson, above).

————, "The Persistent Vegetative State: The Medical Reality (Getting the Facts Straight),"—*Hastings Center Report*, Feb./March, 1988, 27-32.

Donovan, J., "Question Box,"—*The Homiletic and Pastoral Review*, XLIX (August, 1949), 904.

Dulles, Avery, S.J., "Bishops' Conference Documents: What Doctrinal Authority,"—*Origins*, Jan. 24, 1985, 528-534.

"Experts Voice Hope in Alzheimer's Fight,"—*New York Times*, Nov. 17, 1987, C 1 and C 10.

Ford, J., "The Refusal of Blood Transfusions by Jehovah's Witnesses,"—*Linacre Quarterly*, XX (1955), 3-10.

Gannon, P., "La Grève de la Faim,"—*La Documentation Catholique*, 1920, 333-336.

Goodwine, J., "The Physician's Duty to Preserve Life by Extraordinary Means,"—*Proceedings of the Seventh Annual Convention of the Catholic Theological Society of America*, 1952, 125-138.

Grant, Edward R., JD and Forsythe, Clarke D., JD, "The Plight of the Last Friend: Legal Issues for Physicians and Nurses in Providing Nutrition and Hydration,"—*Issues in Law and Medicine*, January, 1987, 277-299.

"Guidelines for Legislation on Life-Sustaining Treatment," NCCB statement in *Origins*, Jan. 14, 1985, 526-528.

Kelly, Gerald, S.J., "The Duty to Preserve Life,"—*Theological Studies*, XII (1951), 550-556.

————, "The Duty of Using Artificial Means of Preserving Life,"—*Theological Studies*, XI (1950), 203-220.

"Hospices, Comfort and Care for the Dying,"—*Mayo Clinic Health Letter*, March, 1988, 6-8.

Kolata, Gina, "Clinical Promise With New Hormones,"—*Science*, May 1, 1987, 517-519.

Landsman, Ron M., JD, "Terminating Food and Water: Emerging Legal Rules,"—*By No Extraordinary Means*, 135-149 (cf. Carson, above).

Levy, David E., MD et al., "Predicting Outcome From Hypoxic-Ischemic Coma,"—*Journal of the American Medical Association*, March 8, 1985, 1420-1426. Editorial comment on this article, *ibid.*, 1215-1216.

Lynn, Joanne, MD, "Elderly Residents of Long-Term Care Facilities,"—*By No Extraordinary Means*, 163-179 (cf. Carson, above).

Lynn, Joanne, MD and Childress, James F., Ph D, "Must Patients Always be Given Food and Water?,"—*Hastings Center Report*, Oct., 1983, 17-21.

"For Macks, 'Miracle' Meant 7 Years of Pain,"—*Minneapolis Star and Tribune*, Nov. 23, 1986, 1 A, 8 A and 9 A. Cf. also Nov. 3, 1986 (1 A and 7 A), and Nov. 7, 1986 (1 B and 2 B) issues of the same newspaper.

Major, David, MD, "The Medical Procedures for Providing Food and Water: Indications and Effects,"—*By No Extraordinary Means*, 21-28 (cf. Carson, above).

McCartney, James J., O.S.A., Ph D, "Catholic Positions On Withholding Sustenance for the Terminally Ill,"—*Health Progress*, Oct., 1986, 38-40.

Meilaender, Gilbert, Ph D, "Caring for the Permanently Unconscious Patient,"—*By No Extraordinary Means*, 195-201 (cf. Carson, above).

————, "The Confused, the Voiceless, the Perverse: Shall We Give Them Food and Drink?,"—*Issues in Law and Medicine*, Sept., 1986, 133-148.

Micetich, Kenneth, MD, Steinecker, Patricia, MD, Thomasma, David, Ph D, "An Emperical Study of Physician Attitudes,"—*By No Extraordinary Means*, 39-43 (cf. Carson, above).

Nevins, Michael, "Perspectives of a Jewish Physician,"—*By No Extraordinary Means*, 99-107 (cf. Carson, above).

"Providing Food and Fluids to Severely Brain Damaged Patients," Brief of the New Jersey Catholic Conference,—*Origins*, Jan. 22, 1987, 282-284.

"Questions de science ecclésiastique,"—*L'Ami du Clergé*, 1920, 529-533.

Ramsey, Paul, Ph D, "Prolonged Dying: Not Medically Indicated,"—*Hastings Center Report*, Feb., 1976, 14-17.

"The Rights of the Terminally Ill," Statement of the National Conference of Catholic Bishops,—*Origins*, Sept. 4, 1986, 222-224.

Rodriquez, Joseph H., Jr., JD, "The Role of the Public Advocate,"—*By No Extraordinary Means*, 256-259 (cf. Carson, above).

Schmitz, Phyllis, RN and O'Brien, Merry, RN, "Observations on Nutrition and Hydration in Dying Cancer Patients,"—*By No Extraordinary Means*, 29-38 (cf. Carson, above).

Strasser, William, JD, "The Conroy Case: An Overview,"—*By No Extraordinary Means*, 245-248 (cf. Carson, above).

Stryker, Jeff, "In re. Conroy: History and Setting of the Case,"—*By No Extraordinary Means*, 227-245 (cf. Carson, above).

Sullivan, C. and Campbell, E., "One Thousand Cesarean Sections in the Modern Era of Obstetrics,"—*Linacre Quarterly*, XXII (1955), 117-126.

Taylor, R., "Consent for Treatment,"—*Linacre Quarterly*. XXII (1955), 131-135.

Vander Heeren, A., "Suicide,"—*The Catholic Encyclopedia*, XIV, 326-328.

Wanzer, Sidney H., MD, etc al., "The Physician's Responsibility Toward

Hopelessly Ill Patients,"—*New England Journal of Medicine,* April 12, 1984, 955–959.

Weisbard, Alan J., JD and Seigler, Mark, MD, "On Killing Patients With Kindness: An Appeal for Caution,"—*By No Extraordinary Means,* 108–116 (cf. Carson, above).

Zerwekh, Joyce V., "Should Fluid and Nutritional Support be Withheld from Terminally Ill Patients?,"—*American Journal of Hospice Care,* July/August, 1987, 37–38.

INDEX

Lugo, J., de
    example of "little" vs "nothing", 188–189
    examples of extraordinary means, 85–88
    oft-quoted by theologians, 156
    on questions of suicide, 47–56
    4, 10, 13, 247–250, 252, 254
Lukashok, Herbert, M.S., 218
Lynn, Joanne, M.D.
    examples of "useless" situations, 187
    when patient is close to death, 196
    193, 206, 266

Macks, Sargeant David
    unusual case of regained consciousness,
      223ff
    effect on family members, 226–228
Magisterium of Church
    address of Pius XII (1957), 157–158
    Declaration on Euthanasia (1980), 153,
      154
    Pontifical agencies (1980 & 1985), 170–174
    "religious assent of soul," 175–176
    statements of National Catholic
      Conference, 180–181
    235, 237, 262
Major, David, M.D.
    various types of artificial feeding, 163–164
Man's responsibility of administration &
    custody, 13ff
Marc-Gestermann
    refers to "moral impossibility", 100
    "virtual impossibility", 201
Maurus, R., 6
Mayo Clinic
    Health Letter on hospice, 218–219
    hospice follow-up programs, 227
Mazzotta, N.
    elements that make means extraordinary,
      64
    refers to "a certain type" of impossibility,
      100
    251
McCartney, James, O.S.A.
    misinterpretation of Pius XII view, 157
McCormick, Richard, S.J., 153–154,
    271–272
McFadden, C.
    hastening death of embryo, 125–126
    view on total parental nutrition, 165

    115, 130
Means of Conserving Life
    according to one's circumstances, 64–65,
      93ff, 107–110
    modesty factor, 45–46, 58, 65–66, 110–111
    artificial means, 78ff, 142
    beneficial, 53–54, 62ff, 80–83, 85ff,
      104–105, 114
    common, 37ff, 55ff, 64–65, 82–83, 92ff
    congruent, 37ff
    convenient, 40
    cost of, 42, 47, 54ff, 63–66, 71ff, 96,
      107ff, 120
    danger, 72ff, 89, 96
    difficult, 53, 94ff, 103–104
    easy, 98, 99
    fear in use of, 72–73, 110ff
    proportionately grave inconvenience in
      use of, 100–101
    repugnance and, 110ff, 120
    risks in use of, 117ff, 144
    supplanting a natural function, 83
    237, 244, 246, 248–262
Medical Treatments
    conflicting views on, 166–170
    expanded in 20th century, 156
    hopes of advancing technology, 219–222
    main focus of Piux XII Address (1957),
      157
    "natural" vs "artificial", 142–143
    often extraordinary means, 231
    235, 238
Medicare, Medicaid
    response to insurance needs, 199–200
    benefit for hospice care, 217
    limited assistance for comatose, 218
    260
Medicine
    per se intended by nature, 79ff
    236, 239, 247, 249, 250–251, 253, 264,
      272
Meilaender, Gilbert
    view on care of patient, 189–190
    example of psychological burden, 192–193
Merkelbach, B.
    meaning of "ordinatio rationis", 101–102
    measures that prolong life, 74
    on human imputability, 204
    "voluntarium in causa", 160

Schmitz, Phyllis
  on variations in feeding, 193-195
Schuster, 12
Science, 235, 240
Seigler, Mark, M.D.
  opposed to equating artificial feeding with
    respirator, 167, 169
  "respirator" vs "tube feeding", 160
Sertillanges, R.P., 17
Society for the Right to Die
  influence in changing "living will" laws,
    178-179
  view on number of comatose, 213-214
  263, 266
Soto, D.
  amputation as mutilation, 38
  taking medicines under obedience, 95
  8, 86
"Spes Salutis"
  meaning of the phrase, 189
Sporer, P.
  precept of self-conservation, 60-61
Sriram, K., M.D.
  reference to "cyclic feeding", 193
"Starting" vs "Stopping" Artificial Feeding
  cf. "Withholding" vs "Withdrawing"
    Artificial Feeding
Starvation, Voluntary
  contrary to Civil and Church law, 151,
    154-155, 182, 208
  as viewed by some authors, 169-170
  considered as suicide, 181
Strasser, William, J.D.
  report on Conroy (Claire) case, 166
Stryker, Jeff
  review of Conroy (Claire) case, 166
  72
Suarez, F.
  obligation to conserve life, 44-45
"Substitute" vs "Supplement" Distinction
  application to intravenous techniques,
    164-165
  in comparing tube-feeding with respirator,
    169-170
  228-229
Suicide
  against American law, 149
  Church teachings, Declaration on
    Euthanasia, 153
  direct vs indirect, 183

malice of, 4, 8, 34, 38
  argument from virtue of charity, 12
  argument from God's dominion, 7ff
  argument from virtue of piety, 12
  moral teaching regarding, 4ff
  negative precept of natural law, 47
  239, 243-244, 263-267, 275
Sullivan, J.
  view on intravenous feeding, 131-132
  108, 256
Surgery
  can be extraordinary means, 74ff, 83-84
  hospital practice, 117ff
  pain factor & extraordinary means, 104ff,
    144
  relative to conserving life, 119ff
  271
Symbolic Aspects of Feeding
  article by Donald Carson, Ph.D., 167
  demand consolidation, 167-168, 205-208
  important for family members, 225ff
  revealed in physicians' survey, 207

Tamburini, T.
  view on amputation, 60
  use of extraordinary foods, 103
Tanquerey, A.
  prolongation of life, 75
Terminal Condition
  defined, 185
  not to be confused with comatose
    condition, 209
  view of Dr. Cranford, 222-223
Theologians, Early Centuries
  no need of treatment/care distinction,
    155-156
Thomas Aquinas, St.
  argument from charity, 16-17
  argument from natural law, 97, 101
  conserving life, 7ff, 18ff
  evil of suicide, 8, 34
  oft-quoted by theologians, 156
  on human imputability, 204
  12, 16, 243-244, 246
Total Parenteral Nutrition
  effective for long periods, 164
Tournely, H.
  view on amputation, 56-57
  view on pain, 96
  on "moral impossibility", 100

Pope John Center Publications

The Pope John XXIII Medical-Moral Research and Education Center has dedicated itself to approaching current and emerging medical-moral issues from the perspective of Catholic teaching and the Judeo-Christian heritage. Publications of the Pope John Center include:

THE AIDS CRISIS AND THE CONTRACEPTIVE MENTALITY by Msgr. Orville N. Griese, S.T.D., J.C.D., and Dr. Eugene F. Diamond with a Pastoral Commentary by The Most Reverend Donald W. Montrose, 1988, 69pp., $3.95. A moral evaluation of potential means of protecting the general population from the scourge of AIDS . . .Using the AIDS crisis to renew dedication to Christian standards of morality.

SEXUALITY: THEOLOGICAL VOICES—Kevin T. McMahon $14.95. A Critical Analysis of American Catholic Theological Thought from 1965 through 1980.

THEOLOGIANS AND AUTHORITY WITHIN THE LIVING CHURCH by Msgr. James J. Mulligan $13.95.
The author's intention is to answer some questions that have been raised about the proper place of authority and theology in the Catholic Church. Using clear and readable language, the author seeks to explain, to clarify and to share with the reader a context within which he thinks there can be peace.

CATHOLIC IDENTITY IN HEALTH CARE By Msgr. Orville N. Griese, S.T.D., J.C.D. $17.95.
This book is a detailed commentary on the *Ethical and Religious Directives for Catholic Health Facilities* approved by the National Conference of Catholic Bishops. The author organized his material around nine core principles upon which the *Directives* rest.

SCARCE MEDICAL RESOURCES AND JUSTICE (Proceedings of the 1987 Bishops' Workshop). $17.95.
These are the Proceedings of the 1987 Bishops' Workshop in which, with the help of appropriate experts, the bishops pondered the respective responsibilities of individuals and various institutions with regards to the equitable distribution of burdens and benefits in the provision of health care.

CONSERVING HUMAN LIFE (The Pope John Center Edition) by The Most Reverend Daniel A. Cronin, $13.95.
Originally written in 1958 before the issue had become emotionally

charged, this updated and edited version of a doctoral dissertation traces the development of the Church's understanding of the moral law in regard to the ordinary and extraordinary means of conserving life. With Commentaries. 1989

THE FAMILY TODAY AND TOMORROW: The Church Addresses Her Future (Proceedings of the 1985 Bishops' Workshop) Edited by Donald G. McCarthy, Ph.D., 1985, 291 pp. $17.95.
One of the family's fundamental tasks is: "to build up the kingdom of God in history by participating in the life and mission of the Church" (Familiaris Consortio, 49). The challenges and obstacles that inhibit the family in this role today are examined, with reflections from the Church's teachings and possible future directions. Fifteen experts in sociology, psychology, medicine and theology have contributed to this volume.

THEOLOGIES OF THE BODY: Humanist and Christian By Benedict M. Ashley, O.P., 1985, 770 pp., $20.95.
With a rare breadth of vision and insightful erudition, this wide-ranging theological study of human materiality compares and contrasts two world viewpoints—the humanist and the Christian. It is an historical, philosophical and theological approach to a non-dualistic anthropology as a foundation for Christian ethics.

MORAL THEOLOGY TODAY: Certitudes and Doubts (Proceedings of the 1984 Bishops' Workshop) 1984, 355 pp., $17.95.
This book presents a concise survey of morals and ethics in their biblical and systematic theology roots, their historical development, and the relationships of theologians to bishops, the tradition and the magisterium. Contemporary challenges in moral methodologies are examined and compared with traditional principles of exceptionless moral norms, totality, double-effect and the moral inseparability of the unitive and procreative meanings of the conjugal act.

SEX AND GENDER: A Theological and Scientific Inquiry Edited by Mark Schwartz, Sc.D., Albert S. Moraczewski, OP, Ph.D. and James A. Monteleone, MD, 1983, 385 pp., $19.95.
This is an attempt to provide in the area of human sexuality the most current scientific data and additional psychological, philosophical and theological reflections upon that data from the viewpoint of the meanings of sexuality as expressed in Catholic teaching.

TECHNOLOGICAL POWERS AND THE PERSON: Nuclear Energy and Reproductive Technologies (Proceedings of the 1983 Bishops' Workshop) 1983, 500 pp., $15.95.
In the 1983 Dallas workshop, the assembled bishops listened, pondered and reacted to scientific and theological experts speaking on the awesome powers of nuclear energy (for peaceful purposes) and reproductive technologies. This book is a collection of the lectures and edited discussions.

HANDBOOK ON CRITICAL SEXUAL ISSUES Edited by Donald G. McCarthy, Ph.D. and Edward J. Bayer, S.T.D., 1983, 230 pp., $9.95.
Taking an historical approach beginning with biblical roots of Catholic teaching developing through early and medieval periods and bringing it

up to post Vatican II, the book attempts to present the roots of sexual norms in Catholic sexual teaching. After discussing the Christian vocation of marriage and natural family planning, the book enters into the second part in which specific sexual issues are considered.

HANDBOOK ON CRITICAL LIFE ISSUES Edited by Donald G. McCarthy, Ph.D. and Edward J. Bayer, S.T.D., 1982, 230 pp., $9.95. This is a carefully edited version of the presentation made by thirty-one experts in medicine, theology, psychology, law and sociology who for twelve days addressed such issues as abortion, defective fetal development, organ transplants, technology for prolongation of life, and brain-related criterion for the determination of a person's death.

MORAL RESPONSIBILITY IN PROLONGING LIFE DECISIONS Edited by Donald G. McCarthy, Ph.D. and Albert S. Moraczewski, OP, Ph.D., 1982, 316 pp., $9.95. This book contains twenty chapters plus two appendizes and discusses the medical, moral and legal aspects of prolonging life decisions. It also examines the specific responsibilities of administrators of health care facilities, physicians, nurses and pastoral care persons.

HUMAN SEXUALITY AND PERSONHOOD (Proceedings of the 1981 Bishops' Workshop) 1981, 254 pp., $9.95. With input from several relevant disciplines, this Bishops' Workshop sought to present a contemporary and balanced theology of human sexuality and marriage in the light of magisterial teaching and a Christian theology of the human person.

GENETIC COUNSELING: The Church and the Law Edited by Gary Atkinson, Ph.D. and Albert S. Moraczewski, OP, Ph.D., 1980, 259 pp., $9.95. An appreciative review in the December 1980 issue of *Theological Studies* (Page 805) describes succinctly: "Highly recommended for genetic counselors, pastors, and students. Its clear common succinct style makes the book a good introduction to biogenetic morality and a valuable survey of the present debate."

NEW TECHNOLOGIES OF BIRTH AND DEATH: Medical, Legal, and Moral Dimensions (Proceedings of the 1980 Bishops' Workshop) 1980, 196 pp., $8.95. Five theologians, two physicians and two lawyers discuss subjects as old as abortion and contraception and as new as in vitro fertilization and the ovulation method of family planning. The book also reviews efforts to determine if human death has occurred even though vital signs are artificially maintained.

A MORAL EVALUATION OF CONTRACEPTION AND STERILIZATION: A Dialogical Study by Gary Atkinson, Ph.D. and Albert S. Moraczewski, OP, Ph.D., 1980, 115 pp., $4.95. The authors of this paper hope it will be a contribution to a more clear understanding of the multifaceted issues of contraception by presenting accurately, clearly, and fairly the principal arguments of this controversy.

ARTFUL CHILDMAKING: Artificial Insemination in Catholic Teaching by John C. Wakefield, Ph.D., 1978, 205 pp., $8.95.

By providing an historical and theological review of the Church's teaching with regard to artificial insemination, the present publication does some of the ground work for an understanding of the Catholic Church's position with regards to technological reproduction.

AN ETHICAL EVALUATION OF FETAL EXPERIMENTATION Edited by Donald G. McCarthy, Ph.D. and Albert S. Moraczewski, OP, Ph.D., 1976, 137 pp., $8.95.

The present study seeks to analyze the ethical issues involved in fetal experimentation and to discover the valid foundations for a broadly based consensus concerning our need as a human, civilized community to protect the fetus. The book also includes a detailed discussion of the issue of delayed hominization and its refutation.

The following books have been published collaboratively with the Catholic Health Association of the United States:

GENETIC MEDICINE AND ENGINEERING: Ethical and Social Dimensions Edited by Albert S. Moraczewski, OP, Ph.D., 1983, 198 pp., $17.50.

This book intends to assist the decision-makers in Catholic Health Ministries, especially in forming appropriate and practical policies in matters concerning these developing technologies in the area of genetic medicine and engineering. It is a collection of articles by experts in the field of genetics and ethics.

ETHICS COMMITTEES: A Challenge for Catholic Health Care Edited by Sister Margaret John Kelly, D.C., Ph.D. and Donald G. McCarthy, Ph.D., 1984, 151 pp., $15.50.

This work treats the various needs which have contributed to the development of the Ethics Committees; reflects on ethical methodologies and legal aspect of such committees and offers models for various types of ethics committees to meet the needs at the institutional, diocesan and multi-institutional system levels.

DETERMINATION OF DEATH: Theological, Medical, Ethical and Legal Issues by Albert S. Moraczewski, OP, Ph.D. and J. Stuart Showalter, JD, MFS, St. Louis, The Catholic Health Association of the U.S. 1982, 39 pp., $2.50.

In a concise manner, this work focuses on the question, "Is the Patient Dead?" In the first section, the biblical and theological roots of the concept of person and the philosophical aspects of life and death are briefly reviewed. In the final section, the statutory and case law aspects are discussed.

As a service to those interested in the meaning of "moral" laws and norms, The Pope John Center is making available a published doctoral dissertation:

THE MEANING OF THE TERM "MORAL" IN ST. THOMAS AQUINAS By Brian Thomas Mullady, OP, S.T.D., Pontifical Academy of St. Thomas, 1986, 142 pp., $12.00.
This work, while probing the meaning of the term moral as used by St. Thomas, looks squarely at some of the contemporary issues especially with regards to the denial of exceptionless moral norms.

These books may be ordered from: The Pope John Center, 186 Forbes Road, Braintree, MA 02184, Telephone (617) 848-6965. Prepayment is encouraged. Please add $1.00 for shipping and handling for the first book ordered and 25 cents for each additional book.

Subscriptions to the Pope John Center monthly newsletter, *ETHICS AND MEDICS*, may be sent to the same address. Annual subscription is $15.00 (domestic) and $18.00 (foreign).